Practical Diagnosis
of
Hematologic Disorders

Authors

Carl Kjeldsberg, MD

Professor of Pathology and Medicine
University of Utah, School of Medicine
Executive Vice President, ARUP, Inc.
Salt Lake City, Utah

Ernest Beutler, MD

Chairman, Department of Basic and Clinical Research
Scripps Clinical Research Foundation
La Jolla, California

Carol Bell, MD

Director of Clinical Laboratories
David Brotman Memorial Hospital
Culver City, California

Cecil Hougie, MD

Professor Emeritus, Pathology
University of California, San Diego
School of Medicine
La Jolla, California

Kathy Foucar, MD

Associate Professor
Department of Pathology
University of New Mexico
School of Medicine
Albuquerque, New Mexico

Richard Savage, MD

Associate Pathologist
Millard Fillmore Hospital
Buffalo, New York

Practical Diagnosis
of
Hematologic Disorders

Carl Kjeldsberg, MD, Editor

ASCP Press
American Society of Clinical Pathologists • Chicago

Library of Congress Cataloging in Publication Data

Practical diagnosis of hematologic disorders.

    Includes bibliographies and index.
    1. Blood—Diseases—Diagnosis.
2. Hematology. I. Kjeldsberg, Carl R. [DNLM:
1. Hematologic Diseases
—diagnosis. WH 100 P8949]
RC636.P72 1989   616.1'5075   88-35068
ISBN 0-89189-235-4

Printed in the United States of America.

93 92 91 90 89   5 4 3 2 1

We dedicate this book to William C. Maslow, MD, former Chairman, Division of Clinical Pathology, City of Hope National Medical Center, Duarte, California. He was the editor of the book *Practical Diagnosis: Hematologic Disease,* upon which the present book is based. Dr. Maslow started his professional career as a skilled and compassionate clinical hematologist. In mid-career he obtained training in clinical pathology, and for the rest of his life he applied his great talents to laboratory aspects of hematology. Thus, he was particularly well-suited to prepare a book that could be of value both to clinicians and to pathologists. We feel very fortunate that Dr. Maslow laid the foundation for the present book prior to his untimely death.

Contents

Common Abbreviations

ACD	anemia of chronic disease
ADP	adenosine diphosphate
AIHA	autoimmune hemolytic anemia
ALL	acute lymphoblastic leukemia
AML	acute myeloblastic leukemia
AMP	adenosine monophosphate
APTT	activated partial thromboplastin time
ATP	adenosine triphosphate
BM	bone marrow
CALLA	common ALL antigen
CAT	cold agglutinin titer
CBC	complete blood count
CGL	chronic granulocytic leukemia
CLL	chronic lymphocytic leukemia
CML	chronic myelogenous leukemia
CMV	cytomegalovirus
DAT	direct antiglobulin test
DIC	disseminated intravascular coagulation

EBV	Epstein-Barr virus
EDTA	ethylenediamine tetraacetic acid, or edetic acid (anticoagulant)
G6PD	glucose-6-phosphate dehydrogenase
Hb	hemoglobin
HMW-K	high–molecular-weight kininogen
IBC	iron-binding capacity
ITP	idiopathic thrombocytopenic purpura
LAP	leukocyte alkaline phosphatase
MCHC	mean corpuscular hemoglobin concentration
MCV	mean corpuscular volume
ML	myelogenous leukemia, or myeloblastic leukemia
PMN	polymorphonuclear (basophils, neutrophils, etc)
PNH	paroxysmal nocturnal hemoglobinuria
PT	prothrombin time
RDW	red cell distribution width
SLE	systemic lupus erythematosus
TdT	terminal deoxynucleotidyl transferase
TIBC	total iron-binding capacity
TT	thrombin time

Tests

Tables

Figures

Preface

Our goal with *Practical Diagnosis of Hematologic Disorders* is to provide an up-to-date, concise source of guidelines to the selection, use, and interpretation of laboratory tests, while at the same time providing an overview of the pathogenesis, clinical features, and treatment of the most common hematologic disorders.

We have attempted to make this book well-organized, practical, and easy to use by structuring information consistently throughout. The introduction considers the hematopoietic system and basic hematologic tests. Each chapter defines a disorder, discusses the relevant pathophysiology, clinical findings, approach to diagnosis, hematologic findings, other laboratory tests, and clinical course and treatment, and provides selected up-to-date references. The chapters contain tables and selected morphologic illustrations. Since most chapters discuss primarily one disorder, the information on each disease should be easy to find. Additional features include an appendix of reference values for various hematologic parameters, and the expression of all laboratory values in both SI and conventional units.

It is our hope that this book be of interest to a large audience, including medical students, residents and fellows in pathology and medicine, pathologists, internists, and medical technologists. It is intended to be a practical book for the nonspecialist, but it may also be a quick source of review for the hematologist/oncologist. The book should also be helpful to those preparing for boards in pathology and internal medicine.

Acknowledgment

I wish to express my deep thanks and appreciation for the excellent job done by all the authors. I am most grateful to Joe Marty, MS, MT (ASCP), for his expertise in photomicrography. I would like to thank Joshua Weikersheimer and staff of the ASCP Press for their assistance in manuscript preparation and production.

Practical Diagnosis
of
Hematologic Disorders

1

Hematopoiesis: Peripheral Blood and Bone Marrow Examination

The development of blood cells involves maturation stages visible on morphologic examination of bone marrow and other stages that are not visible. The earlier stages of hematopoietic maturation or proliferation can be detected only by sophisticated studies such as marrow cell culture techniques. These early undetectable cells are called "stem cells." They are capable of self-renewal and may differentiate to several different cell types, depending on their degree of commitment. The earliest stem cells are multipotential or pluripotential—capable of giving rise to many cell types. The later forms are limited to one or two cell types and are often called "colony-forming units." Production of specific, committed cell types involves differentiation of the precursor cells that can be recognized on morphologic examination. These cells are capable of very limited self-renewal, and their primary role is to develop into functional blood cells in response to maturation agents and modulators such as erythropoietin, thrombopoietin, and colony-stimulating factor—granulocytic/monocytic.

Many hematologic diseases involve failure of maturational mechanisms, abnormal stem cell differentiation, or failure of normal feedback mechanisms to regulate cell proliferation appropriately. Acute leukemia, for example, is a disorder in which proliferation proceeds at a relatively normal rate, but differentiation is totally or nearly totally lacking. As the marrow becomes incapable of producing functional cells in response to proliferative stimuli, proliferation and renewal of the primitive stem cells are essentially unregulated and lead to progressive accumulations of functionless "blasts cells" in both bone marrow and blood. One cause of aplastic anemia is the specific failure of very early, multipotential stem cells to renew themselves. Myelodysplastic states occur when proliferation proceeds but differentiation is abnormal, resulting in production of cells with variable functional and morphologic abnormalities. In chronic granulocytic leukemia, proliferation is unrestrained while differentiation abnormalities are minimal. Thus, large numbers of mature myeloid cells with minimal morphologic and functional abnormalities are produced. The pathophysiology of many blood disorders can be explained by study of the proliferative capacity and the degree of differentiation seen when marrow cells are cultured.

A brief, introductory discussion of the types of blood cells will appear in a subsequent section. The functional cells that are seen circulating in the peripheral blood are the result of many stages of differentiation in the marrow. In addition, cells such as neutrophils can be held "in reserve" in the marrow and are also adherent to vessel walls in the circulation, the "marginal granulocytic pool." Platelets can be sequestered in the spleen in a similar reserve. Thus, release of cells in response to acute stimuli can be immediate from the marrow or a reserve pool, or delayed until the full process of proliferation and differentiation has run its course. The degree of demand, the adequacy of reserves, and the proliferative and differentiation capacity of the marrow govern the number of functional normal and abnormal cells seen in the blood and marrow in various diseases.

Blood Cell Morphology

Virtually all of the formed elements in the blood are end-stage, functional cells. The elements are: erythrocytes or red cells, the functional cell responsible for oxygen transport; granulocytes, the functional cells responsible for phagocytosis and destruction of invading organisms as well as inflammation; lymphocytes, which may be both functional, committed cells or stem cells and are involved in antibody production and cell-mediated immune responses; monocytes; and platelets, the anucleate, formed elements important in blood coagulation. Each major cell class contains several morphologically distinguishable normal and pathologic cell types, and morphologic variations in these cells reflect and are often diagnostic of hematologic diseases. As this introductory chapter is not intended as an atlas, only a brief discussion of the normal cell types is presented, and photomicrographs are not included. The interested reader is referred to any of the several textbooks or atlases cited at the end of this chapter.

Normal and Pathologic Red Blood Cells

The normal red cell is a biconcave disc, 6 to 9 μm in diameter and 1.5 to 2.5 μm thick. Red cells are anucleate and have a dense outer rim and a clearer center, as seen on peripheral smear. The center occupies approximately one third of the diameter of the red cell as seen on a properly prepared blood smear. Red cell cytoplasm is uniformly pink, and no inclusions or areas of rarefaction are seen in normal red cells. Pathologic red cells can be larger or smaller than normal red cells, may contain inclusions, and are often abnormally shaped. Variation in size is referred to as "anisocytosis"; variation in shape is termed "poikilocytosis." Some pathologic red cell forms indicate specific diseases. Table 1–1 summarizes the names and morphologic abnormalities in red cells that may be seen on blood smears.

Normal and Pathologic Leukocytes

In contrast to red cells and platelets, leukocytes or white blood cells are nucleated and capable of a considerable range of metabolic activities and functions. Leukocytes are divided into granulocytes, monocytes, and lymphocytes; each of the subtypes is further divided according to morphologic features.

Granulocytes. Granulocytes contain elongated or segmented nuclei and possess specific granules that vary in their affinity for different dyes in the Romanovsky stains used on blood and marrow. These staining characteristics reflect different functional granules in the mature cells. Those granulocytes whose granules have an affinity for the blue or basic thiazine dyes are termed "basophils," those with an affinity for the reddish dye eosin are termed "eosinophils," and those with granules staining less intensely with either dye are termed "neutrophils." Maturation of granulocytes proceeds in morphologically recognizable stages, from the most primitive form, the myeloblast, through five later stages to the mature cell. Each mature form has a segmented nucleus and specific granules in its cytoplasm. Each of the major cell types plays a different role in physiology and disease. Neutrophilic granulocytes phagocytose bacteria and participate in inflammatory responses. Eosinophils are important in allergic and parasitic disease; increase following stress, shock, and burns; and are sharply modulated and decreased by increasing corticosteroid levels. The role of the basophil is less understood, but it seems to participate in some allergic and inflammatory reactions. Additional details on the role of each

Table 1–1   Pathologic Red Cells in Blood Smears

Red Cell Type	Description
Acanthocyte (spur cell)	Irregularly spiculated red cells with projections of varying length; dense center like spherocytes
Basophilic stippling	Punctuate basophilic inclusions
Bite cell (degmacyte)	Smooth semicircle taken from one edge
Burr cell (echinocyte), or crenated red cell	Red cells with short, evenly spaced spicules and preserved central pallor
Cabot's rings	Circular blue threadlike inclusion with dots
Ovalocyte (elliptocyte)	Elliptically shaped cell
Howell-Jolly bodies	Small, discrete basophilic dense inclusions; usually single
Hypochromic red cell	Prominent central pallor
Leptocyte	Flat, waferlike, thin, hypochromic cell
Macrocyte	Red cells larger than normal (>8.5 μm), well-filled with hemoglobin
Microcyte	Red cells smaller than normal (<7.0 μm)
Pappenheimer bodies	Small, dense basophilic granules
Polychromatophilia	Greyish or blue hue frequently seen with macrocytes
Rouleaux	Red cell aggregates resembling stack of coins
Schistocyte (helmet cell, schizocyte)	Distorted, fragmented cell, 2 or 3 points

Underlying Change	Disease States
Altered lipids in cell membrane	Abetalipoproteinemia, parenchymal liver disease, postsplenectomy
Precipitated ribosomes (RNA)	Coarse stippling-lead intoxication, thalassemia; diffuse stippling—a variety of anemias
Heinz body "pitting" by spleen	G6PD deficiency, drug induced oxidant hemolysis
May be associated with altered membrane lipids	Usually artefactual crenated red cells; seen in uremia, bleeding ulcers, gastric carcinoma
Nuclear remnant	Postsplenectomy, hemolytic anemia, megaloblastic anemia
Abnormal cytoskeletal proteins	Hereditary elliptocytosis; minor degree may be seen in various anemias (especially iron deficiency)
Nuclear remnant (DNA)	Postsplenectomy, hemolytic anemia, megaloblastic anemia
Diminished hemoglobin synthesis	Iron deficiency anemia, thalassemia, sideroblastic anemia
	Obstructive liver disease, thalassemia
Young red cells, abnormal red cell maturation	Increased erythropoiesis, megaloblastic anemia, oval macrocyte. Round macrocytes; liver disease (usually with target cells and sometimes acanthocytes)
	See hypochromic red cell
Iron-containing siderosome or mitochondrial remnant	Sideroblastic anemia; postsplenectomy
Ribosomal material	Reticulocytosis, premature marrow release of red cells
Red cell clumping by circulating paraprotein	Paraproteinemia
Mechanical distortion in microvasculature by fibrin strands, mechanical disruption by prosthetic heart valve	Microangiopathic hemolytic anemia (DIC, TTP) prosthetic heart valves, severe burns

(Continued.)

Table 1-1 *Continued.*

Red Cell Type	Description
Sickle cell (drepanocyte)	Bipolar, spiculated forms, sickle-shaped, pointed at both ends
Spherocyte	Spherical cell, dense appearance, absent central pallor, usually decreased diameter
Stomatocyte	Mouth or cuplike deformity
Target cell (codocyte)	Targetlike appearance, often hypochromic
Teardrop cell (dacryocyte)	Distorted, fragmented drop-shaped cell

ABBREVIATIONS: DIC = disseminated intravascular coagulation; TTP = thrombotic thrombocytopenic purpura.

of these cells are contained in the discussions of the specific diseases.

Lymphocytes.   Lymphocytes are small, round cells with few distinguishing features on morphologic examination. They are vital in cell- and antibody-mediated immunologic responses and form the body's long-term reserves of immunocompetent cells. Lymphocytes "transform" in response to antigenic stimuli in a complex sequence involving other cells, such as monocytes or macrophages. Normal, small lymphocytes have a round nucleus with condensed chromatin, inconspicuous nucleoli, and virtually no cytoplasm. When lymphocytes transform in response to stimuli, their nuclei become larger, with more open chromatin and a greater degree of nuclear folding. The cytoplasm of the transformed lymphocyte is more abundant than a resting lymphocyte and often has a deeply basophilic hue, indicating synthesis of RNA. Occasionally, small granules may be seen. The degree of morphologic changes and transformation is quite variable and, hence, variant, atypical, or reactive lymphocytes (equivalent terms) can have quite different appearances. Malignant lymphoid forms that may be found in the blood include: circulating cells of malignant lymphoma, acute lymphoblastic leukemia, chronic lymphocytic leukemia, and hairy cell leukemia. Detailed discussion of these different morphologic cell types is beyond the scope of this introductory chapter.

Underlying Change	Disease States
Molecular aggregation of HbS	Sickle cell disorders: SS, SC, S-thalassemia, SD disease, etc; not in S trait
Decreased membrane redundancy	Hereditary spherocytosis, immunohemolytic anemia
Membrane defect with abnormal cation permeability	Hereditary stomatocytosis, liver disease
Increased redundancy of cell membrane	Liver disease, postsplenectomy, thalassemia, HbC disease
	Myelofibrosis, myelophthistic anemia (space occupying lesions of marrow)

Monocytes.　The monocyte is important in phagocytosis of infective organisms. Monocytes are larger than neutrophils and often have cytoplasmic protrusions and small pseudopods. The cytoplasm is blue-gray, largely agranular, and may contain small vacuoles. Monocyte nuclei vary considerably in size and shape. They are usually lobulated, indented, or oval. Immature monocytes may be seen in the blood in myeloid leukemias; such cells are termed "promonocytes" and "monoblasts."

Platelets.　The platelet, or thrombocyte, is an anucleate cytoplasmic fragment originating from the megakaryocyte. On light microscopic examination, it possesses a central group of purple-blue granules and usually a clear or hyaline periphery. This morphologic distinction is best seen in large platelets. Platelets may be round or oval and often have long, filiform projections from their borders. A minority of circulating platelets are so-called giant forms, and may be the size of a red blood cell or larger. Platelets often clump on smear, especially when the slides are made from heparinized blood.

Automated Hematology

In both the office and hospital settings, most patients' blood is evaluated using an electronic blood cell counter. A bewildering variety of instruments is available for such testing, but all of them employ one of a few common operating principles to analyze the patient's blood. The two principal analytic mechanisms used today are voltage pulse-impedance analysis and low- or high-angle light scatter from a coherent light source, such as a laser. In an impedance counter, such as those first developed by Coulter Electronics, the passage of a particle through an aperture—an orifice of standard size and thus standard volume—displaces conductive electrolyte solution within the orifice. If an electric current is applied across the orifice, a change in resistivity and conductivity of the electrolyte solution occurs as the particle passes through the orifice. A detector will note the presence of a pulse, indicating that a particle has passed through the orifice, and the pulse will be of a size proportional to the volume of the electrolyte solution displaced by the particle. Thus, the counter is capable of counting and sizing particles simultaneously. In a laser counter, such as the Ortho family of instruments or the Technicon H*1, interruption of the laser beam by a particle produces a pulse, and the angle of light scatter and the intensity of the light scattered at particular angles is proportional to several physical properties of the cell, especially size. All instruments have electronic "screens" to suppress electronically aberrant pulses; all correct for or prevent the presence of the chance occurrence of two particles in the sensing zone or aperture of the instrument at the same time; and all have electronic routines to eliminate noise caused by debris.

Most newer whole blood cell counters keep a record in the instrument's memory of the number of particles passing through the aperture or sensing zone in the predetermined size range, which the instrument's program can evaluate. The instrument can generate a histogram of size distribution on the x axis and relative number of particles on the y axis, and most instruments will be able to plot one for each class of particles that the instrument enumerates, such as red cells, white cells, and platelets. Many instruments display histogram information automatically on a cathode-ray screen and are capable of printing it as hard copy. Visual examination of the histogram of size distribution of the cells can provide useful information, especially when minor populations of red cells are present. In addition, the newer instruments generate an index giving the degree of dispersion of red cell sizes (anisocytosis) compared with a "normal" size distribution histogram. On the Coulter and Technicon instruments, this index of average size dispersion or degree of anisocytosis is referred to as a "red cell distribution width" (RDW); the Ortho family of instruments has a comparable measurement referred to as a "red cell morphology index" (RCMI). Use of an index based on degree of dispersion of red cell size can provide valuable clues to the correct classification of anemia.

White cells and platelets are evaluated in the same way as red cells are. White cells are enumerated and sized in a separate set of apertures or a separate pass through the laser flow cell after the red cells have been removed by osmotic or detergent lysis. Platelets and red cell stroma are ignored by the instrument by setting the sensing threshold or "gates" to a size high enough to exclude these smaller particles. Platelet enumeration and sizing are especially difficult, as the platelet size distribution is skewed to the left or is log-normally distributed rather than following the classic gaussian or bell-shaped curve. In addition, platelets must be enumerated in the presence of a larger number of larger particles, the red cells. Most hospital and many office instruments, however, count platelets directly on unseparated anticoagulated peripheral blood (whole blood counters), and most counters also give an estimation of the mean platelet volume, a measurement that can be useful in the differential diagnosis of thrombocytopenia.

☞ The latest generation of automated instrumentation is capable of sizing and classifying white cells into several different groups. So-called three-part differential cell counts have been developed for most Coulter, Ortho, and Baxter (Sysmex) instruments, which are capable of classifying white cells into small (roughly translated as lymphocytes), large (roughly translated as granulocytes), and intermediate-sized ranges (including monocytes and many abnormal cells). The use of these three-part differential cell count screens for selecting cases that require peripheral smear evaluation is still in its infancy, but data suggest that the use of such screens may cut down considerably the number of cases that require an evaluation by a formal 100- or 200-cell microscopic differential cell count. The newest instrument, the Technicon H*1, performs a full cytochemical differential cell count that is capable of detecting clinically significant numbers of abnormal white cells and alerting the instrument operator to their presence.

Red Blood Cell Indices

The red cell indices, as originally conceived by the late Maxwell Wintrobe, were calculated from manual chamber particle counts, spun microhematocrit, and spectrophotometric hemoglobin determinations, as shown in Table 1–2. They remain the basis of non-morphologic evaluation of red cell abnormalities. The diagnostic significance of the classic Wintrobe indices, however, is very different when the numbers are generated on automated equipment. The decrease in mean corpuscular hemoglobin concentration (MCHC) so characteristic of iron deficiency is now known to be caused by analytic artifact. Microcytic red cells with decreased hemoglobin

Table 1–2   Classic Wintrobe Formulae for Red Cell Indices

$$MCV \ = \frac{Hct \ (\%)}{red \ cell \ (millions/\mu L)} \times 10$$

$$MCH \ = \frac{Hgb \ (g/dL)}{red \ cell \ (millions/\mu L)} \times 10$$

$$MCHC = \frac{Hgb \ (g/dL)}{Hct \ (\%)} \times 100$$

Abbreviations: MCV = mean corpuscular volume; Hct = hematocrit; MCH = mean corpuscular hemoglobin; MCHC = mean corpuscular hemoglobin content.

concentration are less deformable and trap more plasma when spun in a microhematocrit centrifuge than do normally deformable normochromic red cells. Hence, with an MCHC calculated as

$$\frac{Hemoglobin \ Level}{Hematocrit \ Value} \times 100 = MCHC,$$

the artifactually high hematocrit value caused an early decrease in the MCHC in iron deficiency. Modern instrumentation, whether laser or impedance type, derives hematocrit value in a fashion unaffected by plasma trapping. As the MCHC changes very late in the course of any disease process, including iron deficiency, the MCHC has become an index suited only for use in laboratory quality control. The only exception to this general rule appears to be that the MCHC is high in hereditary spherocytosis (>360 g/L or 36 g/dl), but only when the blood is analyzed on Coulter or another impedance counter. The mean corpuscular hemoglobin (MCH), on the other hand, retains some residual utility when calculated by the instrument as hemoglobin level divided by red cells times 10; the fall in hemoglobin concentration may be proportionately greater than the decrease in red cells and produce an MCH value slightly lower than "normal" as the mean corpuscular volume (MCV) decreases. The magnitude of this "MCH sag" is slight, however, and thus the MCH also has a limited utility in the differential diagnosis of anemia.

Since 1974, the increasing utilization of "new indices," especially the Coulter and Technicon RDW, has introduced new information that may be of considerable utility in the differential diagnosis of anemia. In general, variable defects affecting red cell maturation and hemoglobinization, such as iron or vitamin deficiency, as well as those diseases affecting mature red cells in the peripheral blood, such as fragmentation hemolysis, will increase the RDW (or RCMI). Those diseases that have a relatively constant effect on red cell maturation, such as thalassemia or aplastic anemia, produce a decreased or increased MCV and a relatively normal RDW. The patterns commonly encountered on Coulter instrumentation are discussed in chapter 2 (see Table 2-3). Many exceptions to such classification categories do occur, especially in cases of thalassemia and hemoglobinopathy traits, which may have a high RDW as well as a low MCV, and in the anemia of chronic disease, which may likewise have a low or normal MCV and a high RDW. Other analyzers, such as the Technicon H*1, have other, newer analytic features in addition to the RDW, such as the capacity to measure the hemoglobin content of each red cell.

Evaluation of the Peripheral Blood Smear

Examination of the peripheral blood smear by a physician who is aware of the patient's clinical condition is useful in the total evaluation of the anemic patient. Highly skilled laboratory personnel may occasionally overlook subtle changes, such as minimal hypersegmentation of neutrophils in cases of combined folate and iron deficiency (so-called masked macrocytosis), or basophilic stippling in a patient with thalassemia and complicating causes of anemia. Such clues may be useful in the differential diagnosis if they are noted by a physician familiar with the patient. Electronically derived red and white cell indices, although useful, are simply representations of the mean and overall degree of dispersion of the cell distribution and give little information concerning other parameters, especially the shape of the red cells (poikilocytosis), the presence or absence of minor populations of abnormal red cells and subtle changes in white cells. Histogram evaluation is useful in the evaluation of minor red blood cell populations, particularly in the patient who receives a transfusion; smear examination for specific shape variations, such as those listed in Table 1-1, can provide valuable clues to the patient's underlying diseases. Some abnormalities, such as the reticulin skein of the reticulocyte, Heinz bodies, and hemoglobin H inclusions, can be demonstrated only by supravital stains, such as brilliant Cresyl blue or new methylene blue. In addition, smear examination for platelet estimation and detection of clumping, satellitosis, or abnormal white cells is helpful. The platelet-to-red cell ratio is approximately 1:10 to 1:20; each standard oil immersion field ($\times 100$ objective with $\times 10$ oculars) should contain 7 to 21 platelets. Semiquantitation of platelet counts may be estimated for values falling in the low-to-mid normal range by counting the number of platelets in 10 or 20 oil fields, averaging, and multiplying by $20 \times 10^9/L$ ($20 \times 10^3/\mu l$).

The Reticulocyte Count

Reticulocytes are defined as immature red cells seen in the peripheral blood that contain at least two dots of reticulin material reactive with new methylene blue (NMB) in their cytoplasm. More immature forms have multiple dots and small networks of skeins of bluish material. These remnants are residual ribosomal RNA used for hemoglobin synthesis in the developing erythrocyte. The RNA is too finely distributed to form networks on Wright's stain; a supravital stain causes precipitation and aggregation of the RNA and creates the dots and skeins of reticulin. RNA-containing red cells are usually grayish on Wright's stain and contrast well with mature, orthochromic or pink red cells, providing a clue to the presence of a reticulocyte response. Reticulocytes are counted as the number of NMB-reactive cells per 1,000 red cells and expressed as percent reticulocytes (absolute number per 100 red cells). Interobserver variation and uneven distribution of reticulocytes on the new methylene blue smear introduces a high analytic variation in reticulocyte counting; interlaboratory coefficients of variation in the 20% range are common, a degree of imprecision of which every clinician should be aware. Duplicate reticulocyte counts or 3-day average values may help to reduce the imprecision of the raw reticulocyte count.

Effective red cell production is a dynamic process; the number of reticulocytes "born" or released from the marrow should be compared with the number released in a nonanemic patient, who produces 1% of $5 \times 10^{12}/L$ ($5 \times 10^{6}/\mu l$) red cells daily for an absolute reticulocyte production of $50 \times 10^{9}/L$ (50,000/mm^3). Clinicians generally use the corrected reticulocyte count rather than the absolute number or proportion counted by the laboratory.

$$\text{Corrected Reticulocyte Count} = \frac{\text{Raw Percent Observed} \times \text{Patient's Hematocrit Value}}{45}$$

Other variations for reticulocyte correction include correction to a "standard" hemoglobin value of 150 g/L (15 g/dl) or to a "standard" red count of $5 \times 10^{12}/L$ ($5 \times 10^{6}/\mu l$). Use of the red cell count ratio seems less desirable than use of the other two alternatives, as the red cell count can be close to normal in the patient with microcytosis and, if used to correct a reticulocyte count, could produce an impression of a more brisk reticulocyte response than would be calculated if the other formulas were used.

Another complicating factor in reticulocyte count correction is that an anemic patient may release reticulocytes prematurely into the circulation. Reticulocytes are usually present for 1 day in the blood before they extrude the residual RNA and become erythrocytes; however, if they are released early from the bone marrow, they may be present in the reticulocyte form in peripheral blood for 2 or 3 days. The situation is of course most likely to occur in those patients whose severe anemia causes a marked acceleration in erythropoiesis and release. Hence, some authors have advocated a further correction of the reticulocyte count for "shift" reticulocytes, again based on the hematocrit value. This correction is called the "reticulocyte production index" (RPI):

$$RPI = \frac{\text{Percent Reticulocyte} \times \text{Patient's Hematocrit Value}}{45} \times \text{Correction Factor.}$$

The correction factor calculation is as follows:

Patient's Hematocrit Value	Correction Factor (Maturation) (d)
40–45	1.0
35–40	1.5
25–34	2.0
15–24	2.5
<15	3.0

If erythropoiesis flags and erythropoietin values are low (not an unlikely situation in patients with renal or hepatic disease), however, application of an RPI correction may hide a failure of marrow response, as the shift does not take place fully or at all. In general, however, RPI values less than 2 indicate failure of bone marrow red cell production, a hypoproliferative anemia; RPIs of 3 or greater indicate marrow hyperproliferation or an appropriate response to the destruction of red cells in the blood or tissues, a hemolytic anemia.

Examination of the Bone Marrow

Marrow aspiration and biopsy are innocuous procedures in expert hands. Processing and interpretation have significant technical variables and require experienced personnel; marrow examination should be limited to situations where noninvasive procedures do not yield clear answers. Microcytic anemia with a high RDW and low serum ferritin levels in a 65-year-old woman should not require marrow aspiration for "evaluation of storage iron." Obvious hemolytic anemias do not require marrow examination but instead should be worked up by other means. Table 1–3 illustrates the most common indications for marrow examination, which, optimally, includes both a Wright-stained aspirate preparation and a histologic preparation, preferably a core needle biopsy. The false-negative rate

Table 1–3 Indications for Bone Marrow Examination

Based on Blood Count/Peripheral Smear
  Unexplained anemia or thrombocytopenia
  Unexplained leukopenia or leukocytosis
  Presence of teardrop/nucleated red cells without explanation[a]
  Presence of rouleaux or cryoprotein[a]
  Unexplained reticulocytopenia
  Presence of abnormal white cells (lymphoma, immature granulocytes)
    or abnormal platelets[a]

Based on Signs/Symptoms of Systemic Disease
  Evaluation of unexplained splenomegaly, lymphadenopathy, or
    hepatomegaly[a]
  Staging of solid tumor[a]
  Staging of Hodgkin's disease or non-Hodgkin's lymphoma[a]
  Fever of unknown origin[c]
  Monitoring of chemotherapy effect[a]
  Evaluation of trabecular bone in metabolic bone disease[b]

[a] Optimal information requires both aspirate and biopsy
[b] Biopsy using nondecalcified bone necessary; aspirate usually noncontributory
[c] Cultures essential; yield rate for morphologic exam alone <5%

for metastatic carcinoma using aspiration alone is about 25%; for lymphomas it seems to be somewhat higher, 30% to 40%, depending on the cell type.

Several sites in the skeleton have been used for marrow sampling. As active hematopoiesis involves the long bones of the arms and legs in infants under the age of 8 months, aspiration from the anterior aspect of the tibial tuberosity is useful. For adults, the posterior iliac crest is the recommended site. The sternum is aspirated relatively easily, but its structure does not allow biopsy. The occasional dramatic fatal laceration of the heart or internal mammary arteries and the psychological effect on the patient produced by insertion of the sternal needle render sternal aspiration a relatively poor choice for marrow sampling in all but the very elderly. In these patients sternal marrow may be most representative of the patient's hematopoiesis and superior to that of the acellular iliac crest. Sternal aspiration may also be most appropriate for patients who have lesions in the sternum or ribs.

Erythrocyte Sedimentation Rate

A commonly used but widely misunderstood test is determination of the erythrocyte sedimentation rate, first introduced in the early

Table 1−4 Factors Affecting the Erythrocyte Sedimentation Rate

Increases Rate	Decreases Rate
Anemia	Microcytosis
Macrocytosis	Abnormal red cells, especially sickle cells
Hypercholesterolemia	
Pregnancy	Polycythemia
Certain points of menstrual cycle	High white cell counts
Chronic inflammatory diseases, especially collagen-vascular diseases	Cachexia and hypoalbuminemia
Increased fibrinogen, gamma-globulin, beta-globulins	Hypofibrinogenemia
Temporal arteritis	

1920s. The test is employed as a nonspecific indicator of an acute-phase reaction, and it depends on the fact that an erythrocyte suspended in plasma will sediment out at a rate determined by the balance between gravitational force (which is directly proportional to cell mass), the buoyant force of the erythrocyte in proportion to its volume, the ascending flow of plasma in response to gravity, and the macromolecular constituents in the plasma. Erythrocytes normally tend to repel one another because of a net negative surface charge. In the presence of increased quantities of positively charged plasma proteins, however, the repulsive forces are partially or totally counteracted, and the erythrocytes sediment more rapidly because of the formation of red cell aggregates or rouleaux. Macromolecules effective in producing this reaction are the acute-phase proteins such as fibrinogen, betaglobulins, and the pathologic immunoglobulins produced by diseases such as myeloma and cryoglobulinemia. In addition, the number of red cells and their shape and volume directly affect the sedimentation rate. Macrocytes have a small surface-to-volume ratio and have therefore less surface charge and repulsive force in relation to their mass than smaller red cells. Thus, macrocytes sediment more rapidly than normal cells, and microcytes sediment more slowly. In anemic patients, the erythrocyte sedimentation rate is increased because the frictional forces retarding the sedimentation of red cell aggregates are reduced. Sickle cells and other hemoglobinopathies tend to retard sedimentation, as rouleaux form with difficulty because of the abnormal shape of the red cells. Table 1−4 summarizes causes for increases and decreases in erythrocyte sedimentation rate.

The erythrocyte sedimentation rate is very technique dependent.

Commonly used methods include: the Westergren sedimentation rate, which is directly affected by anemia; the Wintrobe sedimentation rate, which is unaffected by anemia but is also less sensitive; and the newer modifications, such as the Zeta sedimentation rate, which are not readily available in many laboratories. In all sedimentation rate determinations, the predictive value of the test as a determinant of specific disease activity is relatively low. In some populations, such as the chronically ill geriatric population, an accelerated erythrocyte sedimentation rate correlates with the presence of underlying chronic infection, connective tissue diseases, and malignant neoplasms. The utility of the test is augmented if anemia and hypoalbuminemia are not present in the population. The yield of the erythrocyte sedimentation rate as a screening test for "nonspecific disease activity," however, is quite low.

References

Koepke JA, (ed): *Laboratory Hematology.* Chapter 1, An Overview of Erythropoiesis, JP Lewis; Chapter 9, *An Overview of Granulopoiesis,* SA Bentley; Chapter 35, Instruments for Quantitative Hematology Measurements, JA Koepke, MD; Chapter 37, Differential Counting, RV Pierre. New York, Churchill Livingstone, 1984.

Schumacher HR, Garvin DF, and Triplett DA: *Introduction to Laboratory Hematology and Hematopathology.* Chapter 1, Peripheral Blood and Bone Marrow; Chapter 13, Anemia: Approach to Diagnosis. New York, Alan R. Liss, 1984.

Wintrobe MM, Lee GR, Boggs DR, (eds): *Clinical Hematology*, ed 8. Chapter 1, The Diagnostic and Therapeutic Approach to Hematologic Problems; Chapter 2, The Principles of Hematologic Examinations; Part II: The Normal Hematopoietic System Basic Cytology. Philadelphia, Lea & Febiger, 1981.

Atlases

1. Diggs LW, Sturm D, Bell A: *The Morphology of Human Blood Cells,* ed 5. Abbott Park, Ill, Abbott Laboratories, 1985.
2. Hyun BH, Gulati GL, Ashton JK: *Color Atlas of Clinical Hematology.* New York, Igaku-Shoin Medical Publishers, 1986.
3. McDonald GA, Dodds TC, Cruickshank B: *Atlas of Haematology,* ed 4. New York, Churchill Livingstone, 1978.

PART
1

Anemias

2

Diagnosis of Anemia

The primary function of the red cell is to provide a mode of transportation for hemoglobin to deliver oxygen to the tissues. The physiologic consequences of anemia result from a decrease in the ability of the blood to deliver oxygen. Theoretically, anemia is correctly defined as a reduction in the total number of red cells, amount of hemoglobin in the circulation, or circulating red cell mass. Because this reduction generally results in a compensatory expansion of plasma volume, measurement of the concentration of red cells or hemoglobin very nearly reflects red cell mass in most cases. Increased plasma volume may cause factitious anemia in pregnancy, and decreased plasma volume caused by dehydration may mask a real decrease in circulating red cell mass.

Anemia is itself not a diagnosis but merely a sign of underlying disease. Hence, the workup of an anemic patient is directed at elucidating the causes for a patient's decreased red cell mass. Tables 2–1 and 2–2 show important features in patient history and physical findings that can yield valuable information, considerably narrowing possible causes for anemia and reducing the necessity of performing expensive tests. An adequate history and physical examination are crucial for an intelligently directed approach to the differential diagnosis of anemia.

Table 2−1   Patient History in Diagnosis of Anemia

Considerations	Related Concerns
Age of onset	History of anemia, jaundice, gall bladder disease
Duration of illness	Results of last medical examination Last known normal blood count Last time accepted or rejected as blood donor Prior prescriptions of hematinics (iron, folate, B_{12})
Suddenness and severity of anemia, symptoms of respiratory and circulatory decompensation	Dyspnea on exertion Palpitation Dizziness Faintness on arising from sitting or lying position Marked fatigue, (may be only symptom with insidious onset)
Chronic blood loss	Excessive menstrual bleeding, frequent pregnancy Black stools, bloody stools Gastrointestinal symptoms
Hemolytic episodes	Episodes of weakness with slight icterus and dark urine
Toxic exposure	Occupation, hobbies, drug use
Dietary history	Milk feeding without supplements for long period in infants (iron deficiency) Chronic alcoholism, dietary idiosyncrasy; folate deficiency in the elderly
Family history	History of anemia, splenomegaly, splenectomy; early gall bladder disease in parents, siblings, or offspring

Examination of the Blood

As discussed in chapter 1, the initial classification of anemia is best accomplished by examination of the data from a hematology analyzer, especially the indices, and by an examination of the peripheral blood smear. Useful morphologic findings seen on blood smear review have been discussed in chapter 1. Very few of these findings

Table 2–2   Physical Examination in Diagnosis of Anemia

Anatomic Location	Finding	Disease
Skin and mucous membrane	Pallor and Scleral icterus Smooth tongue	Hemolytic anemia Pernicious anemia, severe iron deficiency
	Petechiae	Associated thrombocytopenia, eg, leukemia
Lymph nodes	Lymphadenopathy	Infectious mononucleosis, leukemia, lymphoma
Heart	Cardiac dilatation, tachycardia, loud murmur	Severe anemia
	Murmurs	Subacute bacterial endocarditis; anemia, usually mild
Abdomen	Splenomegaly	Infectious mononucleosis, leukemia, lymphoma, subacute bacterial endocarditis
	Massive splenomegaly	Chronic granulocytic leukemia, myelofibrosis with myeloid metaplasia
	Hepatosplenomegaly with ascites	Liver disease
Central nervous system	Subacute combined degeneration of the spinal cord	Pernicious anemia
	Delayed Achilles tendon reflexes	Hypothyroidism

are specific, however, and the physician most commonly classifies anemias initially by the instrument's red cell indices, especially the mean corpuscular volume (MCV). On newer counters, the red cell distribution width (RDW) or red cell morphology index (RCMI) is another useful measurement. Use of these two measurements allows anemia to be classified into six "cells." The anemia may be

Table 2-3   Red Cell Distribution Width and Mean Corpuscular Volume Patterns in Some Disease States

Microcytic States, with Anemia

Normal RDW/Low MCV

Thalassemia minor
Anemia of chronic disease

> anisocytosis

High RDW/Low MCV

✳ Iron deficiency
Fragmentation hemolysis
Hemoglobin H disease
Some thalassemia minor
Hemoglobinopathy traits (AC)
Some ACD

Macrocytic States, with Anemia

Normal RDW/High MCV

Aplastic anemia
Some cases of
   myelodysplasia

High RDW/High MCV

Vitamin B_{12} (folate) deficiency
Autoimmune hemolytic anemia
Cold agglutinin disease

Normocytic States, with Anemia

Normal RDW

Chronic disease
Hereditary spherocytosis
Some hemoglobinopathy
   traits

High RDW

Early iron/vitamin B_{12} or folate
   deficiency
Sickle cell anemia or SC disease

SOURCE: after Bessman JD, Gilmer PR, Gardner FH: Improved classification of anemia by MCV and RDW. *Am J Clin Pathol* 1983; 80:322-26.

ABBREVIATIONS: RDW = red cell distribution width; MCV = mean corpuscular volume; AC = hemoglobins A and C; ACD = anemia of chronic disease; SC = sickle cell.

variously microcytic, normocytic, or macrocytic; anisocytosis (as measured by the dispersion index parameter, RDW or RCMI) may be present or absent. The most common classification scheme using these two parameters is the one developed by Bessman et al (Table 2-3), which generally splits anemias into those caused by a type of deficiency, such as iron, vitamin B_{12}, or folic acid, and those anemias that are caused by genetic defects, such as thalassemia or primary marrow disorders. The deficiency-state anemias tend to have a greater degree of anisocytosis than do those caused by genetic defects or primary marrow disorders. Studies from several different centers have indicated that there are many loopholes in this classification scheme, particularly as they relate to anemia of chronic disease.

Another commonly used approach is to classify the anemia by the degree of reticulocytosis or marrow response present. The reticulocyte count and the correction procedures intended to correct for shift reticulocytes and for the degree of anemia were presented in chapter 1. Thus, the anemia may be classified as hyperproliferative, normoproliferative, or hypoproliferative, depending on the degree of reticulocytosis present. If the degree of reticulocytosis is adequate to correct the loss of red cells, the anemia is said to be "compensated"; if it is not adequate, the anemia is likely to worsen. This classification is less useful, except in certain situations such as hemolytic anemias. Because such classification schemes are not exclusive, incorporation of measurements of both cell volume and dispersion and measurements of the degree of reticulocytosis is possible.

Differential Diagnosis of Anemia

A bewildering variety of laboratory tests is available to evaluate the anemic patient. In some situations, some tests are appropriate; in others, they are inappropriate. All too often, the physician adopts a scatter gun approach by which many tests are ordered in the hope that one will provide an answer. The initial classification schemes using readily available complete blood count (CBC) data and the reticulocyte count, however, allow for appropriate classification of anemias into broad groups. This section presents a series of approaches to the differential diagnosis and proper classification of anemia using data developed from laboratory examinations.

Macrocytic Anemia. Macrocytic anemias are less commonly encountered than normocytic or microcytic anemias. Bessman et al have divided the macrocytic anemias into those with normal RDW, principally those caused by marrow failure states, such as aplastic anemia and myelodysplasia, those caused by deficiencies of vitamin B_{12} or folic acid, and those caused by autoimmune hemolysis or cold agglutinins; however, many exceptions to this classification scheme exist. For example, a mild degree of macrocytosis with a normal RDW is relatively common as a direct effect of alcohol. Macrocytosis is usually modest in this situation, with MCVs in the range of 102 to 105 fL. Likewise, some cases of myelodysplasia may have a high RDW. An alternative is to classify the macrocytic anemias by the presence or absence of a reticulocyte response. Hemolytic anemias, blood loss, and partially treated vitamin B_{12} or folic acid deficiencies will show an increased reticu-

Table 2−4   Classification of Macrocytic Anemias

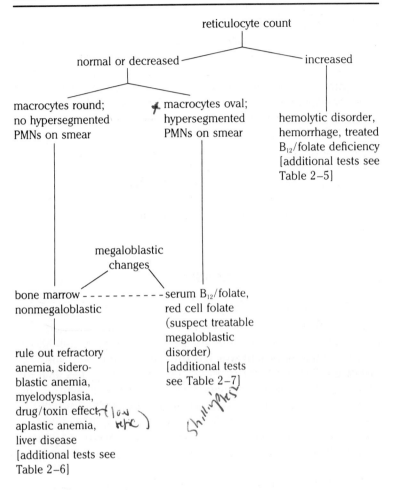

NOTE: MCV > 100 fL

ABBREVIATIONS: MCV = mean corpuscular volume; PMN = polymorphonuclear leukocyte.

locyte count; those caused by untreated vitamin B₁₂ or folic acid deficiencies or caused by the broad variety of toxic drugs, liver disease, thyroid disease, or the myelodysplasias will generally show a low reticulocyte response.

Table 2−4 indicates an effective classification scheme for macrocytic anemias based on the reticulocyte count. For those with an increased reticulocyte count, a search should be made for occult blood loss. If this is not present, autoimmune hemolysis, disorders

Table 2-5 Classification of Normocytic or Macrocytic Hyperproliferative Anemia

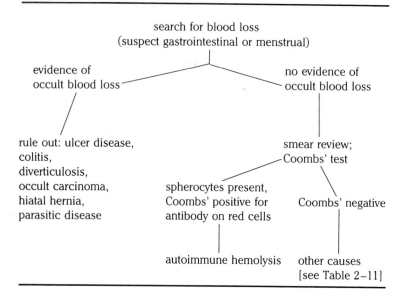

of membrane structural proteins (eg, elliptocytosis), paroxysmal nocturnal hemoglobinuria, and fragmentation hemolysis should be suspected. Not all such anemias are macrocytic; Table 2-5 indicates that some may be normocytic as well. For those patients with a normal or decreased corrected reticulocyte count, a disorder producing decreased marrow function, such as an untreated vitamin deficiency, drugs or toxins, liver or thyroid disease, or primary marrow failure should be suspected. Those patients whose blood smears show morphologic features compatible with megaloblastic anemia may be evaluated by vitamin assays without bone marrow examination, which is usually needed to detect megaloblastic changes in patients whose smears do not suggest vitamin B_{12} or folate deficiency. Further follow-up testing, as indicated in Tables 2-6 and 2-7, may be needed as well.

Microcytic Anemia.   Table 2-8 shows the initial classification protocol for patients who have an automated CBC MCV less than 75 fL. The three most common causes of microcytic anemias are iron deficiency, thalassemia minor, and anemia of chronic disease (ACD). Cases of thalassemia generally (but not invariably) have elevated red counts and lower RDWs than would be expected for the MCV and the degree of anemia. Iron deficiencies are almost always associated with a high RDW. The values seen in ACD are bewildering. Some ACDs may be normocytic; many, particularly in

Table 2−6   Ancillary Tests for Hypoproliferative Macrocytic Anemia Without Marrow Megaloblastosis

---

Thyroid function studies

Iron/iron-binding capacity; ferritin (assess iron stores)

Chromosomes, hemoglobin F/A_2 levels (evaluate myelodysplasia or aplastic anemia)

Table 2−7   Ancillary Tests for Hypoproliferative Macrocytic Anemia with Marrow Megaloblastosis

---

Dietary and drug history

Malabsorption studies

Schilling test if B_{12} deficiency documented

Search for occult tumor or myeloma

Ferritin

---

renal patients, are microcytic. ACD patients with microcytosis do not have decreased iron stores; in these situations, the test results reflective of body iron stores, such as serum ferritin, tend to be normal to high. A step-wise approach ordering noninvasive tests, such as ferritin, serum iron, and serum iron-binding capacity determinations, in patients with microcytosis and an elevated RDW will classify most patients without the necessity of a bone marrow examination. These approaches are outlined in Table 2−9.

Normocytic, Normochromic Anemia.   Normocytic anemic patients with an elevated reticulocyte count are evaluated using the same general approach used for macrocytic patients with an elevated reticulocyte count. Those patients with normal proliferative, normocytic, normochromic anemias generally require bone marrow evaluation. A peripheral smear may provide valuable clues for the differential diagnosis in such patients, as is indicated in Table 2−10.

Normocytic, normochromic anemias with elevated reticulocyte counts can be divided into those with positive antiglobulin test results (Coombs' test) and those lacking evidence of red cell bound antibodies. Coombs'-negative hemolytic anemias are quite heterogeneous. The peripheral blood smear and the history often suggest possible causes for the anemia (Table 2−11).

The differential diagnosis of anemia is often tempered or modified by knowledge of other patient data. All algorithmic classifi-

Table 2–8 Classification Protocol for Microcytic Anemias

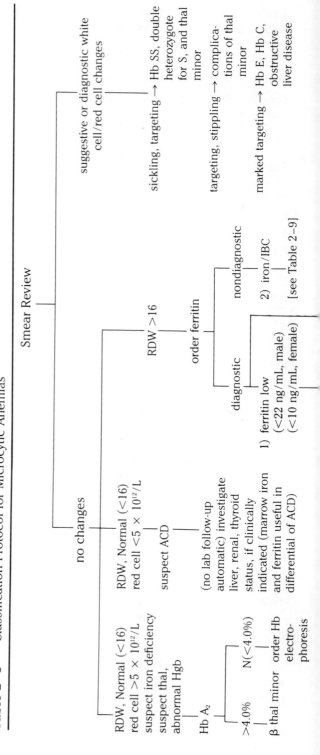

Smear Review

no changes

RDW, Normal (<16)
red cell >5 × 10¹²/L
suspect iron deficiency
suspect thal,
abnormal Hgb

Hb A₂

>4.0% N(<4.0%)

β thal minor order Hb electro-phoresis

RDW, Normal (<16)
red cell <5 × 10¹²/L

suspect ACD

(no lab follow-up automatic) investigate liver, renal, thyroid status, if clinically indicated (marrow iron and ferritin useful in differential of ACD)

RDW >16

order ferritin

diagnostic

1) ferritin low
(<22 ng/mL, male)
(<10 ng/mL, female)

nondiagnostic

2) iron/IBC
[see Table 2–9]

suggestive or diagnostic white cell/red cell changes

sickling, targeting → Hb SS, double heterozygote for S, and thal minor

targeting, stippling → complications of thal minor

marked targeting → Hb E, Hb C, obstructive liver disease

Table 2–9   Iron D

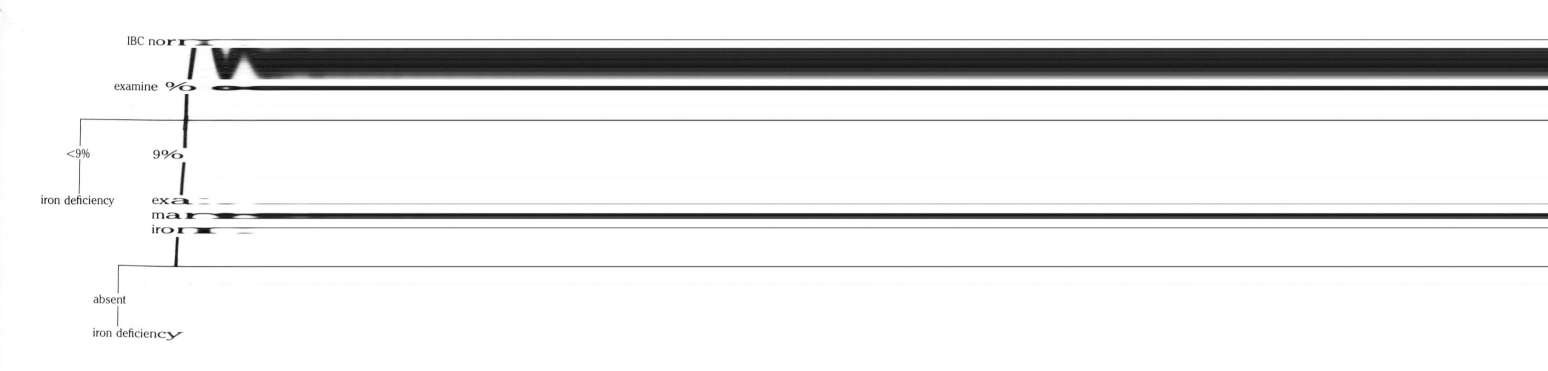

IBC nor

examine %

<9%   9%

iron deficiency   exa
                         mar
                         iro

absent

iron deficiency

ABBREVIATIONS: IBC = iron-bi
TIBC = total iron-binding ca

Table 2–10   Worku
Without Hyperprolifera

leukoerythroblastosis

perform bone marrow cult
save cells for leukemia/
lymphoma studies

red cell fragments, polychromatism → unsuspected hemolysis

rouleaux → increase in globlulins or decrease in albumin (benign or malignant)

neutrophils → hypersegmentation, with or without macrocytes

iron deficiency

2) ferritin high

examine bone marrow to rule out sideroblastic anemia, aplastic anemia (complicated), other causes of marrow failure

NOTE: automated MCV <75 fL.

ABBREVIATIONS: MCV = mean corpuscular volume; RDW = red cell distribution width; thal = thalassemia; ACD = anemia of chronic disease; IBC = iron-binding capacity.

Table 2–9   Iron Deficiency v Anemia of Chronic Disease

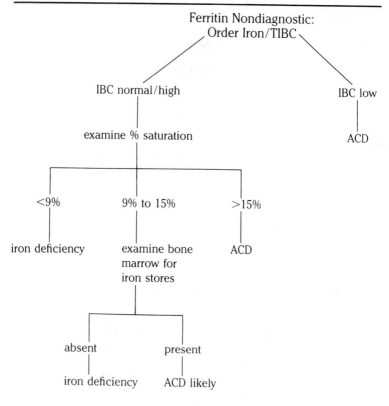

ABBREVIATIONS: IBC = iron-binding capacity; ACD = anemia of chronic disease; TIBC = total iron-binding capacity.

Table 2–10   Workup of Normocytic, Normochromic Anemia Without Hyperproliferative Response

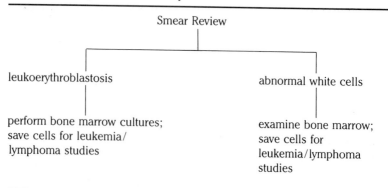

Table 2-11   Workup of Coombs' Negative Hemolytic Anemia

Is hemolysis episodic?

    Rule out G6PD deficiency (other enzymopathy if G6PD normal).

    Rule out PNH (sucrose hemolysis followed by Ham test if sucrose positive).

Does the smear suggest red cell fragmentation?

    Rule out DIC and TTP (haptoglobin, plasma hemoglobin, tests for unstable hemoglobin and Heinz bodies plus coagulation tests for DIC).

Does the smear contain morphologically abnormal red cells?

    Stippling suggests lead poisoning, pyrimidine 5'nucleotidase deficiency or thalassemia.

    Abnormal red cell shapes or increased target cells suggest abnormal hemoglobin.

    Spherocytes or family history suggests hereditary spherocytosis; perform *incubated* osmotic fragility.

    Other forms (elliptocytes, acanthocytes, etc) may be detected.

ABBREVIATIONS: G6PD = glucose-6-phosphate dehydrogenase; PNH = paroxysmal nocturnal hemoglobinuria; DIC = disseminated intravascular coagulation; TTP = thrombotic thrombocytopenic purpura.

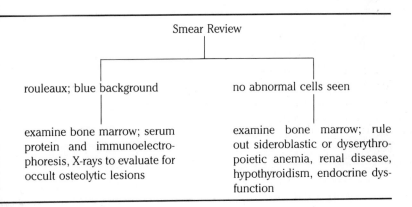

Smear Review

rouleaux; blue background	no abnormal cells seen
examine bone marrow; serum protein and immunoelectrophoresis, X-rays to evaluate for occult osteolytic lesions	examine bone marrow; rule out sideroblastic or dyserythropoietic anemia, renal disease, hypothyroidism, endocrine dysfunction

cation schemes should be tempered with the pragmatic knowledge of the physician considering the probable causes for anemia in an individual patient or patient group. For example, because 98% or more of the anemias in children under the age of 4 years are caused by iron deficiency, many pediatricians simply treat all anemic children in this group with iron supplementation and work up only those failing to respond to iron therapy. Likewise, in an elderly man with evidence of renal disease, directly ruling out plasma cell myeloma and performing tests to evaluate renal function would be the most cost-effective and appropriate way of working up such an anemic patient, regardless of classification algorithms. In many situations, clinical knowledge can suggest several possible causes of anemia; classification algorithms are suggested paths for physicians to follow in test utilization and should not be considered required routes.

References

1. Van Assenfeldt OW: Anemia and polycythemia: Interpretation of laboratory tests and differential diagnosis, in Koepke JA (ed): *Laboratory Hematology*. New York, Churchill Livingstone Inc, 1984, pp 865–902.

2. Schumacher HR, Garvin DF, Triplett DA (eds): Anemias: Approach to diagnosis, in *Introduction to Laboratory Hematology and Hematopathology*. New York, Alan R Liss Inc, 1984, pp 253–272.

3. Wintrobe MM, Lee GR, Boggs DR, et al (eds): The approach to the patient with anemia, in *Clinical Hematology*, ed 8. Philadelphia, Lea & Febiger, 1981, pp 529–558.

4. Williams WJ, Beutler E, Erslev AJ, et al (eds): The patient with hematologic disease, in *Hematology*, ed 3. New York, McGraw International Book Co, 1983, pp 37–53.

3

Iron Deficiency Anemia

Hypochromic microcytic red cells seen in the blood film of an anemic patient suggest a defect in the rate of hemoglobin synthesis. Such a defect may arise because insufficient iron is present; because of hereditary abnormalities in globin synthesis, such as the thalassemias or the unstable hemoglobins (see chapter 11); or as a result of inhibition of heme synthesis by toxic materials, such as lead. It may occur as a consequence of neoplastic disorders, or as a hereditary or idiopathic disorder in which increased numbers of sideroblasts are present in the bone marrow. The most common types of hypochromic anemia are listed in Table 3–1.

Pathophysiology

Iron deficiency is the most common cause of anemia and ranks among the most common of all diseases in humans. In infants and children, a negative iron balance may occur because the dietary intake of iron is inadequate to meet the requirements for growth. In adults, iron deficiency may be the result of pregnancy or of blood loss, and because losses of iron are otherwise very small, dietary intake plays at most a contributory role in the etiology of the disease. Physicians must identify the cause of iron deficiency, because it may be the first sign of a malignant lesion of the gastrointestinal or genitourinary tract.

Table 3–1   Causes of Hypochromic Anemia

Iron deficiency

Thalassemias
  Alpha-thalassemias
  Beta-thalassemias

Sideroblastic anemias
  Hereditary (sex-linked)
  Acquired
    Drug-induced (eg, lead, alcohol, isoniazid [INH])
    Idiopathic (myelodysplastic syndromes)

Chronic disorders
  Chronic infections
  Chronic inflammatory states
  Neoplastic diseases

Thalassemia is also very common in many populations and rivals iron deficiency in frequency of occurrence.

Clinical Findings

The clinical findings of hypochromic anemias depend on the severity of the anemia and its underlying cause. Severe anemia is associated with pallor, weakness, palpitations, and even dyspnea. These symptoms are more prominent in iron deficiency anemia, where the deficiency state contributes to the symptomatology, than they are in mild thalassemia. Mild to moderate chronic anemia is well tolerated by most patients, particularly in the younger age groups.

Approach to Diagnosis

Hypochromic, microcytic anemias may be evaluated as follows:

1. Examination of red cell morphology, red cell indices, the size distribution of the red cells, and, occasionally, the bone marrow.

2. Estimation of serum iron levels and total iron-binding capacity or ferritin levels. The measurements reflect iron stores and help

to distinguish iron deficiency from other causes of microcytic, hypochromic anemia.

3. Measurement of free erythrocyte protoporphyrin, which is of particular value as a screening test for distinguishing iron deficiency from thalassemia minor.

4. Examination of aspirated bone marrow for stainable iron, the most direct assessment of iron stores.

5. Hemoglobin electrophoresis, particularly to determine levels of HbA_2, which are increased in most patients with beta-thalassemia.

6. Determination of globin chain synthetic ratios, which is often the only means of making a positive diagnosis of mild forms of alpha-thalassemia.

7. Documentation of the hematologic response to therapy, which confirms the diagnosis of iron deficiency.

Hematologic Findings

In well-developed iron deficiency anemia, hypochromia, microcytosis, and anisocytosis are usually present. No morphologic abnormalities of the red cells however, may be present in mild iron deficiency. Hypochromia and microcytosis are found uniformly in the thalassemias, and the reductions in MCV and MCHC are generally greater than those observed in iron deficiency anemia of the same degree. Microcytosis with significant elevations of the red cell count to $>6 \times 10^{12}/L$ $(6 \times 10^6/\mu l)$ are common in thalassemia minor. Stippled red cells are seen commonly on the blood film in thalassemia but are unusual in iron deficiency. Hypochromia is often present in patients with sideroblastic anemia, but it is by no means a universal finding. It also occurs in patients with chronic inflammatory or neoplastic disorders. Changes in the size distribution of the red cells are determined best with automated cell-counting equipment. Characteristically, the variability of red cell size is increased in iron deficiency, but not in thalassemia.

Blood Cell Measurements.   When anemia is severe, the MCV is decreased. The reticulocyte count may be modestly decreased, normal, or modestly increased. Indices are often normal in patients with hemoglobin levels >100 g/L (10g/dl).

Peripheral Blood Smear Morphology.   Hypochromia and microcytosis are present (Figure 3–1). Other changes are noted in Table 3–2.

Table 3–2 Blood Smear Findings in Hypochromic Anemia

Cause of Hypochromic Anemia	Anisocytosis and Poikilocytosis	Basophilic Stippling
Iron deficiency	Yes	No
Thalassemia minor	No	Yes
Sideroblastic anemias		
Hereditary	Yes	Yes
Acquired	Variable	Yes
Chronic disease	No	No

Bone Marrow Examination. Erythroid hyperplasia is often present, but it is not as prominent as it is in the hemolytic anemias. The only specific findings in this group are decreased or absent stainable storage iron in iron deficiency anemia and the presence of ring sideroblasts in sideroblastic anemias.

Other Laboratory Tests

3.1 Serum Iron Quantitation and Total Iron-Binding Capacity

Purpose. Serum iron and total iron-binding capacity (TIBC) determinations are particularly useful in mild iron deficiency anemia, in which decreased serum iron levels may precede changes in red cell morphology or in red cell indices, and in distinguishing iron deficiency anemia from other microcytic hypochromic anemias.

Principle. All transport iron in the plasma is bound in the ferric form to the specific iron-binding protein, transferrin. Serum iron refers to this transferrin-bound iron. TIBC, the concentration iron necessary to saturate the iron-binding sites of transferrin, is a measure of transferrin concentration. Saturation of transferrin is calculated by the following formula:

$$\% \text{ Transferrin Saturation} = \frac{\text{Serum Iron (mol/L)}}{\text{TIBC (}\mu\text{mol/L)}} \times 100.$$

Normal mean transferrin saturation is approximately 30%. Unsaturated iron-binding capacity (UIBC) is the difference between TIBC and serum iron.

Specimen.   A specimen of blood should be drawn in the morning. Serum is used for the determination.

Procedure.   Serum iron is freed from transferrin by acidification of the serum and is then reduced to the ferrous form. After the protein has been precipitated, the filtrate is reacted with a chromogen, such as 3-(2-pyridyl)-5,6 bis (4-phenylsulfonic acid), and the color formed is measured. The colorimetric determination of TIBC involves addition of iron to serum followed by removal of excess, unbound iron by absorption. The bound iron is then released from transferrin and reduced, and its concentration is measured as in the serum iron test. The TIBC also can be determined by measuring transferrin by immunodiffusion.

Interpretation.   The representative normal range of values for serum iron is 12.7 to 35.9 μmol/L (60 to 180 μg/dl); for TIBC, 45.2 to 77.7 μmol/L(250 to 410 μg/dl); and for percent saturation, 20% to 50%. The serum iron level is low, and percent saturation is characteristically reduced in both iron deficiency anemia and the anemia of chronic disease. Although the value for percent saturation is often reduced to levels <16% in iron deficiency anemia and is more frequently >16% in anemia of chronic disease, values overlap in the two conditions. The TIBC is uniformly increased in severe uncomplicated iron deficiency anemias and is decreased or normal in the microcytic anemia of chronic disease. In mild iron deficiency anemia, both the serum iron and TIBC may be normal. Serum iron concentration is increased in the sideroblastic anemias and in some cases of thalassemia (Table 3–3).

Notes and Precautions.   Because of diurnal variations in serum iron levels (maximum, 7 to 10 AM), and the fact that stated ranges are for morning normal levels, specimens should be drawn in the morning. Iron therapy should be withdrawn 24 hours before the blood sample is drawn. Iron dextran administration causes plasma iron levels to be elevated for several weeks. A normal plasma iron level and iron-binding capacity do not rule out the diagnosis of iron deficiency when the hemoglobin level of the blood is above 90 g/L (9 g/dl) (females) and 110 g/L (11g/dl) (males).

Table 3–3 Serum Iron, Iron-Binding Capacity, and Storage Iron in Hypochromic Anemias

Cause of Hypo-chromic Anemia	Serum Iron	TIBC	(%) Saturation	Bone Marrow Storage Iron
Iron deficiency	Decreased[a]	Decreased[a]	Decreased[a]	Decreased
Thalassemias	Increased or normal	Decreased or normal	Increased or normal	Increased or normal
Sideroblastic anemias	Increased	Decreased or normal	Increased	Increased
Chronic disease	Decreased	Decreased	Decreased	Increased

ABBREVIATIONS: TIBC = total iron-binding capacity.

[a] Serum iron and TIBC occasionally normal in iron deficiency

3.2   Stainable Bone Marrow Iron

Purpose.   The most direct means for assessing body iron stores is by histochemical examination of aspirated bone marrow for storage iron.

Principle.   Iron is stored in reticuloendothelial cells, and iron granules are formed in developing normoblasts. Normoblasts that contain one or more particles of stainable iron are known as sideroblasts. Iron is stored as ferritin, in which iron is complexed to the protein, apoferritin, and as hemosiderin, which consists of iron-protein complexes with a high iron content, at least partially, and of ferritin-denatured aggregates. Hemosiderin is the stainable form of storage iron that appears blue when treated with an acid potassium ferrocyanide solution used in the Prussian-blue reaction.

Specimen.   Either sectioned bone marrow fragments or particle smears are used for the assessment of reticuloendothelial iron, but marrow films must be used to detect sideroblasts.

Procedure.   The bone marrow aspirate is stained using the Prussian-blue reaction. Heating the staining mixture to 56°C increases its sensitivity. The search for sideroblasts is aided by a counterstain, such as basic fuchsin.

Interpretation. Normally, hemosiderin granules are seen in reticuloendothelial cells in every third or fourth oil-immersion field. With reduced iron stores, either no or only a few hemosiderin granules are seen in the entire preparation. With increased iron stores, hemosiderin granules are seen in every oil-immersion field, often deposited in clumps. The appraisal of reticuloendothelial iron is extremely helpful in the differential diagnosis of anemia (Table 3–3). Since iron from breakdown of red cell heme cannot be excreted and is diverted to the storage compartment, increased amounts of iron are generally present in the marrow of anemic patients who are not iron deficient. An exception may exist in myeloproliferative disorders in which bone marrow iron stores may be absent without other evidence of iron deficiency; this may result from impaired storage function. Since stainable marrow iron is occasionally absent in healthy subjects, the presence of such iron is more diagnostic than its absence. When storage iron is present in the marrow, anemia cannot be a result of iron deficiency, unless the patient has been treated with parenterally administered iron.

Normally, 20% to 40% of red cell precursors are sideroblasts. Although a sideroblast count is not ordinarily necessary for the diagnosis of iron deficiency anemia, it may be useful when an inadequate number of marrow particles was obtained and in patients who have received parenterally administered iron. Loss of sideroblasts from the marrow is seen in iron deficiency anemia, after acute blood loss when reticuloendothelial stores have not yet been depleted, and in chronic inflammatory disease. Sideroblastic anemia is characterized by the presence of ring sideroblasts. These are normoblasts that contain iron granules surrounding at least three fourths of the nuclear circumference.

Notes and Precautions. Some practice is required to distinguish stainable reticuloendothelial iron from artifacts. When a patient has received iron by the parenteral route, either as an iron carbohydrate complex, such as iron dextran (Imferon), or in the form of blood transfusions, histochemically stainable iron stores may be seen in the marrow in the presence of iron deficiency anemia. Particles on a marrow film represent a larger volume of marrow than do sections of fixed marrow particles; thus, iron is more likely to be seen on marrow films. A well-prepared marrow film is essential for the detection of iron granules in normoblasts.

3.3   Serum Ferritin Quantitation

Purpose.   Minute amounts of the iron storage compound ferritin or the antigenically equivalent apoferritin normally circulates in the plasma. Estimating serum ferritin levels provides a semi-quantitative, less invasive test for iron store determination than the histochemical examination of aspirated marrow.

Principle.   Ferritin is a complex of the protein apoferritin and iron. It serves principally as an iron storage compound. The largest quantities of ferritin are found in the liver and reticuloendo-thelial cells. Ordinarily, serum ferritin concentration reflects the amount of stored iron.

Specimen.   Serum is obtained.

Procedure.   Reliable estimation of serum ferritin levels has been achieved with a sensitive radioimmune method using a sandwich technique. Ferritin is removed from the serum by solid-phase antiferritin antibodies, and radioactively labeled antiferritin antibodies are then permitted to bind to the removed ferritin.

Interpretation.   The normal concentration of serum ferritin varies in a broad range from 10 to 500 $\mu g/L$ (10 to 500 ng/mL). In iron deficiency anemia, serum ferritin level is diminished and appears to be a relatively sensitive and reliable indicator of the presence of iron deficiency. Serum ferritin levels may be low in iron deficiency that is not associated with anemia, while elevated levels are common in iron-overload states, including sideroblastic anemia.

Serum ferritin levels are elevated in patients with inflammatory disease and, for poorly understood reasons, in patients with Gaucher disease. Ferritin levels are increased in hemochromatosis.

Notes and Precautions.   When iron deficiency and inflammatory disease coexist, serum ferritin levels may be in the normal range.

3.4   Free Erythrocyte Protoporphyrin

Purpose.   Free erythrocyte protoporphyrin (FEP) levels are elevated in anemias associated with failure of iron incorporation into heme.

Principle.   When insufficient iron is available for developing erythroblasts, some protoporphyrin that was destined to be converted to heme accumulates as FEP. This substance is elevated both with depleted iron stores and in conditions associated with an internal block in iron utilization, as in certain chronic disorders, lead poisoning, and sideroblastic anemias.

Specimen.   Whole blood is collected in anticoagulant. There is also a spot test for blood specimens collected on filter paper.

Procedure.   FEP is extracted from red cells with ethyl acetate/acetic acid and is quantitated fluorometrically.

Interpretation.   FEP is normally <1.7 $\mu mol/L$ (100 $\mu g/dl$) packed red cells. Elevated levels are seen in iron deficiency, in chronic disease states associated with decreased transferrin saturation, and in acquired idiopathic sideroblastic anemia. Marked elevation of FEP is seen in sideroblastic anemia secondary to lead intoxication with FEP values of about 17 $\mu mol/L$ (1000 $\mu g/dl$) packed red cells. In microcytic anemias associated with abnormal globin synthesis rather than abnormal heme synthesis, such as thalassemia minor, FEP levels are normal. Because iron deficiency anemia and thalassemia minor are the first and second most common causes, respectively, of hypochromic, microcytic anemia, measurement of FEP may be particularly useful as a screening test to distinguish these two disorders.

Course and Treatment

In the final analysis, the correctness of the diagnosis of iron deficiency depends on demonstration of an adequate response to iron therapy. Treatment usually consists of the oral administration of a ferrous iron salt, such as ferrous sulfate, in a dosage providing 0.06 to 0.12 g of iron three times a day. Under some circumstances, the parenteral administration of iron may be preferred. Although reticulocytosis and a significant rise in blood hemoglobin concentration may occur as early as the third or fourth day after treatment, particularly in children, a reticulocyte response often is not observed for 7 or 8 days, and the hemoglobin concentration in the blood may not rise significantly during the first 10 days of treatment. Thereafter, however, restoration of the hemoglobin level to normal should be rapid and essentially complete by the sixth week after institution of therapy, regardless of the initial severity of the anemia. Infection, inflammatory disease, or neoplastic disease may prevent an adequate response, and continued bleeding may blunt the apparent therapeutic effect. The most common cause of failure to respond, however, is an incorrect diagnosis. It is important to identify the cause of the iron deficiency (almost always blood loss or pregnancy in adults) to correct it, if possible. Iron deficiency can be an early warning of gastrointestinal cancer.

References

1. Fairbanks VF, Beutler E: Iron in medicine and nutrition, in Shils ME, Young VR (eds): *Modern Nutrition in Health and Disease.* Philadelphia, Lea & Febiger, 1988, pp 193–226.
2. Fairbanks VF, Beutler E: Iron deficiency, in Williams WJ, Beutler E, Erslev A, et al (eds): *Hematology,* ed 3. New York, McGraw-Hill International Book Co, 1983, pp 466–489.
3. Finch CA, Cook JD: Iron deficiency. *Am J Clin Nutr* 1984; 39:471–477.
4. Finch CA, Huebers H: Perspectives in iron metabolism. *N Engl J Med* 1982; 306:1520–1528.
5. Lipschitz DA, Cook JD, Finch CA: A clinical evaluation of serum ferritin as an index of iron stores. *N Engl J Med* 1974; 290:1213–1216.

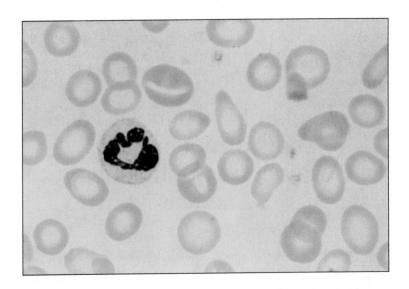

Figure 3–1   Iron deficiency anemia. The red blood cells are hypochromic and microcytic.

4

Anemia of Chronic Disease and Normochromic, Normocytic Nonhemolytic Anemias

Anemia occurring in patients with chronic diseases is often caused by multiple simultaneously acting mechanisms, including nutritional deficiencies, blood loss, and anemia of chronic disease (ACD). ACD is defined by a constellation of clinical, morphologic, and laboratory features (Table 4–1) and is second only to iron deficiency anemia in incidence. In a tertiary care setting, chronic disease may be the most frequently encountered cause of anemia. Affected patients usually develop normocytic, normochromic (hemolytic or nonhemolytic) anemia that is mild and nonprogressive 1 to 2 months after the onset of chronic disease. This anemia is associated with multiple iron-related abnormalities, including: decreased serum iron level, decreased transferrin level, decreased transferrin saturation, and normal-to-increased storage iron level. The bone marrow examination reveals that erythroid precursors are generally present in normal numbers, but the erythroid iron is decreased, while the storage iron is increased.

A variety of inflammatory, infectious, and neoplastic disorders (Table 4–2) are associated with ACD. Because the etiologies of anemias are considerably more complex in patients with renal, hepatic, and endocrine disorders, these will be discussed separately at the end of the chapter.

Table 4–1   Characteristics of Anemia of Chronic Disease

Clinical

   Development of anemia 1–2 months after onset of chronic disease

Blood

   Usually normocytic, normochromic anemia with normal MCV, MCHC, and RDW

Iron Studies

   Decreased serum/plasma iron

   Decreased transferrin (TIBC)

   Decreased transferrin saturation

   Normal-to-increased storage iron

Bone Marrow

   Normal numbers of erythroid precursors

   Decreased sideroblasts

   Increased storage iron

ABBREVIATIONS: MCV = mean corpuscular volume; MCHC = mean corpuscular hemoglobin concentration; RDW = red cell distribution width; TIBC = total iron-binding capacity.

Pathophysiology

Three separate pathophysiologic defects are responsible for ACD. Failure of erythropoiesis, lack of iron for hemoglobin synthesis, and decreased red cell survival together produce this disorder. The major defect is thought to be a failure of sufficient erythropoiesis to compensate for the decreased red cell survival, although erythroid precursors are present in the bone marrow. The decreased availability of iron for hemoglobin synthesis further aggravates this inadequate erythropoiesis. Erythroid precursors normally acquire from transferrin the iron necessary for hemoglobin synthesis. The decrease in serum iron level, serum transferrin level, and stainable iron in erythroid precursors indicates that insufficient iron is available for hemoglobin synthesis. The mildly decreased red cell survival is caused by extracorpuscular abnormalities rather than any intrinsic red cell defect; in patients with ACD, the marrow is unable to compensate for this survival defect.

    Current evidence suggests that the three pathophysiologic defects responsible for the development of ACD can be attributed

Table 4–2   Diseases Associated with Anemia of
Chronic Disease

Chronic inflammatory disorders

    Rheumatoid arthritis

    Systemic lupus erythematosis

    Sarcoidosis

    Trauma

Chronic infections

    Tuberculosis

    Pyelonephritis

    Osteomyelitis

    Chronic fungal infections

    Subacute bacterial endocarditis

Neoplasms

    Malignant lymphoma

    Carcinoma

---

largely to sustained interleukin-1 secretion. This monocyte-macrophage-secreted hormone (also designated as leukocyte endogenous mediator or endogenous pyrogen) mediates rapid host response to inflammation and infection and produces a wide variety of systemic and local effects by its action on numerous cell types throughout the body (Table 4–3). Several of these local and systemic effects, sustained over a prolonged period, appear to cause ACD. For example, chronic interleukin-1 production decreases plasma iron level, elevates body temperature, causes secondary granule release by neutrophils, and activates T-cells and monocytes (Table 4–4). Because T-cells and monocytes participate in the regulation of hematopoiesis, their activation causes some alteration in this regulatory process and may be responsible for the marrow's failure to compensate for anemia. Secondary granules of neutrophils contain lactoferrin that, when released, has a major impact on the availability of iron for erythropoiesis, because lactoferrin competes with transferrin for iron binding within the blood. This competition is exacerbated if the blood pH level is decreased in an infectious or inflammatory process, because at low pH the binding of iron to lactoferrin is enhanced. Once iron has bound to lactoferrin, it is delivered exclusively to macrophages and is therefore not available for erythropoiesis. Iron is also an important nutritional factor for

Table 4–3   Characteristics of Interleukin-1

Definition:
Hormone primarily produced by monocytes and macrophages. Mediates rapid host response to inflammation and infection.

Acute Phase

    Hepatic synthesis of proteins

Reactions Mediated by IL-1

    Decreased plasma iron

    Fever

    Neutrophilia

    Neutrophil migration to tissues enhanced by increased endothelial cell adhesiveness

    Secondary granule release by neutrophils

    T-cell activation

    B-cell activation with immunoglobulin synthesis

    Decreased appetite

    Attraction of neutrophils, monocytes, and lymphocytes to tissue sites of inflammation

    Monocyte activation

Cells with IL-1 receptors

    T and B lymphocytes

    Neutrophils

    Macrophages

    Fibroblasts

    Endothelial cells

    Natural killer cells

    Hepatocytes

    Osteoclasts

    Chondrocytes

    Synovial cells

    Muscle cells

ABBREVIATIONS: IL-1 = interleukin-1.

Table 4–4   Mechanisms by which Interleukin-1 May Cause Anemia of Chronic Disease

---

Indirect suppression of erythropoiesis

  IL-1 regulates lymphoid cells and monocytes that in turn regulate hematopoiesis

Lactoferrin release from secondary granules of neutrophils

  Lactoferrin competes with transferrin for iron

  Lactoferrin delivers iron exclusively to macrophages, rendering it unavailable for erythropoiesis

Indirect responsibility for the mild red cell survival defect

  Fever may cause shortened red cell survival

  Activated macrophages more readily ingest erythrocytes

ABBREVIATIONS: IL-1 = interleukin-1.

---

microorganisms, so that a low serum iron level limits their proliferation. Sustained interleukin-1 production also may contribute to the mild red blood cell survival defect noted in patients with ACD. Fever, induced by interleukin-1 secretion, has been shown to decrease red blood cell survival. In addition, enhanced ingestion of erythrocytes by macrophages activated by interleukin-1 decreases red cell survival.

Clinical Findings

Because ACD is generally mild, the patient's symptoms are related largely to the underlying disease. There are no physical examination findings unique to ACD.

Approach to Diagnosis

In a patient with anemia *and* a chronic illness, the contribution of ACD to this anemia can vary from major to insignificant. Because multiple underlying causes of anemia in such a patient population is the rule rather than the exception, the patient's evaluation should also establish the diagnosis of other types of anemia. For example, a patient with a neoplasm may suffer from iron deficiency anemia secondary to chronic blood loss, myelophthistic anemia secondary to bone marrow replacement by tumor, hypoplastic anemia sec-

Table 4–5   Causes of Anemia in Patients with Malignancies

Anemia of chronic disease

Blood loss

Bone marrow replacement by tumor

Bone marrow suppression by chemotherapy

Chemotherapy-related myelodysplasia

Hypersplenism

Microangiopathic hemolytic anemia secondary to drug treatment (eg, mitomycin C)

Microangiopathic hemolytic anemia secondary to intravascular mucin released from certain widespread adenocarcinomas

Immune-mediated hemolysis (autoantibody produced by certain B-cell neoplasms)

---

ondary to bone marrow suppression by chemotherapeutic agents, or even microangiopathic hemolytic anemia secondary to drug treatment or mucin production by the tumor. Table 4–5 lists these and other possible factors that contribute to the anemias that occur in patients with neoplasms. During the course of the clinical and hematologic evaluation of the patient, it is often readily apparent that one or more of these additional causes of anemia is present. In clinical practice, the distinction between ACD and iron deficiency anemia is the most frequent diagnostic dilemma.

The laboratory evaluation of patients for possible ACD usually includes the following:

1. Measurement of standard hematologic parameters with reticulocyte count.

2. Evaluation of peripheral blood smear for "clues" suggesting other types of anemia.

3. Iron studies, including assays of serum iron, transferrin, and iron stores.

4. Appropriate laboratory testing to establish or exclude diagnoses of other types of anemia.

5. Bone marrow aspiration, with iron stains, and biopsy in selected cases that are not clear-cut after other studies.

The laboratory approach to the evaluation of these patients must always be correlated with the patient's clinical findings. The approach should be tailored to each case using clues from the patient's history and physical examination to direct the sequence of tests utilized.

Hematologic Findings

There are no pathognomonic findings in the peripheral blood in patients with ACD. These patients generally have a mild-to-moderate anemia that is not associated with an increase in the reticulocyte count.

Blood Cell Measurements. In ACD, the hemoglobin level ranges from 70 to 110 g/L (7 to 11 g/dl). These cells vary little in size as indicated by their normal or near-normal red cell distribution width (RDW). The mean corpuscular volume (MCV), mean corpuscular hemoglobin (MCH), and mean corpuscular hemoglobin concentration (MCHC) are generally normal, although the MCV and MCHC may be mildly decreased. Although the reticulocyte count is usually within the normal range, it is decreased when corrected for the degree of anemia. White blood cell and platelet count are usually normal.

Peripheral Blood Smear Morphology. Erythrocytes are generally normocytic and normochromic without significant anisopoikilocytosis or polychromasia. These cells occasionally are mildly hypochromic, and there are usually no abnormalities of white blood cells or platelets.

Bone Marrow Examination. Erythroid elements in the bone marrow are generally morphologically normal and present in normal numbers. Sideroblasts are decreased, while the storage iron is increased substantially. Myeloid and megakaryocytic elements are generally unremarkable.

Other Laboratory Tests

While no single laboratory test is specific for ACD, a well-established laboratory profile includes serum iron, iron transport protein, and storage iron measurements that can aid in this diagnosis.

4.1   Serum Iron Quantitation

Purpose.   The determination of serum iron, in conjunction with other iron studies described below, is important in distinguishing ACD from other types that may develop in these patients.

Principle, Specimen, Procedure, Notes, and Precautions.
See Test 3.1.

Interpretation. A prompt decline in serum iron level is associated with infection and other types of tissue injury. This decrease precedes the development of anemia, which occurs only if the infection or injury is sustained. Low serum iron level is seen also in iron deficiency anemia.

4.2 Transferrin Measurement (Total Iron-Binding Capacity)

Purpose, Principle, Specimen, Procedure, Notes, and Precautions. See Test 3.1.

Interpretation. Transferrin is characteristically decreased in patients with ACD in contrast to the substantial elevation of this protein level that occurs in patients with iron deficiency anemia. This test, however, is neither specific nor sensitive enough to consistently distinguish between these two types of anemia.

4.3 Transferrin Saturation

Purpose. The percent saturation of transferrin reflects the availability of iron for erythropoiesis and can be calculated by dividing the transferrin level by the serum iron level.

Interpretation. The percent saturation of transferrin is generally decreased in patients with ACD, in whom a range of 10% to 25% saturation is usually found. Although in iron deficiency anemia the percent saturation of transferrin is usually less than 15%, there is some overlap between the percent saturation ranges found in these two disorders.

4.4 Ferritin Quantitation

Purpose. The serum ferritin level is a measure of the patient's total body iron stores.

Principle, Specimen, Procedure, Notes, and Precautions.
See Test 3.3.

Interpretation.   The serum ferritin level is characteristically normal to increased in patients with ACD, reflecting their abundant storage iron. The serum ferritin level in patients with iron deficiency anemia is generally markedly decreased.

Notes and Precautions.   Because ferritin is an acute-phase reactant, it may be elevated spuriously in patients' acute inflammatory processes. Despite this problem, serum ferritin levels are still of value in patients with possible ACD because they can help distinguish these patients from those with iron deficiency anemia. If results of serum ferritin assays are correlated with erythrocyte sedimentation rate, the distinction between ACD and iron deficiency anemia is enhanced.

Ancillary Tests

The free erythrocyte protoporphyrin level is elevated in ACD because the iron available for hemoglobin synthesis is decreased. This test, however, is not generally used in the initial evaluation of patients for this disorder.

Course and Treatment

Treatment and management of the underlying disease is of paramount importance in the care of patients with ACD. Eradication of the underlying disorder results in improvement of the anemia. ACD is often mild and usually does not require specific treatment. Therapies that have been tried and have been generally unsuccessful in these patients include iron and androgen treatment. Transfusion results in temporary improvement but is not recommended unless the patient has symptoms of anemia.

Anemia with Chronic Renal Disease.   The anemia that often occurs in patients with chronic renal disease is similar to ACD. The anemia in these patients is generally normocytic and normochromic, and its severity roughly parallels the severity of the underlying renal disease. As in ACD, multiple factors contribute to the development of anemia in patients with renal disease. Some important pathophysiologic differences exist between these two disorders, however. The primary pathophysiologic mechanism for anemia in these patients is decreased erythropoiesis secondary either to decreased erythropoietin level or nonfunctional erythropoietin. In these patients, the bone marrow usually shows erythroid hypoplasia. Azotemia also exacerbates the anemia, because it directly suppresses the bone marrow, and because it causes decreased red blood cell survival. Other manifestations of the anemia associated with chronic renal disease include burr cells in the blood, decreased serum iron level, and decreased transferrin level. Sustained secretion of interleukin-1 may be responsible for these iron and transferrin abnormalities. Several additional factors can contribute to a patient's anemia. These patients may have chronic blood loss because of both platelet and vessel defects secondary to the underlying renal disease. Patients undergoing chronic hemodialysis can readily become folate deficient. Finally, patients with renal disease are very prone to fluid overload, which can further decrease the hematocrit value.

The management and treatment of the underlying renal disease is of primary importance in these patients. Transfusion is generally not recommended, unless patients have significant symptoms from the anemia. Treatment with synthetic erythropoietin has recently become a therapeutic option.

Anemia with Chronic Endocrine Disease.   The anemias seen in patients with chronic endocrine disorders are similar to ACD. The major difference between these two disorders is the pathophysiologic mechanisms. Anemia in patients with chronic endocrine disorders is thought to be caused primarily by the decreased oxygen requirements of tissues that result from decreased thyroid hormone secretion. Decreased erythropoietin production, however, may also occur in these patients, because its production is indirectly modulated by pituitary and thyroid hormones. In these patients, other types of anemia may develop simultaneously with the anemia secondary to endocrine abnormalities. For example, some patients with hypothyroidism develop pernicious anemia, or iron deficiency anemia in addition to the decreased tissue oxygen requirement.

Treatment of the underlying endocrine disorder is of primary importance in the care of these patients. The anemia generally does not require treatment.

Anemia Associated with Alcoholism.   Anemia is a very common finding in patients with acute and chronic alcoholism. Although this anemia is generally mild to moderate, it can periodically become more severe in proportion to the patient's alcohol ingestion and the severity of the patient's liver disease.

Although ACD may occur in patients with alcoholism, the anemia in these patients frequently has multiple causes, including:

direct toxic effects of alcohol, various nutritional deficiencies, red cell survival defects, abnormal iron metabolism, or all of these. The predominant mechanism causing anemia may vary with time. The pathogenesis and morphologic features of the various causes of anemia in patients with alcoholism are shown in Table 4–6. Alcohol, especially when ingested in large amounts, has a direct toxic effect on hematopoietic elements, resulting in decreased bone marrow cellularity and vacuolization of erythroid precursors. Nutritional deficiencies often found in patients with chronic alcoholism include folate and iron deficiency. Folate deficiency is particularly common in these patients because of decreased ingestion, impairment of folate absorption by alcohol, and antagonism of folate by alcohol. Although typical morphologic features of megaloblastic anemia may be identified in the blood and bone marrow of patients with alcoholism, these changes are often masked by concurrent red cell abnormalities from iron deficiency, hemolysis, or both. Iron stores may be decreased in patients with chronic alcoholism because of decreased ingestion and chronic gastrointestinal blood loss. Hypochromasia is generally present, but the microcytosis of iron deficiency may be masked by the macrocytosis caused by liver disease, folate deficiency, or both. Decreased red cell survival is seen frequently in alcoholic patients with significant hepatic disease. The target cells, spherocytes, spur cells, and microspherocytes that may be identified in the peripheral blood of patients with chronic alcoholism are secondary to extracorpuscular red cell defects caused by congestive splenomegaly, lipoprotein abnormalities in the blood, and severe hypophosphatemia. In addition to iron deficiency, patients with chronic alcoholism frequently have abnormal iron metabolism that is manifested by ring sideroblasts in the bone marrow. Although the etiology of this phenomenon is not completely understood, the ring sideroblasts are caused in part by decreased functional pyridoxine and decreased activity of the enzymes involved in hemoglobin synthesis. Finally, portal hypertension is often associated with an increase in plasma volume that leads to dilutional anemia.

It is beyond the scope of this chapter to detail the clinical findings and laboratory features of patients with acute and chronic alcoholism. Details of the laboratory evaluation of patients (alcoholic or otherwise) with iron deficiency and folate deficiency can be found in chapters 3 and 6, respectively. Except for patients with pronounced spur cell formation, marked nutritional deficiency, or gastrointestinal tract bleeding, the anemia associated with chronic alcoholism is generally mild to moderate and does not require treatment. Management of the portal hypertension and congestive splenomegaly is important in ameliorating the red cell survival defects.

Table 4–6 Pathogenesis and Morphologic Features of Anemia in Patients with Alcoholism[a]

Mechanism	Morphologic Features	Etiology/Cause
Toxic suppression	Hypocellular bone marrow with vacuolated erythroid precursors	Alcohol toxic to hematopoietic elements
Folate deficiency[b]	Megaloblastic anemia with oval macrocytes and hypersegmented neutrophils Macrocytosis perhaps masked by concurrent iron deficiency	Decreased ingestion, impaired absorption, and antagonistic action of alcohol v folate
Iron deficiency[c]	Hypochromia present but microcytosis often masked by concurrent macrocytosis from hepatic disease	Decreased ingestion of iron and chronic blood loss via GI tract
Decreased red cell survival	Target cells, spherocytes, sometimes spur cells and microspherocytes	Extracorpuscular red cell defects due to: Congestive splenomegaly and portal hypertension Lipoprotein abnormalities causing target and spur shapes Severe hypophosphatemia
Abnormal iron metabolism	Ring sideroblasts in bone marrow	Complex etiology, not completely known Caused in part by decreased functional pyridoxine and inhibition of enzymes involved in hemoglobin synthesis
Hemodilution	None	Portal hypertension associated with fluid overload leading to dilutional anemia

[a] See earlier discussion on anemia of chronic disease
[b] See chapter 6 for more details
[c] See chapter 3 for more details

References

1. Cartwright GE, Lee GR: The anaemia of chronic disorders. *Br J Haemotol* 1971; 21:147–152.

2. Colman N, Herbert V: Hematologic complications of alcoholism: Overview. *Semin Hematol* 1980; 17:164–176.

3. Erslev AJ: Anemia of chronic disorders, in Williams WJ, Beutler E, Erslev AJ, et al (eds): *Hematology*, ed 3. New York, McGraw-Hill International Book Co, 1983, pp 522–528.

4. Erslev AJ: Anemia of chronic renal failure, in Williams WJ, Beutler E, Erslev AJ, et al (eds): *Hematology*, ed 3. New York, McGraw-Hill International Book Co, 1983, pp 417–425.

5. Erslev AJ: Anemia of endocrine disorders, in Williams WJ, Beutler E, Erslev AJ, et al (eds): *Hematology*, ed 3. New York, McGraw-Hill International Book Co, 1983, pp 425–429.

6. Eschbach JW, Egrie JC, Downing MR, et al: Correction of the anemia of end-stage renal disease with recombinant human erythropoietin. *N Engl J Med,* 1987; 316:73–78.

7. Larkin EC, Watson-Williams EJ: Alcohol and the blood. *Med Clin North Am* 1984; 68:105–120.

8. Le J, Vilcek J: Tumor necrosis factor and interleukin-1: Cytokines with multiple overlapping biological activities. *Lab Invest* 1987; 56:234–248.

9. Lee GR: The anemia of chronic disease. *Semin Hematol* 1983; 20:61–80.

10. Lewis JP, Feldman BF: The anemia associated with chronic disease, in Koepke JA (ed): *Laboratory Hematology.* New York, Churchill Livingstone Inc, 1984, pp 29–41.

11. Loughlin KR, Gittes RF, Partridge D, et al: The relationship of lactoferrin to the anemia of renal cell carcinoma. *Cancer* 1987; 59:566–571.

12. McGonigle RJS, Boineau FG, Beckman B, et al: Erythropoietin and inhibitors of in vitro erythropoiesis in the development of anemia in children with renal disease. *J Lab Clin Med* 1985; 105:449–458.

13. O'Brien RT: Hematologic manifestations of chronic systemic disease, in Miller DR, Baehner RL, McMillan CW (eds): *Blood Diseases of Infancy and Childhood,* ed 5. St Louis, 1984, pp 468–482.

14. Oppenheim JJ, Kovacs EJ, Matsushima K, et al: There is more than one interleukin-1. *Immunol Today* 1986; 7:45–56.

5

Aplastic, Hypoplastic, and Miscellaneous Types of Anemia

For clarity, this chapter is organized into three divisions: "Aplastic and Hypoplastic Anemias," "Bone Marrow Replacement Disorders," and the "Congenital Dyserythropoietic Anemias."

Aplastic and Hypoplastic Anemias

There are several types of aplastic or hypoplastic bone marrow disorders associated with variable blood cytopenias (Table 5–1), some of which are hereditary, eg, Diamond-Blackfan anemia, Fanconi's anemia, and dyskeratosis congenita. These rare hereditary disorders are often associated with other abnormalities, predominantly bony and neurologic, which are detailed in Table 5–1. In some of these inherited disorders, only the red cell line is reduced, while in others, such as Fanconi's anemia, all hematopoietic cell lines are reduced.

In children, the acquired disorders of erythropoiesis include transient erythroblastopenia of childhood (TEC) and acquired aplastic anemia. TEC is a self-limited disease of childhood usually associated with a preceding viral or allergic illness. In contrast, aplastic anemia can occur at any age and can be associated with drug treatment, pregnancy, radiation exposure, and infections, although the majority of cases are idiopathic (Table 5–2). Patients with acquired aplastic anemia have variable, but often profound, blood

Table 5–1   Features of Aplastic/Hypoplastic Anemias

Type	Usual Clinical Features	Blood/Bone Marrow Morphology
Diamond-Blackfan (congenital hypoplastic) anemia	Often present at birth, onset prior to 2 years of age One-third of patients have associated abnormalities such as short stature, hypertelorism, mental retardation, etc Autosomal recessive and dominant types of inheritance	Erythrocytes normochromic macrocytic (MCV 100–140 fL) Platelets usually increased Mild neutropenia may be present Bone marrow shows marked erythroid hypoplasia with normal granulocytic and megakaryocytic elements
Fanconi's anemia	May be congenital, usually presents in infancy Associated with hyperpigmentation of skin, short stature, bone abnormalities, microcephaly, and renal abnormalities Autosomal recessive	Gradual development of hematologic abnormalities Thrombocytopenia usually first cytopenia Pancytopenia usually present by 6–9 years of age Erythroid elements in bone marrow initially increased but aplasia gradually develops May evolve to myelodysplasia or leukemia
Dyskeratosis congenita	Very rare, congenital Associated with hyperpigmentation, dystrophic nails, leukoplakia, mental retardation X-linked recessive	Pancytopenia may develop Bone marrow aplasia may develop
Transient erythroblastopenia of childhood	Onset 1 month – 6 years Often associated with recent viral illness or allergic episode No physical abnormalities	Normocytic, normochromic anemia with unremarkable granulocytes and platelets

Pathophysiology	Comments

Multiple defects suggested:
  Stem cell defect
  T-cell abnormality
  Disorder of differentiation
	Fetal hemoglobin increased
	Red cell i present
	Spontaneous remission in 25%;
	  most others respond to corti-
	  costeroids

Stem cell disorder with karyotypic
  abnormalities
	Cytogenetic abnormalities in-
	  clude increased chromo-
	  somal breaks, sister chroma-
	  tid exchange
	Fetal hemoglobin increased
	Red cell i present
	Most patients respond to andro-
	  gens

Possible stem cell disorder	Many similarities with Fanconi's
	  anemia
	Increased incidence of squa-
	  mous cell carcinoma

Transient immunosuppression of
  erythropoiesis secondary to hu-
  moral or cellular immunoregu-
  latory abnormality
	Fetal hemoglobin normal
	No i on red cells
	Spontaneous recovery in 2–8
	  weeks; no treatment needed

(Continued.)

Table 5-1 *Continued.*

Type	Usual Clinical Features	Blood/Bone Marrow Morphology
	Negative family history	Absent erythroid precursors in bone marrow; normal granulocytic and megakaryocytic elements
Acquired aplastic[a] anemia	Can occur at any age, more frequent in elderly No cytogenetic abnormalities	Pancytopenia; all elements morphologically normal Markedly reduced bone marrow cellularity
Acquired pure red[b] cell aplasia	Usual onset from puberty to adulthood Association with thymoma (50%), toxin or drug (25%), neoplasms (lymphoreticular and carcinomas), infections (usually viral), and autoimmune disease	Normocytic, normochromic anemia; neutrophils and platelets normal Absent erythroid precursors in bone marrow; other elements normal

ABBREVIATIONS: MCV = mean corpuscular volume.
[a] See Table 5–2 for more details
[b] See Table 5–3 for more details

cytopenias and a markedly hypocellular bone marrow (Figure 5–1). Acquired aplastic anemia is the most common type of hypoplastic bone marrow disorder, featuring an incidence of about 15 cases per 1 million population.

The other type of acquired hypoplastic anemia, pure red cell aplasia, occurs in both adolescents and adults. This acquired disorder is associated with thymomas, various drug treatments, a number of immune disorders, and certain infections (see Tables 5–1 and 5–3).

Pathophysiology	Comments
May be related to drug or toxin exposure or infection Stem cell, immunoregulatory, and microenvironment defects described	Fetal hemoglobin normal or increased Some patients spontaneously recover Severe cases require bone marrow transplant Multiple other treatment modalities efficacious in some patients
Humoral or cellular immune defect resulting in suppression of erythropoiesis	Variety of treatment modalities described including thymectomy, plasmapheresis, corticosteroids, cyclophosphamide, and antithymocyte globulin

Pathophysiology

For erythropoiesis to occur, the necessary components include: adequate stem cells that are capable of renewal and differentiation, erythropoietin and other growth factors, appropriate immunoregulation of hematopoiesis, and adequate microenvironment.

Deficiencies or defects of all of these components have been suggested in the pathophysiology of the diverse spectrum of congenital and acquired disorders of erythropoiesis (Table 5–1).

Table 5–2   Causes of Acquired Aplastic Anemia

Drugs

    Chloramphenicol

    Phenylbutazone

    Anticonvulsants

    Sulfonamides

    Gold

Toxins

    Benzene

    Insecticides

    Solvents

Infections

    Hepatitis

    EBV infection

    Influenza

Other conditions/exposures

    Pregnancy

    Radiation exposure

    PNH

    Graft-versus-host disease[a]

ABBREVIATIONS: EBV = Epstein-Barr Virus; PNH = Paroxysmal nocturnal hemoglobinuria.

[a] Occurs in patients with immunodeficiency disorders who receive blood products

The congenital hypoplastic anemias may represent stem cell disorders, while acquired anemias such as TEC are probably caused by a self-limited, infection-induced, immunoregulatory abnormality.

The most extensive pathophysiologic studies have been performed on patients with acquired aplastic anemia. The apparent defect in most patients with this disorder is deficient or suppressed stem cells, although humoral and cellular immunoregulatory defects and microenvironmental abnormalities have been described in some cases. Increased circulating suppressor T-cells that may be responsible for suppressed hematopoiesis have been identified in some patients with aplastic anemia. Several viral infections have

Table 5–3   Conditions and Drug Treatments Associated with Acquired Red Cell Aplasia

---

Thymoma (50% of cases)

Drug or toxin (25% of cases)

    Chlorpropamide

    Diphenylhydantoin

    Gold

    Halothane

    Isoniazid

    Penicillin

    Phenobarbitol

    Phenylbutazone

    Sulfathiazol

    Tolbutamide

Neoplasms (few cases)

    Carcinoma

    Acute Lymphoblastic Leukemia

    Non-Hodgkin's Lymphoma

    Chronic Lymphocytic Leukemia

Autoimmune disorders (few cases)

Viral infections (few cases)

---

been linked to aplastic anemia, notably hepatitis and infectious mononucleosis. One theory regarding viral-induced aplasia states that the stem cells are directly suppressed or damaged by these agents. Another theory suggests that these viruses attach to stem cells and act as a hapten to initiate an autoimmune response in which these stem cells are "attacked" by the patient's own lymphocytes. Many drug treatments and some toxic exposures have been associated with acquired aplastic anemia caused by either a dose-related or idiosyncratic host response to the drug or toxin (Table 5–2).

Abnormal immunoregulation appears to be the primary pathophysiologic defect in cases of pure red cell aplasia. The frequent association between red cell aplasia and thymoma supports this interpretation.

Clinical Findings

Depending on its severity, patients with hypoplastic or aplastic anemia can present with weakness, fatigue, or tachycardia. If pancytopenia is present, additional findings can include petechiae and purpura secondary to thrombocytopenia, and fever and infection secondary to neutropenia. As described earlier, some congenital types of hypoplastic anemias have associated phenotypic abnormalities, such as bony defects, mental retardation, and skin and nail abnormalities (Table 5–1). On physical examination, other abnormalities are not usually present, nor are hepatosplenomegaly and lymphadenopathy.

Approach to Diagnosis

The diagnosis of hypoplastic anemia requires an approach that both identifies the specific type of disorder and excludes other diseases that can be manifested by blood cytopenias. This approach to diagnosis generally follows these steps:

1. Determine the types and severity of the blood cytopenias.
2. Assess the patient for hepatosplenomegaly and lymphadenopathy on physical examination.
3. Evaluate infants and young children for other manifestations of the hereditary hypoplastic disorders, including physical and radiographic defects (Table 5–1).
4. Carefully investigate for evidence of toxin or drug exposure; infectious diseases, such as hepatitis or infectious mononucleosis; and recent blood loss.
5. Document bone marrow hypocellularity and rule out an infiltrative or fibrotic process.
6. Use clinical history and other clinical evidence of chronic hemolytic anemia to exclude an aplastic crisis of an underlying disorder, such as hereditary spherocytosis or sickle cell anemia.
7. Evaluate adults with pure red cell aplasia for thymoma, other tumors, drug exposure, or infection (Tables 5–1 and 5–3).

Hematologic Findings

In some types of hypoplastic anemia, only erythropoiesis is reduced; in others, all bone marrow cell lines are affected. Therefore, the hematologic manifestations of these cases can range from isolated anemia to pancytopenia.

Blood Cell Measurements. Patients with hypoplastic anemias generally have a moderate to severe normochromic anemia that may be normocytic or macrocytic. An elevated mean corpuscular volume (MCV) is characteristic of Diamond-Blackfan anemia and may also be present in some cases of acquired aplastic anemia. Erythrocytes generally show little anisopoikilocytosis, as evidenced by a normal red cell distribution width (RDW). The corrected reticulocyte count is reduced. In patients with acquired aplastic anemia and Fanconi's anemia, thrombocytopenia and neutropenia are also present.

Peripheral Blood Smear Morphology. In the various hypoplastic disorders, erythrocytes, neutrophils, and platelets are generally morphologically unremarkable.

Bone Marrow Examination. Patients with Diamond-Blackfan anemia, TEC, and acquired pure red cell aplasia show a marked decrease of erythroid precursors in the bone marrow with essentially normal granulopoiesis and megakaryopoiesis. Erythroid precursors may be totally absent, or only the earliest red cell precursors may be identified. A marked lymphocytosis with many hematogones may be present. Early in their disease course, patients with Fanconi's anemia may have a hypercellular bone marrow with megaloblastic changes. In acquired aplastic anemia and advanced Fanconi's anemia, however, all 3 cell lines are usually markedly reduced. There are no specific morphologic abnormalities of the hematopoietic elements in these patients.

Other Laboratory Tests

5.1 Fetal Hemoglobin Quantitation

Purpose. Fetal hemoglobin levels in erythrocytes can be used to distinguish between TEC and constitutional disorders, such as Diamond-Blackfan and Fanconi's anemias.

Principle, Specimen, Procedure, Notes, and Precautions. See Test 7.2.

Interpretation. Fetal hemoglobin level is characteristically increased in Diamond-Blackfan and Fanconi's anemias, while it is normal in patients with TEC. Fetal hemoglobin level may be increased in some cases of acquired aplastic anemia. Usually, only a small population of erythrocytes contains substantial amounts of fetal hemoglobin, and the remainder of erythrocytes contain more.

Ancillary Tests

Other tests that can be used selectively to distinguish among the various types of aplastic and hypoplastic anemias include the red cell i antigen test and cytogenetic studies. Although not available in most laboratories, red cell i antigen can be detected in patients with Diamond-Blackfan and Fanconi's anemia; i antigen is not present on erythrocytes in patients with TEC.

Cytogenetic studies generally reveal chromosomal defects in bone marrow cells of patients with Fanconi's anemia, including increased chromosomal breakages, translocation, sister chromatid exchange, and increased sensitivity to mitomycin C. Karyotypic abnormalities are not usually found in the other types of hypoplastic and aplastic anemias.

Family studies may be helpful in identifying inheritance patterns associated with constitutional disorders.

Since erythropoietin level is generally increased in all aplastic and hypoplastic anemias, it is not a useful test in distinguishing between these disorders.

Course and Treatment

The clinical course of hypoplastic and aplastic anemias is diverse. Some patients, such as children with TEC, have brief, self-limited episodes of red cell aplasia that require no treatment. Other children and most adult patients with these disorders require treatment that ranges from transfusion to bone marrow transplantation. Any drug treatment that the patient is receiving should be discontinued, if possible. Suspected toxins should be removed from the patient's environment. In general, blood product transfusions should be reserved for life-threatening situations. Because these transfusions can have a negative effect on the outcome of bone marrow transplantation, they should be used very judiciously in patients likely to require a bone marrow transplant. In addition, the morbidity from repeated transfusions may include iron overload, hepatitis, and cytomegalovirus infection.

Androgen treatment is recommended for patients with Fanconi's anemia, although it must be given continuously since relapses occur when therapy is discontinued. Some patients also respond to corticosteroid therapy. Bone marrow transplantation has been successful in some patients, while other transplant recipients have suffered from toxic drug effects or lethal graft-versus-host disease.

The clinical course of patients with acquired aplastic anemia depends on the severity of the pancytopenia, the patient's age, and the patient's response to treatment. These patients must be monitored carefully for evidence of infection or bleeding. Various drugs that have been utilized successfully to treat some patients with acquired aplastic anemia include: corticosteroids, androgens, lithium carbonate, and cyclophosphamide. Bone marrow transplantation is recommended for those young patients with severe acquired aplastic anemia who have an HLA-matched donor. Survival rates for bone marrow transplantation approach 70% in this patient population.

The bone marrow of patients with pure red cell aplasia often responds to corticosteroid therapy. If this fails, however, other effective treatments include: plasmapheresis, thymectomy, splenectomy, an alkylating agent, azathioprine, cyclosporine, antithymocyte globulin, and danazol therapies.

There is an increased incidence of acute leukemia in patients who recover from any type of bone marrow hypoplastic disorder.

Bone Marrow Replacement Disorders

Patients with bone marrow replacement disorders suffer from a failure of hematopoiesis because the medullary portion of the bone marrow has been replaced by fibrosis, neoplastic cells, or nonneoplastic cells (Table 5–4). Even if the neoplastic cells are of hematopoietic origin, they are incapable of producing normal peripheral blood elements. Therefore, patients with bone marrow replacement disorders generally present with cytopenias, ranging from isolated anemia to pancytopenia.

Pathophysiology

Despite the bone marrow's ability to compensate, hematopoiesis will fail once a significant portion of the bone marrow medullary space is replaced by tumor or fibrous tissue. This failure of normal hematopoiesis is the primary cause of cytopenias in patients with bone marrow replacement disorders. As described in chapter 4, however, patients with neoplasms can develop other types of anemia. For example, these patients can suffer from chronic blood loss,

Table 5–4   Causes of Bone Marrow Failure Secondary to Replacement

---

Neoplastic disorders replacing bone marrow parenchyma

   Acute and chronic leukemias

   Malignant lymphoma (Hodgkin's disease and non-Hodgkin's lymphoma)

   Multiple myeloma

   Metastatic carcinoma and sarcoma

Disorders/therapy causing bone marrow fibrosis

   Agnogenic myeloid metaplasia

   Radiation

Miscellaneous disorders replacing bone marrow parenchyma

   Storage diseases

   Other histiocytic disorders

   Angioimmunoblastic lymphadenopathy

---

anemia of chronic disease, bone marrow suppression by chemotherapy, hypersplenism, and even immune-mediated hemolysis (Table 4–5).

Clinical Findings

The clinical findings in patients with bone marrow replacement disorders are as diverse as the types of disorders themselves. Most patients with significant bone marrow replacement develop symptoms of cytopenia, most notably malaise and fatigue secondary to anemia. Manifestations of leukopenia and thrombocytopenia, such as infection or bleeding, may also be present. Patients with acute and chronic leukemias, malignant lymphomas, storage diseases, and agnogenic myeloid metaplasia often have significant splenomegaly, which can cause left upper quadrant pain and early satiety. Lymphadenopathy is also present in some of these patients.

Hematologic findings

Although most patients with bone marrow replacement disorders have cytopenias, some of these patients also have specific morphologic abnormalities that suggest a certain type of bone marrow replacement disorder.

Blood Cell Measurements. A normocytic, normochromic anemia is the most common cytopenia in patients with bone marrow replacement disorders. Although these erythrocytes generally show little anisopoikilocytosis, as manifested by a normal red cell distribution width (RDW), some patients, such as those with agnogenic myeloid metaplasia, exhibit marked anisopoikilocytosis. The reticulocyte count is often reduced in these patients, while the white blood cell and platelet counts are highly variable. Patients with leukemias or agnogenic myeloid metaplasia tend to have elevated white blood cell counts. Thrombocytopenia is generally present in patients with bone marrow replacement disorders.

Peripheral Blood Smear Morphology. Most bone marrow replacement disorders have no specific morphologic abnormalities of red blood cells, white cells, or platelets. Patients with certain hematopoietic replacement disorders, however, such as agnogenic myeloid metaplasia, have pronounced anisopoikilocytosis with teardrop forms, a leukoerythroblastic blood picture, basophilia, and large platelets. A leukoerythroblastic blood picture may also be seen in patients with bone marrow involvement by other neoplasms. If the hypoproliferative anemia is complicated by a red cell survival defect, additional morphologic abnormalities will be present. Leukemic or lymphoma cells may be identified in the peripheral blood in patients with this type of replacement disorder.

Bone Marrow Examination. There is a wide spectrum of bone marrow morphologic abnormalities in patients with bone marrow replacement disorders. In some patients, the bone marrow parenchyma is packed with infiltrating tumor cells, while in others it is replaced by collagen. In histiocytic disorders, such as storage diseases, the bone marrow may be replaced by distinctive large, benign-appearing macrophages.

Other Laboratory Tests

Because this group of disorders is so diverse, there are few individual laboratory tests that can distinguish types of replacement disorders. Many tests can be utilized on a selective basis, however, to help establish the diagnosis of specific bone marrow replacement disorders (see chapters 31, 32, 35).

Course and Treatment

Fibrotic and benign histiocytic bone marrow replacement disorders tend to exhibit gradually progressive bone marrow infiltration, while neoplasms generally progress more rapidly. The treatment and disease course vary for each type of replacement disorder.

Congenital Dyserythropoietic Anemias

The congenital dyserythropoietic anemias (CDAs) are rare disorders initially described in 1951 and characterized by profound blood and bone marrow red cell morphologic abnormalities and ineffective erythropoiesis. Other features common to this group of disorders include: a low corrected reticulocyte count, a mildly elevated indirect bilirubin level, and an elevated LDH level. In some patients with CDA, an autosomal recessive pattern of inheritance has been determined. Patients with CDA generally have a mild to moderate anemia, with markedly dyspoietic erythrocytes.

At least 3 types of CDA have been described based on specific morphologic features within the bone marrow. In type I, the erythroid elements within the bone marrow show megaloblastic changes with internuclear chromatin bridges. Type II CDA is characterized by binuclearity and multinuclearity of erythroid precursors. In type III CDA, the multinuclearity is pronounced with up to 12 nuclei present in some erythroid precursors. In all types of CDA, mature erythrocytes are often macrocytic.

The bone marrow in patients with CDA shows erythroid hyperplasia, with asynchrony of nuclear-cytoplasmic maturation. Nuclear abnormalities include variations in size and structure as well as shape abnormalities described above for the CDA subtypes. In addition, mitotic abnormalities, such as lobulation, budding, fragmentation, and karyorrhexis, have also been described. Cytoplasmic abnormalities include vacuolization, basophilic stippling, and excess iron within erythroid precursors.

The pathogenesis of CDA is uncertain, but theories include some primary defect in mitosis or a nuclear or cell membrane defect. Because this type of anemia is mild, these patients are frequently asymptomatic and do not require treatment.

References

1. Alter BP: Childhood red cell aplasia. *Am J Pediatr Hematol Oncol* 1980; 2:121–139.

2. Appelbaum FR, Fefer A: The pathogenesis of aplastic anemia. *Semin Hematol* 1981; 18:241–257.

3. Camitta BM, Storb R, Thomas ED: Aplastic anemia: Pathogenesis, diagnosis, treatment, and prognosis. *N Engl J Med* 1982; 306:645–652, 712–718.

4. Clark DA, Dessypris EN, Krantz SB: Studies on pure red cell aplasia: XI. Results of immunosuppressive treatment of 37 patients. *Blood* 1984; 63:277–286.

5. Freedman MH, Saunders EF: Transient erythroblastopenia of childhood: Varied pathogenesis. *Am J Hematol* 1983; 14:247–254.

6. German J, Schonberg S, Caskie S, et al: A test for Fanconi's anemia. *Blood* 1987; 69:1637–1641.

7. Lewis SM, Path FRC, Verwilghen RL: Dyserythropoiesis and dyserythropoietic anemias, in Brown EB (ed): *Progress in Hematology,* ed 3. New York, Grune & Stratton, 1973; pp 99–129.

8. Lipton JM, Kudisch M, Gross R, et al: Defective erythroid progenitor differentiation system in congenital hypoplastic (Diamond-Blackfan) anemia. *Blood* 1986; 67:962–968.

9. Lipton JM, Nathan DG: Aplastic and hypoplastic anemia. *Pediatr Clin North Am* 1980; 27:217–235.

10. Young NS, Leonard E, Platanias L: Lymphocytes and lymphokines in aplastic anemia: Pathogenic role and implications for pathogenesis. *Blood Cells* 1987; 13:87–100.

11. Zoumbos NC, Gascon P, Djeu JY, et al: Circulating activated suppressor T lymphocytes in aplastic anemia. *N Engl J Med* 1985; 312:257–265.

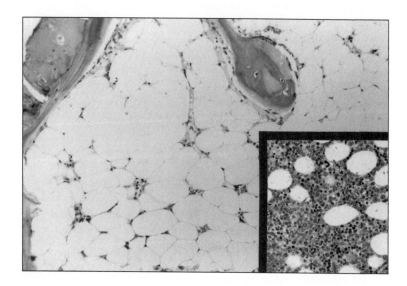

Figure 5-1   Photomicrographs of normal (inset) and aplastic bone marrow biopsy sections highlight the profound loss of cellularity in patients with aplastic anemia.

6

Megaloblastic Anemias

Megaloblastic anemia occurs when the coenzyme forms of folate and vitamin B_{12} necessary for normal DNA synthesis are deficient. The resultant defective DNA synthesis impairs the ability of all proliferating cells to synthesize enough DNA per unit time to allow for mitosis; as a consequence, there are increased numbers of cells in the DNA synthesis phase of the cell cycle. Since RNA synthesis is not dependent on these coenzymes, an asynchrony between nuclear and cytoplasmic maturation occurs, resulting both in "giantism" of all proliferating cells and in cell nuclei that appear less mature than the cytoplasm. While impaired proliferation of hematopoietic elements is the major clinical manifestation of vitamin B_{12} and folate deficiency, other disorders, such as malabsorption caused by defective production of intestinal epithelial cells, can also develop.

Characteristics of vitamin B_{12} and folate, including dietary sources, recommended daily requirements, normal blood levels, and amounts of stored vitamins, are shown in Table 6–1. Vitamin B_{12} circulates in the peripheral blood bound to various binder proteins. Except in infants, total body stores of vitamin B_{12} are abundant and are sufficient to adequately supply the host for 2 to 5 years. Folate is very heat labile and is destroyed readily in the cooking process. Small amounts of folate derivatives circulate largely unbound in the blood; greater concentrations of these derivations are present intracellularly. Except in infants, total body stores of folate are moderate and are sufficient to maintain normal cellular proliferation for

Table 6–1   Characteristics of Vitamin B_{12} and Folate

	Vitamin B_{12}		Folate
Origin	Synthesized exclusively by bacteria		Synthesized by plants and micro-organisms
Dietary source	Meat, fish, dairy products (heat stabile)		Vegetables (especially green leafy vegetables) and fruits (heat labile)
Parent compound	Cyanocobalamin		Pteroglutamic acid
Recommended daily requirements	Infants	0.3 μg	60 μg
	Children	0.5–1.0 μg	100 μg
	Adults	1–2 μg	200 μg
	Pregnant Women	2.5–3 μg	400 μg
	Lactating Women	2.5–3 μg	300 μg
Normal blood levels	150–1,000 pg/mL		>3.7 ng/mL (Red cell: 130–640 ng/mL)
Normal total stores (major storage site)	3,000–5,000 mg[a] (liver)		20–70 mg[a] (liver)
Storage duration on deficient diet	2–5 years		3–5 months

[a]Total stores much smaller in infants

approximately 3 to 5 months. Because of the relatively short duration that folate stores will meet host needs, the incidence of folate deficiency is substantially greater than that of vitamin B_{12} deficiency.

Pathophysiology

The physiology and biochemistry of vitamin B_{12} and folate are detailed in Tables 6–2 and 6–3. In patients with vitamin B_{12} deficiency,

Table 6–2   Physiology of Vitamin B_{12} and Folate

	Vitamin B_{12}	Folate
Compounds in food	Several cobalamin forms	Several polyglutamate forms
Physiology of absorption	Vitamin B_{12} released from food by gastric acid, gastric enzymes & small bowel enzymes → free vitamin B_{12} bound to R-binders primarily; some also binds to IF → pancreatic enzymes degrade R-binder–B_{12} complexes → released B_{12} is then bound to IF	Polyglutamate deconjugated by conjugase enzymes in bile and small bowel lumen
Site of absorption	Vitamin B_{12}–IF complex adheres to receptors on brush border of ileum (pH and calcium-dependent process)	Deconjugated folate absorbed in jejunum
Physiology of circulation	30% of Vitamin B_{12} binds to TCII, which delivers it to liver, bone marrow, and other sites 70% Vitamin B_{12} binds to TCI, TCIII & R-binders, which deliver it exclusively to liver	Folate circulates unbound in blood as 5-methyl THF
Entry into cells	TCII-B_{12} attaches to specific membrane receptors Vitamin B_{12} transfered across plasma membrane. (TCII degraded in this process)	Vitamin B_{12} necessary for folate (THF form) to pass across plasma membranes and be retained in cell
Function	2 active forms, methylcobalamin and 5-deoxyadenosyl cobalamin, which facilitate formation of methionine and succinate, respectively	THF essential for all 1-carbon transfer reactions in mammalian cells THF required for both purine and pyrimidine synthesis
Excretion	Bile, urine	Urine, sweat, saliva, feces

ABBREVIATIONS: IF = intrinsic factor; TC = transcobalamin; R-binder = found in every tissue in body named for rapid mobility on electrophoresis; THF = tetrahydrofolate.

Table 6–3   Biochemistry of Vitamin B_{12} and Folate Activity

	Vitamin B_{12}	Folate
Biologically active form(s):	Coenzyme B_{12} (5-deoxyadenosyl cobalamin) and methylcobalamin	5-methyl THF
Reactions requiring Vitamin B_{12} and/or folate cofactors	I. Homocysteine $\xrightarrow{\text{methylcobalamin}}$ Methionine 5-methyl THF $\nearrow$ THF Failure in this pathway results in megaloblastosis; reaction also important in CNS methylation, and for incorporation of folate into cells II. Methylmalonate $\xrightarrow{\text{Coenzyme } B_{12}}$ Succinate Failure of this reaction *not* involved in neurologic disease or megaloblastosis	I. Required for both purine and pyrimidine synthesis II. Rate limiting step in DNA synthesis (pyrimidine synthesis) dUMP $\longrightarrow$ dTMP, THF, DHF III. Folate also essential in amino acid synthesis

ABBREVIATIONS: THF = tetrahydrofolate; CNS = central nervous system; dUMP = deoxyuridine monophosphate; dTMP = deoxythymidine monophosphate; DHF = dihydrofolate.

Table 6–4   Probable Sequence in Development of
Vitamin B_{12} Deficiency

Time Interval After Onset of Intake Failure	Pathologic Abnormality
1–2 years	Vitamin B_{12} level in serum decreased Early blood and bone marrow abnormalities including hypersegmentation and macrocytosis Early myelin damage to nerves
2–3 years	Vitamin B_{12} level markedly decreased Vitamin B_{12} binders 10% saturated Florid megaloblastosis in blood and bone marrow Decreased red cell folate, normal to increased serum folate Severe damage to myelin

both the megaloblastic anemia and the neurologic complications appear to be secondary to the defective formation of methionine (Table 6–3). The rate-limiting step in DNA synthesis that requires folate is the conversion of deoxyuridine monophosphate to deoxythymidine monophosphate in pyrimidine synthesis.

The sequence of events in the development of vitamin B_{12} and folate deficiency is listed in Tables 6–4 and 6–5, respectively. Although folate stores are depleted much more rapidly than vitamin B_{12} stores, the sequence of events in the development of blood and bone marrow abnormalities as deficiency evolves is similar for both

Table 6–5   Sequence in Development of Folate Deficiency

Time Interval After Onset of Intake Failure	Pathologic Abnormality
3 weeks	Decreased serum folate
5–7 weeks	Hypersegmentation of neutrophils in bone marrow and blood
10 weeks	Mild megaloblastic changes in bone marrow
17–18 weeks	Macro-ovalocytes, decreased red cell folate
19–20 weeks	Florid megaloblastosis with anemia

Table 6–6   Mechanisms of Vitamin B_{12} Deficiency

	Example	Condition/Disorder
Inadequate intake	Dietary deficiency	Strict vegetarianism
Increased requirement	Growth, development	Pregnancy, lactation
Defective absorption	Decreased IF	Pernicious anemia, congenital IF deficiency
	Decreased pancreatic enzymes	Pancreatitis
	Lack of calcium or abnormal pH	Zollinger-Ellison syndrome
	Defective ileal mucosa	Sprue, regional enteritis, surgical reaction
	Parasitic or bacterial overgrowth	Tapeworm, blind loop
	Drug interference with absorption	Alcoholism, colchicine treatment, PAS treatment
Defective transport	Decreased TCII	Congenital deficiency of TCII
Disorders of metabolism	Suppression or inhibition of metabolic enzymes	Nitrous oxide administration enzyme deficiencies

Abbreviations: IF = intrinsic factor; TC = transcobalamin; PAS = para-amino salicylic acid.

vitamins. Hypersegmentation of neutrophils appears early in the development of megaloblastic anemia, while actual anemia is a late event associated with florid megaloblastic morphologic changes. Damage to myelin in peripheral nerves occurs progressively throughout the evolution of vitamin B_{12} deficiency.

There are 5 basic mechanisms leading to vitamin B_{12} deficiency, including inadequate intake, increased requirement, defective absorption, defective transport, and disorders of B_{12} metabolism (Table 6–6). By far, the most common mechanism for vitamin B_{12} deficiency is defective absorption. For vitamin B_{12} absorption to occur, there must be normal amounts of intrinsic factor, sufficient pancreatic enzymes to degrade the vitamin B_{12}–R-binder complexes, appropriate calcium and hydrogen ion concentrations to facilitate the transfer of vitamin B_{12} across plasma membranes, an intact ileal

Table 6–7   Mechanisms of Folate Deficiency

	Example	Condition/Disorder
Inadequate intake	Dietary deficiency	Alcoholism, drug addiction, poverty
	Inactivation of folate	Overcooking of food
Increased requirement	Growth, development	Pregnancy, lactation, infancy
	States of increased cell turnover	Chronic hemolytic anemias, malignancies
Defective absorption	Defective jejunal mucosa	Sprue, amyloidosis, lymphoma, surgical resection
	Drug-induced malabsorption	Anti-convulsant, antituberculous, oral contraceptive drug therapy, alcoholism
Disorders of metabolism	Suppression or inhibition of metabolic enzymes	Methotrexate, pyrimethamine treatment, alcoholism
		Congenital disorders of folate metabolism

mucosal surface, and lack of competing parasites or bacteria for the ingested vitamin B_{12}. Although abnormalities in any of these components can result in defective absorption, the one most commonly encountered in clinical practice is decreased intrinsic factor in patients with pernicious anemia. Intrinsic factor is secreted by gastric parietal cells stimulated by gastrin and histamine. The antibodies directed against intrinsic factor commonly detected in patients with pernicious anemia may be the cause of the decreased intrinsic factor. Other disorders associated with defective absorption are listed on Table 6–6.

Although vitamin B_{12} deficiency may occur secondary to a lack in dietary intake, a stringent diet deficient in all meat, egg, and milk products must be followed. Because vitamin B_{12} stores are so abundant, the increased requirement for this vitamin during pregnancy and lactation is rarely associated with megaloblastic anemia. Vitamin B_{12} deficiency secondary to transport or metabolic defects is extremely rare.

The major causes of folate deficiency include dietary deficiency and increased requirement, although defective absorption and disorders of metabolism have occasionally been responsible for folate deficiency (Table 6–7). Dietary deficiency of folate is common in chronic alcoholics, drug addicts, and patients of low socioeconomic class who consume inadequate diets. Excessive cooking destroys folate. Increased folate is required by infants, pregnant and lactating women, and patients with malignancies or chronic hemolytic anemias. Premature infants have very low folate stores and are highly susceptible to folate deficiency. Disorders and drug treatment associated with defective absorption of folate and abnormal folate metabolism are listed in Table 6-7.

Clinical Findings

Patients with megaloblastic anemia characteristically present with moderate to severe fatigue and malaise of several months' duration. Their skin may be lemon-yellow because of the combined effects of a moderately increased bilirubin level and the marked pallor of the underlying anemia. Because the defective DNA synthesis affects all proliferating cells, these patients have atrophy of the mucosal surfaces of the tongue, gastrointestinal tract, and vagina. This can cause pain in the mouth and vagina and can lead to a secondary malabsorption in the gastrointestinal tract.

Although the neurologic manifestations of pernicious anemia have been well described, patients with folate deficiency can also develop neuropsychiatric disorders that include: irritability, forgetfulness, and sleepiness. Occasionally, patients with folate deficiency will manifest peripheral neuropathy similar to that described in patients with vitamin B_{12} deficiency. In pernicious anemia, this peripheral neuropathy is secondary to defective myelin synthesis and is insidious in onset, beginning first in peripheral nerves and gradually progressing to involve the posterior and lateral columns of the spinal cord. The clinical manifestations of peripheral nerve involvement include paresthesias, such as numbness and tingling in the hands and feet; decreased vibration sense; and decreased position sense. With progression to spinal cord involvement, the patient may experience ataxia and eventually symmetrical paralysis. If the megaloblastic anemia is untreated, the patient may eventually develop cerebral involvement, which has been called "megaloblastic madness" and is manifested by mental changes, paranoia, and depression.

Approach to Diagnosis

The approach to the diagnosis of megaloblastic anemia includes:

1. Establishing the presence of a macrocytic anemia.
2. Distinguishing between the various causes of macrocytic anemia.

3. Determining if the patient is vitamin B_{12} or folate deficient.

4. Identifying and treating the underlying disease responsible for the megaloblastic anemia.

In addition to megaloblastic anemia, peripheral blood macrocytosis may be seen in patients with alcoholism, liver disease, reticulocytosis, myelodysplastic disorders, and chemotherapeutic effect. Clinical history and a review of the blood smear help exclude these alternate diagnoses. The clinical history should also include: questions regarding family history (some very rare types of megaloblastic anemia are secondary to hereditary disorders), drug ingestion, intestinal function, and prior surgical procedures. Evidence of peripheral neuropathy and other neurologic manifestations of vitamin B_{12} or folate deficiency should be assessed on physical examination. Once the diagnosis of megaloblastic anemia has been established, the specific vitamin deficiency causing this anemia must be determined via laboratory tests discussed below. Finally, the cause of the vitamin deficiency must be identified and treated appropriately.

Hematologic Findings

The hematologic findings can be virtually diagnostic in patients with full-blown megaloblastic anemia in whom characteristic abnormalities of erythrocytes and neutrophils can be identified readily. In patients suffering from concurrent iron deficiency anemia, however, the hematologic findings are less predictable.

Blood Cell Measurements. A patient with megaloblastic anemia typically has a moderate to severe normochromic macrocytic anemia with mean corpuscular volumes (MCV's) ranging from 100 to 150 fL, while the mean corpuscular hemoglobin concentration (MCHC) is normal. Although MCVs at the lower end of this spectrum can be seen in a variety of disorders, a patient with an MCV exceeding 120 fL is very likely to have megaloblastic anemia. Some patients with vitamin B_{12} or folate deficiency will have a normal MCV because these patients also have iron deficiency, inflammatory disorders, or renal failure. The red cell distribution width (RDW) is characteristically markedly elevated in megaloblastic anemia caused by extreme anisopoikilocytosis. The reticulocyte count is very low; in severe cases, the neutrophil and platelet counts are decreased.

Peripheral Blood Smear Morphology. The peripheral blood smear characteristically contains numerous oval macrocytes as well as schistocytes of various sizes, broken erythrocytes, and even spherocytes (Figure 6–1). Red blood cell fragmentation occurs because of the increased fragility of these large erythrocytes, which probably are damaged during their passage through the spleen. Basophilic stippling and Howell-Jolly bodies have also been described in red cells. When the hematocrit value drops below (20%), nucleated red blood cells may be found in the blood. Hypersegmentation of mature neutrophils is a characteristic feature that appears very early in the development of megaloblastic anemia and is a reflection of the nuclear maturation defect. Hypersegmentation can be manifested by cells with 6 or more nuclear lobes or by an elevation in the mean neutrophil lobe count.

Bone Marrow Examination. The bone marrow in patients with megaloblastic anemia is characteristically hypercellular with erythroid and granulocytic hyperplasia. Mitotic activity is abundant, but there is significant intramedullary cell death secondary to the nuclear maturation defect. The proliferating erythroid and myeloid cell lines show megaloblastic changes. In the erythroid elements, the major morphologic manifestation is nuclear-cytoplasmic asynchrony, in which the nuclei are large with finely dispersed chromatin, while the cytoplasm is more mature with hemoglobinization (Figure 6–1). The dominant myeloid abnormality is giantism of bands and metamyelocytes and nuclear hypersegmentation of mature granulocytes. Large megakaryocytes have also been described.

Masking of erythroid megaloblastosis can occur because of concomitant iron deficiency, such as may be seen in pregnant women, patients with various malabsorption disorders, patients with chronic alcoholism, and in approximately one third of patients with pernicious anemia. In these patients, the peripheral blood and bone marrow erythroid picture may be intermediate between that described in iron deficiency and in megaloblastic anemia, although the megaloblastic changes in the granulocytic cell line persist.

Other Laboratory Tests

The primary laboratory tests utilized in the diagnosis of megaloblastic anemias include measurements of serum vitamin B_{12}, serum folate, and red blood cell folate. Some features of these and other ancillary laboratory tests are shown in Table 6–8.

6.1 Serum Vitamin B_{12} Quantitation

Purpose. The level of vitamin B_{12} in the blood is a useful measure of the patient's vitamin B_{12} stores.

Principle.   Most laboratories currently utilize a competitive protein-binding assay for this determination. In this assay, the patient's vitamin B_{12} competes with radiolabeled vitamin B_{12} for a fixed number of binding sites. The amount of radiolabeled vitamin B_{12} that is bound is inversely proportional to the patient's vitamin B_{12} level.

Specimen.   Either serum or plasma (EDTA) is suitable for this test. Specimen must be separated and frozen if the test cannot be performed within 3 or 4 hours of collection.

Procedure.   In competitive protein-binding assays, the patient's serum or plasma is heated to destroy nonspecific binding proteins and is then mixed with a constant amount of radiolabeled vitamin B_{12} before purified intrinsic factor covalently coupled to magnetic particles is added. In general, a series of tubes containing standards, controls, and patient samples are used. After appropriate mixing and incubation, the specimens are placed in a magnetic separation unit. The tubes are then decanted and counted in a gamma counter for 1 minute.

Interpretation.   Decreased vitamin B_{12} levels are seen in patients with pernicious anemia and any other type of megaloblastic anemia caused by vitamin B_{12} deficiency.

Notes and Precautions.   The assay must utilize purified intrinsic factor to avoid falsely elevated results secondary to the binding of inactive cobalamin analogues to other binding proteins. In patients with pernicious anemia and coexisting disease, such as iron deficiency, liver disease, hemoglobinopathy, or myeloproliferative disorders, the vitamin B_{12} level may be normal or increased. Falsely low levels may be seen in patients with folate deficiency, pregnant women, women taking oral contraceptives, and patients with transcobalamin deficiency.

6.2   Serum Folate Quantitation

Purpose.   Assays of serum folate, in conjunction with red blood cell folate, are useful in determining the status of the patient's folate stores.

Principle.   Serum folate is currently measured using a competitive protein-binding assay analogous to that used for vitamin B_{12}. The

Table 6–8   Laboratory Tests for Diagnosis of
Megaloblastic Anemia

Test[a]	Specimen	Procedure
Vitamin B_{12}[a]	Serum/plasma	Competitive protein-binding assay using radiolabeled B_{12} and purified IF
Folate[a]	Serum/plasma	Competitive protein-binding assay using radiolabeled folate and folate-binding proteins
Red cell Folate[a]	Lyzed red cells	Same assay as for folate except that lyzed red cells used
LDH	Serum/heparinized plasma	LDH catalyzes oxidation of lactate to pyruvate with reduction of NAD to NADH Absorbance of NADH measured
Iron, IBC	Serum/heparinized plasma	See chapter 3
IF antibodies	Serum	Competitive protein-binding assay
Parietal cell antibodies	Serum	Immunofluorescent test using sections of rat stomach and appropriate control tissues

Interpretation	Notes and Precautions
Decreased in PA and other anemias secondary to vitamin B_{12} deficiency	Test should use purified IF as binding protein, otherwise may get false normal results
Decreased in anemias due to folate deficiency; normal or increased in PA	False normal results in some patients with severe iron deficiency Levels fluctuate with diet Falsely elevated level with hemolyzed specimen
Since red cells metabolically inactive, red cell folate level reflects patient folate status at time these cells formed; level is decreased in folate and Vitamin B_{12} deficiency	Because vitamin B_{12} required for folate to enter cell, level is decreased in both B_{12} and folate deficiency
LDH is markedly elevated in megaloblastic anemia due to intramedullary destruction of cells	Hemolysis falsely elevates results
Serum iron, storage iron, and IBC all increased in megaloblastic anemias due to decreased iron utilization in erythropoiesis	See chapter 3
Present in 50% of cases of pernicious anemia	Very specific for PA but present in only about 50% of cases
Fluorescence of parietal cells in stomach sections (with negative controls) indicates that patient has parietal cell antibodies	Sensitive for PA (Positive in 90% cases) but also found in other disorders

(Continued.)

Table 6–8   *Continued.*

Test[a]	Specimen	Procedure
Indirect bili- rubin	Serum	See chapter 7
Gastrin	Serum	Competitive protein- binding assay

ABBREVIATIONS: IF = intrinsic factor; PA = pernicious anemia; IBC = iron-binding capacity; LDH = lactate dehydrogenase; NAD = nicotinamide adenine dinucleotide; NADH = reduced nicotinamide adenine dinucleotide.

[a]Tests should be performed in all cases of suspected megaloblastic anemia; other tests are helpful in selected clinical settings

amount of labeled folate that binds to folate-binding proteins is inversely proportional to the amount of the patient's folate.

Specimen.   Either serum or plasma (EDTA) can be used for this test. The specimen must be separated and frozen if the test cannot be performed within 3 or 4 hours of collection.

Procedure.   A constant amount of radiolabeled folate and folate-binding proteins is added to the patient sample. The same magnetic separation and counting of radioactivity with a gamma counter is performed for this assay, as described above for vitamin B_{12}.

Interpretation.   Decreased serum folate levels are detected in patients with megaloblastic anemia secondary to folate deficiency, while normal or increased levels of serum folate are found in patients with pernicious anemia.

Notes and Precautions.   Because serum folate shows significant fluctuation with diet, a patient can have a normal serum folate level and actually be folate deficient. Folate deficiency can also be masked by a more severe iron deficiency in which the serum and red cell folate levels may be within normal limits despite the fact that the patient is folate deficient. The reason for this phenomenon is unknown. Hemolyzed samples will give markedly elevated serum folate levels because of the large amounts of folate normally present in erythrocytes. Patients receiving methotrexate or leucovorin

Interpretation	Notes and Precautions
Mildly increased in megaloblastic anemia due to hemolysis of some abnormal red cells	See chapter 7
Markedly increased in PA	

treatment will have falsely elevated folate levels secondary to the binding of these drugs to the folate-binding proteins used in the competitive protein-binding assay.

6.3 Red Blood Cell Folate Quantitation

Purpose. Red blood cell folate determination is a more stable measurement of the status of the patient's folate stores than is serum folate. Since red blood cells are metabolically inactive, the red cell folate levels reflect the patient's folate status at the time these cells were produced.

Principle. Red blood cell folate is measured by a competitive protein-binding assay analogous to that utilized for measuring serum folate.

Specimen. Whole blood is collected in EDTA, which can be frozen or processed immediately. Red blood cells are lyzed with ascorbic acid.

Procedure. The procedure for the quantitation of red cell folate is the same as that used for serum folate. (see Test 6.2.)

Interpretation. Because vitamin B_{12} cofactor is necessary for folate to enter and be retained within red blood cells, decreased red blood cell folate is found in patients with either folate or vitamin B_{12} deficiency. Table 6–9 compares the serum vitamin

Table 6–9   Serum Vitamin B_{12}, Serum Folate, and Red Cell
Folate Levels in Megaloblastic Anemia

Disorder	Serum Vitamin B_{12}	Serum Folate[a]	Red Cell Folate
Vitamin B_{12} deficiency	Decreased	Normal or Increased	Decreased
Folate deficiency	Normal	Decreased	Decreased
Deficiency of both vitamin B_{12} and folate	Decreased	Decreased	Decreased

[a] Fluctuates with changes in dietary folate

B_{12}, serum folate, and red blood cell folate levels in patients
with vitamin B_{12} deficiency, folate deficiency, or both.

Ancillary Tests

Several additional laboratory tests, including measurements of serum LDH, bilirubin, serum and storage iron, intrinsic factor antibody, parietal cell antibody, gastrin, and Schilling and deoxyuridine
(dU) suppression tests can be useful in evaluating patients with
megaloblastic anemia. The expected values for these tests, along
with the reason they are abnormal in megaloblastic anemia, are
detailed in Table 6–8.

Parietal Cell and Intrinsic Factor Antibodies.   Most patients with pernicious anemia have parietal cell and intrinsic factor
antibodies. Although parietal cell antibodies are more sensitive for
pernicious anemia, they are also seen fairly frequently in patients
with chronic gastritis. Antibodies to intrinsic factor are more specific
for pernicious anemia but they are found only in about half of these
patients.

Gastrin Test.   Gastrin stimulates parietal cells to secrete intrinsic factor and hydrochloric acid, and serum gastrin levels are
typically markedly elevated in patients with pernicious anemia. Recent evidence suggests that some parietal cell antibodies may be
directed against the gastrin receptor on these cells, which explains
the failure of parietal cells to respond to gastrin. The achlorhydria

in gastric juices is secondary to the failure of the production of hydrochloric acid by parietal cells.

Schilling Test. Although the three-part Schilling test is not used consistently today in the initial diagnosis of megaloblastic anemia, it may help to determine the etiology of a megaloblastic anemia in patients with ambiguous results on other tests. The first part of this test measures only the patient's ability to absorb vitamin B_{12}. Intrinsic factor and vitamin B_{12} are given to the patient in the second part of the Schilling test; the third part utilizes antibiotics to destroy bacteria and is designed to detect patients with bacterial overgrowth disorders. The patient ingests radiolabeled vitamin B_{12}, followed by an injection of a loading dose of unlabeled vitamin B_{12}. A 24-hour urine sample is collected, and the amount of radioactivity in this sample is measured. In patients with pernicious anemia, the urinary excretion of labeled vitamin B_{12} will be normal only when intrinsic factor is given.

Several problems are common in performing the Schilling test. First, the collection of a 24-hour urine sample is cumbersome, and often an incomplete sample is submitted for evaluation. The patient must have normal renal function and normal intestinal mucosa for the test to be valid. In addition, some patients who cannot absorb dietary vitamin B_{12} can absorb the crystalline vitamin B_{12} that is used, giving a falsely normal result.

dU Suppression Test. A recently developed test of intra-nuclear vitamin B_{12} and folate levels, referred to as the dU suppression test, is based on studies of thymidine synthesis. This test of cultured blood or bone marrow cells is designed to distinguish between the primary and salvage pathways utilized in thymidine synthesis. It assesses both vitamin B_{12} and folate levels, because cofactors of both of these vitamins are required in the primary metabolic pathway of thymidine synthesis. The salvage pathway is favored, however, when a deficiency of either folate or vitamin B_{12} exists. It is possible to test which one of these pathways is operating in the nucleus of the cell, because the salvage pathway can utilize a radioactive deoxyuridine substrate while the primary pathway cannot. If nucleated blood cells are deficient in either vitamin B_{12} or folate, the salvage pathway will be favored, resulting in increased incorporation of radioactive label into the cell's nucleus. With the addition of the deficient vitamin, the metabolic pathway reverts back to the primary synthetic pathway, and the radioactivity within the nucleus decreases. The nuclei of long-lived cells, such as lymphocytes, can be studied to determine the patient's vitamin B_{12} or folate status at the time these cells were last mitotically active. This information can be useful in selected cases when other test results fail to confirm a vitamin B$_{12}$ or folate deficiency. Recent vitamin B$_{12}$ or folate therapy will not "mask" this test result, because long-lived cells can be studied.

Course and Treatment

Correction of the vitamin deficiency by either parenteral injections of vitamin B$_{12}$ or oral doses of folate results in prompt improvement of the patient's hematologic abnormalities, with normalization of the hemogram within 4 to 8 weeks. Occasionally, patients with folate deficiency will need parenteral therapy until the gastrointestinal tract epithelium has regenerated. Patients with megaloblastic anemia should be evaluated carefully to determine the underlying cause of the vitamin deficiency.

Because the slow development of the anemia has allowed for some compensation, patients with megaloblastic anemia usually do not require transfusion; however, rare patients may present with cardiovascular decompensation requiring immediate treatment. Transfusion in this clinical situation must be considered very carefully because of possible further cardiac decompensation and death secondary to volume overload. Plasmapheresis with red blood cell infusions may prevent volume overload. Another cardiac complication that occurs in small numbers of patients receiving treatment for megaloblastic anemia is cardiac arrhythmia, which may result in sudden death. The postulated mechanism for this catastrophic complication is the precipitous decrease in potassium level that occurs following vitamin B$_{12}$ therapy. Patients with megaloblastic anemia undergoing therapy may also develop thrombotic complications because of changes in platelet activity associated with restoration of normal vitamin B$_{12}$ or folate levels in platelets.

Following vitamin therapy, there is a rapid and marked decline in the LDH and plasma iron levels as well as a normalization of the serum bilirubin level. The megaloblastic changes in bone marrow erythroid precursors revert to normal within several days of treatment, followed by reversal of the megaloblastic changes within myeloid precursors a few days later. Reticulocytes can be identified in the peripheral blood within 3 to 5 days after treatment is begun, and they generally peak within 7 to 10 days. The height of the reticulocyte count is inversely proportional to the degree of anemia. Within 1 to 2 months, all peripheral blood parameters will have returned to normal.

In patients with pernicious anemia, the neurologic manifestations of this disorder generally improve substantially with vitamin B$_{12}$ therapy, although they may not resolve entirely. There should be no progression of these neurologic defects, however, while the patient continues to receive parenteral vitamin B_{12} therapy. In patients with pernicious anemia, large doses of folate can reduce the hematologic abnormalities, but the neurologic disease will progress.

Prognosis is good for patients with megaloblastic anemia, provided the vitamin deficiency is adequately treated and the underlying disorder that led to the vitamin deficiency is identified and managed appropriately.

References

1. Aizpurua HJD, Ungar B, Toh B-H: Autoantibody to the gastrin receptor in pernicious anemia. *N Engl J Med* 1985; 313:479–483.

2. Beck WS: Erythrocyte disorders: Anemias related to disturbance of DNA synthesis (megaloblastic anemias), in Williams WJ, Beutler E, Erslev AJ, et al (eds): *Hematology,* ed 3. New York, McGraw-Hill International Book Company, 1983, pp 434–465.

3. Beck WS: Metabolic aspects of vitamin B_{12} and folic acid, in Williams WJ, Beutler E, Erslev AJ, et al (eds): *Hematology,* ed 3. New York, McGraw-Hill International Book Company, 1983, pp 311–331.

4. Fairbanks VG: Tests for pernicious anemia: The 'Schilling test.' *Mayo Clin Proc* 1983; 58:541–544.

5. Herbert V: Biology of disease: Megaloblastic anemias. *Lab Invest* 1985; 52:3–19.

6. Herbert V: Making sense of laboratory tests of folate status: Folate requirements to sustain normality. *Am J Hematol* 1987; 26:199–207.

7. Lindenbaum J: Status of laboratory testing in the diagnosis of megaloblastic anemia. *Blood* 1983; 61:624–627.

8. Meyers PA, Miller DR: Megaloblastic anemias, in Miller DR, Baehner RL, McMillan CW, et al (eds): *Blood Diseases of Infancy and Childhood,* ed 5. St Louis, The CV Mosby Co, 1984, pp 147–170.

9. O'Grady LF: The megaloblastic anemias, in Koepke JA (ed): *Laboratory Hematology,* ed 1. New York, Churchill Livingstone Inc, 1984, pp 71–83.

10. Stebbins R, Scott J, Herbert V: Drug-induced megaloblastic anemias. *Semin Hematol* 1973; 10:235–251.

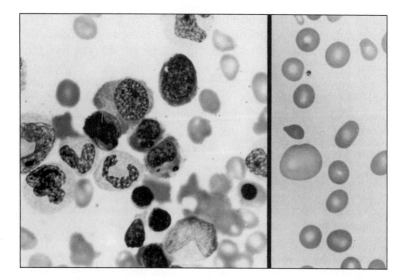

Figure 6–1   Side-by-side photomicrographs of peripheral blood and bone marrow illustrate marked anisocytosis of erythrocytes with oval macrocytes and fragmented erythrocytes in peripheral blood. The bone marrow shows nuclear-cytoplasmic asynchrony of erythroid precursors with open sievelike chromatin. Giant band neutrophils are present.

PART 2

Hemolytic Anemias

7

Accelerated Erythrocyte Turnover

Accelerated erythrocyte turnover in the absence of blood loss is a characteristic of hemolysis. A wide variety of hereditary and acquired diseases associated with hemolysis (Table 7–1) will be discussed in succeeding chapters. In general, diagnosis of hemolysis requires evaluation of the various phases of erythrocyte turnover (Figure 7–1), including bone marrow production phase, circulating phase, and final removal of senescent or damaged cells. Although the actual mechanisms for each phase are not known, their sequence and elapsed time have been determined, allowing normal ranges to be established.

Pathophysiology

Erythropoiesis derives from a marrow stem cell that requires approximately 5 days to progress from erythroblast to marrow reticulocyte. The daily production of red cells is estimated at 3×10^9 cells per kilogram and normally equals the rate of red cell destruction (1% per day). Marrow reticulocytes expel the nucleus before passing through marrow sinusoids into the peripheral blood to become circulating reticulocytes, subsequently requiring 1 or 2 days to shed the reticular network to become mature erythrocytes. The spleen briefly sequesters a small percentage of reticulocytes and then releases them back into the circulation. Mature red cells cir-

Table 7–1   Diseases of Accelerated Erythrocyte Turnover

Etiologic Basis of Hemolysis	Classification of Disorder	Cause of Disorder
Hereditary	Red cell membrane defects	Hereditary spherocytosis, hereditary elliptocytosis
	Red cell enzyme defects	G6PD deficiency
		Pyruvate kinase deficiency
		Glutathione stabilizing enzyme deficiency
		Other deficiencies of the pentose pathway
	Red cell hemoglobin defects	Amino acid substitutions: HbS, HbC, etc
		Alpha-chain production defects: alpha thalassemia, HbH
		Beta-chain production defects: beta thalassemia
Acquired	Infection	Bacterial: *Clostridium perfringens*
		Protozoal: malaria
		Viral: immune mechanisms—mycoplasma, infectious mononucleosis
	Physiochemical	Burns
		Benzene derivatives
	Mechanical	Heart valve prosthesis (aortic)
		Ulcerative colitis
		Hemolytic-uremic syndrome, TTP, DIC
	Drugs	Interaction with G6PD deficiency
		Immune complexes
	Antibody	Alloantibody: incompatible transfusion; erythroblastosis fetalis
		Autoantibody: idiopathic, secondary to lymphocytic neoplasms, associated with collagen diseases, associated with viral infection, secondary to drugs
	Membrane defects	PNH

ABBREVIATIONS: G6PD = glucose-6-phosphate dehydrogenase; TTP = thrombotic thrombocytopenic purpura; DIC = disseminated intravascular coagulation; PNH = paroxysmal nocturnal hemoglobinuria.

Figure 7–1   Laboratory evaluation of phases of red cell production and breakdown. The most useful tests for each phase are underlined. Sequestration is considered an abnormal intermediate step in red cell breakdown and is shown as red cell release from the spleen, diagramatically separate from normal red cell breakdown. RES indicates reticuloendothelial system.

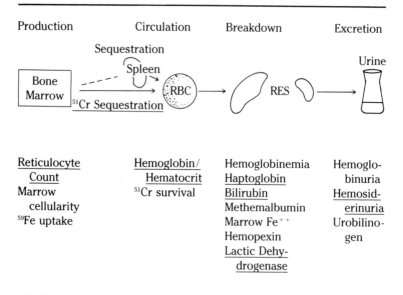

Production	Circulation	Breakdown	Excretion
Reticulocyte Count	Hemoglobin/ Hematocrit	Hemoglobinemia	Hemoglobinuria
Marrow cellularity	⁵¹Cr survival	Haptoglobin	Hemosiderinuria
⁵⁹Fe uptake		Bilirubin	Urobilinogen
		Methemalbumin	
		Marrow Fe⁺⁺	
		Hemopexin	
		Lactic Dehydrogenase	

culate for 120 days and are finally sequestered in the spleen by unknown mechanisms. Splenomegaly, therefore, would be expected to alter red cell circulation and survival. Red cells with defective membranes or with membranes damaged by physicochemical or immune mechanisms are removed more rapidly than normal by the spleen, as well as by the other parts of the reticuloendothelial system including Kupffer's cells in liver sinusoids. The spleen removes marginally damaged red cells, the liver removes more severely damaged red cells, and intravascular hemolysis occurs with the most severe cell damage. There is a limited number of conditions so damaging to the red cell as to cause almost certain intravascular hemolysis. Commonly encountered causes are summarized in Table 7–2.

Red cell destruction releases heme, globin, and iron. Heme is broken down into biliverdin, reduced to bilirubin by biliverdin reductase in the reticuloendothelial system, conjugated to soluble mono- and diglucuronides in the liver, and excreted in the feces as urobilin, urobilinogen, and stercobilinogen. Minimal amounts of the soluble urobilinogen are reabsorbed from the portal circulation and excreted in the urine. Heme iron is taken up by the reticuloendothelial cells and reappears in marrow synthesis of new red cells, or is stored in the reticuloendothelial cells as ferritin or hemosiderin. The globin peptide chains are degraded to component amino acids that return to the metabolic pool. Accelerated red cell turnover results in increased amounts of all breakdown products, many of which can be measured with relative ease.

Substances normally present within red cells are released with red cell destruction; increases in serum levels of such substances, eg, lactic dehydrogenase, imply hemolysis if other causes for serum elevation are excluded.

When intravascular hemolysis occurs, free hemoglobin (Hb) is released into the bloodstream; it is bound by the $alpha_2$-globulin, haptoglobin. The Hp:Hb complex is then metabolized directly by the reticuloendothelial system. If the binding capacity of haptoglobin is exceeded, hemoglobinuria results. Other plasma proteins that bind free hemoglobin include transferrin and albumin. Oxidation of the ferrous ion of the albumin-heme complexes produces the brown pigment, methemalbumin.

Clinical Findings

Clinical findings depend on the rate of hemolysis and the degree of anemia produced. Symptoms may be minimal in well-compensated hemolytic anemia as in the hemoglobinopathies and chronic cold antibody autoimmune hemolytic anemia, or may be severe in acute hemolysis of glucose-6-phosphate dehydrogenase (G6PD) deficiency, ABO group–incompatible transfusion, or warm autoimmune hemolytic anemia. The most common symptoms of anemia are pallor and fatigue. Fever, chills, and headache are symptoms of more acute hemolytic episodes. In compensated hemolysis there is no jaundice and no hemoglobinemia or hemoglobinuria as there is in acute hemolytic anemia. Splenomegaly is variable depending on the cause of increased erythroid turnover. Chronic hemolysis may not be associated with splenomegaly, whereas acute hemolysis with increased reticuloendothelial activity may be associated with mild-to-moderate splenomegaly. Hepatomegaly is less common but is usually associated with long-standing increase in erythroid turnover, reticuloendothelial hyperplasia, and iron deposition. Lymphadenopathy is not characteristic of hemolytic anemia unless there is an underlying lymphoproliferative disorder. Bone pain may be present with long-standing hemolysis and resultant marrow erythroid hyperplasia.

Table 7–2   Causes of Intravascular Hemolysis[a] and Tests for Identification

Disease	Mechanism	Diagnostic Test
Antibody		
Alloantibody ABO incompatible transfusion	Anti-A, anti-B Acute hemolysis	Recheck blood groups and clerical work
Anti-Kidd (anti-Jk[a])	Delayed hemolysis	Antibody screening with enzyme-treated red cells
Anti-Kell, anti-Duffy[a] anti-Lewis[a]	IgG antibody with complement activation	Antibody screening
Antipenicillin	IgG antibody	DAT; test serum v drug-treated red cells
Autoantibody-cold autoimmune hemolytic anemia (mycoplasma)	Anti-I	Cold agglutinin titer; DAT
Infections		
Clostridium perfringens	Hemolysin	Blood cultures
Escherichia coli sepsis	Hemolysin	Wound cultures
Cholera	Hemolysin	Stool cultures
Malaria	Mechanical	Red cell smear
Inherited red cell defects		
G6PD deficiency	Drug interaction	G6PD assay
Hemoglobinurias		
PNH	C′ sensitive red cell membrane	Acid hemolysis sucrose lysis
PCH	IgG antibody	Donath-Landsteiner test
Physicochemical agents		
Third-degree burns	Heat damage to red cell membrane	Red cell morphology

(Continued.)

Table 7–2 *Continued.*

Disease	Mechanism	Diagnostic Test
Prosthetic valves	Mechanical	Red cell morphology
Cardiac bypass surgery	Mechanical	Pump-hemoglobin
Distilled water-prostate resection	Osmotic hemolysis	Urine sediment
Snake bites	Lecithinase	History

ABBREVIATIONS: DAT = direct antiglobulin test; G6PD = glucose-6-phosphate dehydrogenase; PNH = paroxysmal nocturnal hemoglobinuria; PCH = paroxysmal cold hemoglobinuria.

ªCauses that are most likely to be encountered, not single case reports

Approach to Diagnosis

Accelerated erythrocyte turnover can be determined by evaluation of marrow production, calculation of circulating red cell survival, and measurement of breakdown products of cell destruction. Increased marrow production is estimated by the following:

1. Hematologic findings characterize the anemia by red cell indices as normochromic and an elevated reticulocyte count establishes accelerated release to the peripheral blood. Bone marrow aspiration that includes stains for marrow iron is useful in documenting accelerated marrow erythroid production and breakdown. Where the cause of a normochromic anemia is clearly hemolysis (eg, in hemoglobinopathies), marrow aspirate may be unnecessary.

2. Plasma and urinary pigments, can be measured because with increased destruction of red cells, levels of each of the degradation products increase. Tests for these products and their relative usefulness are summarized in Table 7–3. In acute hemolysis, bilirubin (total and fractionated), and plasma and urine hemoglobin are most commonly measured. In less acute or chronic compensated hemolysis, urine hemosiderin may indicate long-term occult red cell degradation. Determination of bilirubin in compensated hemolytic anemia is of limited usefulness. Tests for urobilin and fecal and urine urobilinogen are unsatisfactory and unnecessary.

Table 7–3 Urine and Serum Pigments in Accelerated Erythrocyte Turnover

Pigment	Normal Range	Comments
Bilirubin, serum	0.5–2.0 mg/dL	Limited significance; in non-jaundiced patients level is <3.0 mg/dL; in jaundiced patients fractionation may not be diagnostic
Indirect bilirubin, serum	<0.5 mg/dL	Increased early in hemolysis Nonhemolytic elevation in hereditary disorders of conjugation (Crigler-Najjar syndrome, Gilbert's disease)
Hemoglobin, plasma	≤10 mg/dL	Significant above 50 mg/dL Cherry-red plasma >150 mg/dL Binds to haptoglobin, transferrin, or albumin
Hemoglobin, urine	None present	Appears after haptoblobin saturation Hematuria must be excluded Myoglobinuria gives false-positive dip-stick test
Methemalbumin, serum	None present	Qualitative determination in haptoglobin electrophoresis Spectrophotometric qualitative test (Schumm test)
Hemopexin	80–100 mg/dL	Radial immune diffusion measurement not readily available and requires 24–28 hours
Urobilinogen, fecal or urine		No longer used
Urobilin, fecal		Not used

3. Serum haptoglobin, which is easily measured, is a useful test in the absence of intravascular hemolysis when its consumption would be immediately predictable.

4. Lactic dehydrogenase (LD) is released to the plasma as red cells are rapidly destroyed, whether intravascular, intramedullary, intrasplenic, or within body cavities. LD_1 is an isoenzyme found

predominantly in red cells and myocardium. Isoenzyme determinations are useful if the source of total LD elevation is not clearly red cell–derived.

5. Radioisotope tracer studies are usually limited to chromium-51 (^{51}Cr), which estimates survival of circulating red cells and site of cell sequestration and destruction, and to iron-59 (^{59}Fe), which is incorporated into precursor erythrocytes and evaluates rate of production, site of production, rate of red cell release, and site of sequestration. Chromium-51 red cell survival studies require 3 weeks, but abbreviated tests of 1 hour are also performed. Chromium-51 red cell sequestration studies can determine the site of red cell destruction, which is helpful in evaluating the potential benefit of splenectomy.

6. Ferrokinetics using ^{59}Fe is not commonly available, but can be combined with ^{51}Cr sequestration studies to determine sites of production, marrow or extramedullary, and is helpful if splenectomy is being considered. Since ^{59}Fe has a longer half-life than ^{51}Cr, ^{59}Fe studies should follow chromium studies.

7. Ancillary screening tests, as summarized in Table 7–4, are used to document the cause of accelerated erythrocyte turnover once its presence has been established. These tests are discussed at greater length in subsequent chapters.

Hematologic Findings

Increased red cell turnover stimulates increased marrow production and leads to premature release of marrow reticulocytes before they are stripped of nuclear fragments or their reticular network. These cells are seen on Wright's-stained peripheral smears as polychromatophilic macrocytes. Nucleated red cells may also be seen. With a competent bone marrow, the reticulocyte count is persistently elevated, differing from acute blood loss, in which reticulocytosis is of brief duration and usually less than 5%. Reticulocytosis varies with severity and duration of hemolysis. Marrow turnover may increase 4 to 6 times permitting reticulocyte counts as high as 60% to 70%. Chronic hemolysis may deplete marrow levels of folic acid, diminishing production so that reticulocytosis is inadequate for the degree of hemolysis.

The spleen may be enlarged as a result of increased phagocytosis and, in some cases, particularly hereditary hemolytic anemias, the liver is also enlarged. Depending on the rate of red cell destruction and the ability of the liver to conjugate and excrete the degradation products, variable degrees of jaundice may be present.

Table 7–4   Common Screening Tests for Causes of
Accelerated Erythrocyte Turnover

Etiologic Basis of Hemolysis	Classification of Disorder	Test
Hereditary	Red cell membrane defects	Red cell morphology, osmotic fragility
	Red cell enzyme defects	G6PD screening, pypuvate kinase screening
	Red cell hemoglobin defects	Hemoglobin electrophoresis, Heinz body test, HbA_2 and HbF quantitation
Acquired	Infection—protozoal	Red cell morphology, malarial smears
	Physicochemical—burns	Red cell morphology—spherocytes
	Mechanical—intravascular fibrin, prosthetic valves	Red cell morphology—fragments
	Drugs—interaction with enzyme defect	G6PD screening
	Antibody	
	Alloantibody or autoantibody	DAT
		Serum antibody screening; cold agglutinin titer, Donath-Landsteiner test
	Drug-induced antibody	Antibody screening with drug-treated cells
	Miscellaneous membrane defects—PNH	Acid hemolysis test or sucrose lysis test

ABBREVIATIONS: G6PD = glucose-6-phosphate dehydrogenase; PNH = paroxysmal nocturnal hemoglobinuria; DAT = direct antiglobulin test.

Blood Cell Measurements.   Anemia can be severe (Hb 20 g/L or 2 g/dl) to mild (115 g/L or 11.5 g/dl). Mean corpuscular volume (MCV) is 80 to 110 fL; reticulocytes produce a mild macrocytosis. An MCV greater than 115 fL suggests macrocytic anemia or, rarely, secondary folate depletion. An MCV less than 70 fL in a normochromic anemia suggests hemolysis is due to hemoglobin-opathy or paroxysmal nocturnal hemoglobinuria (PNH).

Peripheral Blood Smear Morphology. Morphology generally includes polychromatophilia, macrocytes, and nucleated red cells. Specific morphology is variable depending on etiology of red cell turnover:

1. Spherocytes—hereditary spherocytosis, autoimmune hemolytic anemia.

2. Target cells—hemoglobinopathies, jaundice, postsplenectomy.

3. Cell fragments—hemolytic uremic syndrome, disseminated intravascular coagulation (DIC), prosthetic valves.

4. Microspherocytes—HbC disease, ABO erythroblastosis, burns.

Bone Marrow Examination. Bone marrow is hypercellular with marked normoblastic erythroid hyperplasia reversing the myeloid/erythroid (M/E) ratio from the normal $3:1$ or $4:1$ to $1:2$. Dyssynchronous nuclear and cytoplasmic maturation creates "megaloblastoid" cells without giant metamyelocytes or other stigmata of megaloblastic dyscrasias. If folic acid or vitamin B_{12} are relatively depleted by prolonged rapid turnover, a true megaloblastic cell population may appear; marrow exhaustion with aplasia can eventually result. Special staining of particle smears with ferroferricyanide (Prussian blue) shows increased iron in marrow histiocytes, termed "marrow siderosis." Stainable iron seen in mitochondria of orthochromic normoblasts produces a ring effect present only when ineffective erythropoiesis is present. In hemolysis, if normoblasts contain granules, they are larger and cover the nucleus. Absence of stainable iron in hemolysis suggests PNH.

Other Laboratory Tests

7.1   Serum Bilirubin, Total and Fractionated

Purpose. Increases in indirect bilirubin in the jaundiced patient support the diagnosis of hemolysis.

Principle. Hyperbilirubinemia indicates increased red cell destruction, failure of liver conjugation, or block of excretory pathways. In hemolysis, an increased bilirubin load is presented to the liver faster than conjugation can proceed so that non–water-soluble (indirect) fraction of bilirubin is increased. In liver failure or obstructive jaundice, conjugation does occur, and hyperbilirubinemia is predominantly direct.

Specimen. Serum specimens are stable for days at refrigeration temperatures.

Procedure. Bilirubin is measured by an internationally standardized test, generally using the Evelyn-Malloy method or a modification of it. Bilirubin is coupled with a diazo dye, and the color is quantitated spectrophotometrically at 1 minute. The quick reacting fraction is considered to be direct (or conjugated) bilirubin. The total bilirubin is measured after the addition of alcohol, and the indirect fraction is calculated by subtracting the amount of direct bilirubin from the total.

Interpretation. Normal ranges for total bilirubin are 0 to 25.65 μmol/L (0 to 1.5 mg/dl), and for indirect bilirubin, less than 5.13 μmol/L (0.3 mg/dl). Levels of total bilirubin above 42.75 μmol/L (2.5 mg/dl) are usually associated with clinical jaundice. The level depends on the ability of the liver to compensate. Initially, more than half the bilirubin will be indirect or unconjugated fraction. If liver function is adequate, after several days the rate of glucuronide conjugation is increased so that direct and indirect fractions are nearly equal, and bilirubin fractionation is no longer diagnostic.

In well-compensated hemolytic anemia, levels of total bilirubin may be less than 51.3 μmol/L (3 mg/dl) and no clinical jaundice is seen. Thus, bilirubin levels should not be used to exclude the diagnosis of accelerated red cell turnover.

In hemolytic disease of the newborn, lipid-soluble, indirect-fraction bilirubin is deposited in the striate nucleus producing kernicterus. In the newborn, a shift in conjugation from indirect to direct bilirubin usually occurs at 7 to 10 days as liver function matures.

Notes and Precautions. Misleading elevations of indirect bilirubin can be seen in hereditary disorders of conjugation (Crigler-Najjar syndrome, Gilbert's disease) and secondary to steroids found in breast milk that interfere with conjugation of bilirubin.

7.2 Plasma Hemoglobin Quantitation

Purpose. Increased plasma hemoglobin indicates intravascular hemolysis. Qualitative assessment is usually satisfactory in acute intravascular hemolysis. Quantitation is useful in sera where other pigments (eg, bilirubin) make interpretation of plasma color uncertain.

Principle. Massive red cell injury results in intravascular hemolysis, which is seen macroscopically as cherry-red plasma. Free hemoglobin can be quantitated by a modified benzidine reaction.

Specimen. Five milliliters of blood is collected in heparin or EDTA. A clot is not a desirable specimen because mechanical hemolysis of red cells during clot formation does not allow for the most accurate measurement. Blood must be drawn atraumatically, and plasma should be separated within 1 to 2 hours.

Procedure. A modified benzidine (see Notes and Precautions section) reaction oxidizes a colorless dye to blue in the presence of hemoglobin, as shown in the following reactions:

$$Hb\text{-}Fe^{++} + 2H_2O_2 \rightarrow Hb\text{-}Fe^{+++} + O_2 + 2H_2O$$
$$O_2 + \underset{\text{(Colorless)}}{\text{Benzidine}} \rightarrow \underset{\text{(Blue)}}{\text{Benzidine}}$$

The color is measured spectrophotometrically. The test lacks accuracy below 0.3 g/L (30 mg/dl) but free hemoglobin at that level is not clinically important; the method also measures methemalbumin. Quantitation is not available in all hospital laboratories.

Interpretation. The normal level of plasma hemoglobin is less than 0.1 g/L (10 mg/dl). At low levels, test variability is great, and thus the test is only reliable above 0.5 g/L (50 mg/dl), which is the threshold for visual estimation. Free hemoglobin levels less than 0.3 g/L (30 mg/dl) are technically inaccurate, and may be seen with difficult venipuncture, mechanical destruction of red cells by Vacutainer tubes, or during clotting of specimen. Hemoglobinemia above 1.5 g/L (150 mg/dl) results in hemoglobinuria. At levels above 2.0 g/L (200 mg/dl) plasma becomes clear cherry red.

Notes and Precautions. Ortholidine (*o*-tolidine) is substituted for benzidine as a result of federal regulations limiting potentially carcinogenic agents in the environment.

7.3   Serum Haptoglobin Quantitation

Purpose.   Absence of haptoglobin indicates hemolysis, liver failure, or, rarely, an hereditary variant.

Principle.   Haptoglobin (Hp) is an $alpha_2$-globulin produced in the liver that binds free hemoglobin on a molecule-for-molecule basis. The entire Hp:Hb complex is metabolized in the reticuloendothelial system, a normal mechanism of regulating the renal threshold of hemoglobin. With intravascular hemolysis haptoglobin is completely saturated; excess hemoglobin is then bound by other serum proteins, hemopexin, transferrin, and albumin, before spilling into the urine as hemoglobinuria. Absence of haptoglobin implies saturation and degradation as in hemolysis, or, alternatively, failure of production (ie, liver failure). Hp° is a genetic variant found in some black individuals that does not bind hemoglobin; however, it is of no clinical significance.

Haptoglobin is an acute-phase reactant, increasing 3 to 4 times in inflammation, infection, or tissue necrosis (eg, pneumonia or myocardial infarction). Such increases may mask increased binding of hemoglobin in hemolysis.

Specimen.   Fresh serum is obtained atraumatically. To avoid extraneous hemolysis serum should not be allowed to remain on red cells. Testing specimens with macroscopic hemoglobinemia is superfluous.

Procedure.   The haptoglobin molecule has separate sites for antibody and for hemoglobin binding. Haptoglobin is quantitated by turbidometric methods using a nephelometer. Antihaptoglobin is added to the patient's serum; immune complexes are formed with serum Hp 1:1, and light is scattered proportionate to the concentration of complexes. Most larger hospitals have nephelometers.

Interpretation.   The normal range for haptoglobin is 0.4 to 1.8 g/L (40 to 180 mg/dl). Less than .25 g/L (25 mg/dl) of haptoglobin is consistent with hemolysis, while greater than 0.2 g/L (200 mg/dl) is consistent with inflammation and not helpful in the diagnosis of hemolysis.

Spectrophotometric results may be falsely high if the serum contains peroxidases or other oxidants that increase development of color in the benzidine reaction.

Molecular sites for hemoglobin binding are not those

for antibody binding by antihaptoglobin. With radial immunodiffusion false elevations of haptoglobin may appear because haptoglobin bound to hemoglobin retains antigenic determinants for antibody. Thus saturated Hp:Hb complexes are also measured if not removed by the reticuloendothelial system.

Haptoglobin is decreased or absent in liver failure, after recent massive transfusion due to removal of senescent transfused red cells, and in some blacks who genetically lack binding sites on the haptoglobin molecule, Hp°.

7.4   Direct Antiglobulin Test (DAT)—Direct Coombs' Test

Purpose.   Detection of globulin adsorbed to the patient's red cells suggests immune mechanisms may be an underlying cause of hemolysis (see chapter 6).

Principle.   Antihuman globulin reagent produced in rabbits agglutinates human red cells that are coated with human globulin. Broad-spectrum reagents agglutinate cells coated both with gamma globulin (IgG, IgM), beta globulin (complement), or both, whereas monospecific serums agglutinate only red cells coated with the specific globulin to which the reagent is directed.

Specimen.   Using the red cells from EDTA specimens prevents nonspecific absorption of complement in specimens with strong, but not pathologic, cold agglutinins. Specimens must be maintained at 37°C until cells and serum have been separated.

Procedure.   Patient's saline washed red cells are centrifuged with antiglobulin reagent and agglutination is graded 0 to 4+. Adsorbed globulin must be eluted and tested for activity against red cells before it is classified as antibody.

Interpretation.   Weakly positive results $(+/-)$ are not usually clinically significant and eluates are usually not successful. Strongly positive tests (2 to 4+) due to antibody do not correlate with the degree of hemolysis. Common causes of nonantibody globulin attached to red cells are multiple myeloma and cephalosporin therapy.

A negative DAT does not exclude hemolysis if red cell destruction has been massive and complete, as in incompatible transfusions.

Notes and Precautions. Refrigeration of blood specimens containing cold agglutinins causes false-positive results or exaggerates true-positives by the resultant cold absorption of the agglutinin and complement.

7.5 Other Serum Pigments

Principle. The presence of methemalbumin indicates chronic or continuing hemolysis. Free hemoglobin dissociates into $\alpha\beta$ dimers, and binds to plasma proteins, haptoglobin, transferrin, and albumin. Ferrous iron of hemoglobin bound to albumin oxidizes to ferric iron of methemalbumin, giving a distinctive rusty appearance to serum. Free hemoglobin in the presence of chloride ion produces hematin, which is bound by the protein hemopexin. Tests for methemalbumin are available in reference laboratories. Tests for hemopexin are not generally available.

Methemalbumin is not present in the normal patient. Methemalbumin clears within 4 or 5 days of the cessation of hemolysis. Hemopexin has a normal range of 0.8 to 1.0 g/L (80 to 100 mg/dl); levels less than 0.4 g/L (40 mg/dl) indicate hemolysis.

Ancillary Tests

Urine Hemoglobin and Hemosiderin. Hemoglobinuria indicates concurrent or recent hemoglobinemia above the excretion threshold of 1.5 g/L (150 mg/dl). It is usually seen as cloudy, smoky, dark-red, or cola-colored urine. In the absence of detectable hemoglobin, hemosiderin indicates ongoing hemolysis. Qualitative analysis of free hemoglobin is made by peroxidase reaction of o-tolidine or benzidine, which produces a blue color. (This reaction is the basis of Hemastix Ames Co., Division Miles Laboratories, Inc., Elkhart, IN 46515.) Hemoglobin, even in occult hemolysis, deposits heme in renal epithelial cells, where it is oxidized to hemosiderin.

In the normal patient, no hemoglobin or hemosiderin is detectable. Urinary sediments that contain significant numbers of red cells usually produce some free hemoglobin in hypotonic or alkaline urines. Other causes of a positive Hemastix reaction are hematuria or myoglobinuria. Myoglobinuria cannot be distinguished from hemoglobinuria by Hemastix and is identified by electrophoresis (it migrates in hemoglobin C zone) or by solubility in 80% ammonium sulfate (hemoglobin precipitates). Hemosiderin granules must be intracellular to have significance.

Total Lactic Dehydrogenase (LD). LD increases whenever there is cell destruction, whether normal or pathologic, as cytoplasmic glycolytic enzymes which include LD are relased to the plasma.

Total LD is usually measured by spectrophotometric kinetic analysis. LD in the patient's serum catalyzes the reaction.

$$\text{Lactate} \; + \; \text{NAD} \; \xrightarrow{\text{LD}} \; \text{Pyruvate} \; + \; \text{NADH}$$

Lactate	+	NAD		Pyruvate	+	NADH
(Substrate)		(Coenzyme)		(Product)		(absorbance
		(no absorbance				at 340 nm)
		at 340 nm)				

Radioactive Labeling with ^{51}Cr

Chromium-51 survival and sequestration studies provide objective information about red cell survival and site of red cell destruction or sequestration. Radioactive survival studies are not generally available except in hospitals with well-developed nuclear medicine departments.

Red cells from the patient or from the potential donor unit are incubated with 50 μCi ^{51}Cr, which binds to the cell membrane and the beta chains of hemoglobin. Ascorbic acid is added to the mixture to oxidize chromium to prevent further tagging, and the labeled sample is injected into the patient. Serial blood samples of equal volume are drawn in the first 60 minutes for the abbreviated test, followed by frequent sampling during the first 48 hours, and then over a 3-week period for the complete test. Samples are counted, and the counts are plotted against time so that a straight line is achieved on linear, semilog, or log-log paper, and the half-life is determined. Chromium-51 elutes from the red cell at a rate of 0.5% to 1.2% daily, so that corrections derived from published charts are calculated before plotting. Beginning on day 2 and periodically over a 14-day period, external counting is performed over the patient's precordium, liver, and spleen to determine the site of red cell destruction. The patient's blood volume must remain stable for the 2 to 3 weeks of the test. Other gamma-emitting labels used in nuclear medicine for lung scans, brain scans, and so forth, must not be given until the ^{51}Cr study is completed.

Chromium-51 red cell survival has a normal half-life of 25 to 32 days, but each laboratory must determine its own normal range. For sequestration studies, spleen:liver ratios are calculated. The normal range is 1.0 to 1.5, the range for hyper-splenism is 1.5 to 2.0, for hemolytic anemia, greater than 3; and for hereditary spherocytosis, 4 to 5. Excessive sequestration in the liver suggests severe red cell damage either by the ^{51}Cr label or by complement lysis. Splenic sequestration occurs in hyper-splenism or when red cells are marginally damaged as with IgG antibodies.

Radioactive Labeling with ^{59}Fe. Ferrokinetics using ^{59}Fe can evaluate the rate of red cell synthesis and identify sites of production. These studies require sophisticated nuclear medicine departments.

In ferrokinetics 10 μCi of injected ^{59}Fe binds to unsaturated transferrin, is transported to the marrow and incorporated into maturing erythrocytes. Serial blood samples are drawn over the first 2 hours and sporadically over the next 10 days to 2 weeks. External body counting is done over the precordium, which acts as the baseline, and over the liver, spleen, sacral, and sternal marrow, and other bones as indicated. External counts are plotted against days for each organ site. The hematocrit is monitored to assess plasma iron turnover.

In healthy individuals, ^{59}Fe is cleared rapidly by incorporation into red cells. Splenic uptake gradually increases reflecting blood flow; liver radioactivity is much less because of a lesser blood flow. Sacral and sternal bone marrow reflect initial uptake, with gradual decrease as red cells containing radioactive hemoglobin are released. Steadily increasing splenic uptake is consistent with hemolysis; initial high levels of radioactivity that remain constant correlate with blood flow, as in hypersplenism.

Plasma iron turnover measures plasma iron clearance in relation to hematocrit. The normal range is 0.04 to 0.08 g/L/24 h (0.4 to 0.8 mg/dl/24 h). Plasma iron turnover is increased with rapid cell turnover or marrow hyperplasia. Red cell utilization of ^{59}Fe can be 90% in healthy individuals. The normal range is 0.03 to 0.07 g/L/24 h (0.3 to 0.7 mg/dl/24 h). Decreased utilization is present in hemolysis, ineffective erythropoiesis, or aplasia.

References

1. Berlin NI: Erythrokinetics, In Williams WJ, Beutler E, Erslev AJ, et al (eds): *Hematology*, ed 3. New York, McGraw-Hill International Book Co, 1983, pp 395–406.
2. Mollison PL, Engelfriet CP, Contreras M: Labelling of red cells with ^{51}Cr:

Blood Transfusion in Clinical Medicine, ed 8. London, Blackwell Scientific, 1987, pp 807–808.

3. Mollison PL: op. cit. (ed 8) pp 102–106.

4. Zimmerman JH, Henry JB: Clinical enzymology, *In* Henry JB (ed): Todd-Sanford-Davidsohn *Clinical Diagnosis and Management by Laboratory Methods,* ed 17. Philadelphia, WB Saunders Co, 1984, pp 266–269.

8

Hereditary Erythrocyte Membrane Defects

Hereditary spherocytosis and hereditary elliptocytosis (ovalocytosis) are hereditary abnormalities of red cell shape. They are generally believed to be caused by an inherited defect of the red cell membrane, and many proposals have been made concerning their nature. Nonetheless, in most cases, the underlying cause of these disorders is not known.

Pathophysiology

Hereditary spherocytosis is probably the most common type of hereditary hemolytic anemia among individuals of Northern European origin, but it occurs in all races throughout the world. The inheritance is autosomal dominant. Therefore, it is to be expected that one of the patient's parents will be affected and that each of the patient's children will have a 50% chance of inheriting the disorder. Although a variety of abnormalities have been described in hereditary spherocytosis, including defects in sodium permeability, increased lipid loss, and decreased aldolase activity, none of these alterations is the primary cause of the disorder. A quantitative decrease in the amount of spectrin can be documented in most patients with hereditary spherocytosis, and this finding may be closer to the basic etiology of the disorder.

   Hereditary elliptocytosis exists in several genetically distinct forms. Although hemolytic anemia is present in some of these, approximately 90% of patients with this abnormality show no clinical evidence of hemolysis. Abnormalities of membrane proteins have been identified in a small minority of patients with hereditary hemolytic elliptocytosis and include a deficiency in membrane protein band 4.1 and a shift in the spectrin tetramer-dimer equilibrium toward the dimer conformation.

Clinical Findings

The chronic hemolytic state in hereditary spherocytosis may vary widely in severity, ranging from an asymptomatic compensated hemolysis to a moderately severe chronic anemia. The age at diagnosis depends on the severity of the hemolytic process; the more severe forms of the disease are diagnosed early in life. Clinical manifestations are most often first noted in children or adolescents. Typical complaints include mild jaundice and nonspecific manifestations of anemia, such as weakness. Because of an increased turnover of bilirubin, patients with this condition have a high incidence of gallstones. Some patients report a history of intermittent jaundice, dark urine, and weakness, often triggered by an infection. Patients in whom an aplastic crisis occurs may have symptoms of rapidly developing anemia with lessening jaundice. The most consistently positive physical finding is splenomegaly, which may be marked. A variable degree of jaundice is frequently seen, and slight scleral icterus is usually present.

The most consistent and therapeutically important feature of hereditary spherocytosis is the clinical cure by splenectomy of hemolytic anemia. Red cell life-span after this procedure is restored to normal or near normal. In patients with hemolytic anemia, splenectomy has usually been found to relieve the hemolysis. Hereditary elliptocytosis, like hereditary spherocytosis, is inherited in an autosomal dominant manner.

Approach to Diagnosis

A diagnosis of hereditary spherocytosis should be suspected in patients with chronic hemolytic anemia, especially when spherocytes are seen on the blood film. Because hereditary spherocytosis is inherited in an autosomal dominant manner, attempted confirmation of this mode of inheritance by family studies is an important part of the diagnostic evaluation. Sometimes examination of the blood of family members reveals the presence of laboratory stigmas of hereditary spherocytosis, even when there is no history of anemia, jaundice, or gallstones. This is not surprising, since the expression of hereditary spherocytosis may be very mild in some affected individuals. Occasionally, even careful examination of the parents of an affected individual fails to reveal the presence of hereditary spherocytosis. Although this should cause the physician to consider the possibility that the diagnosis of hereditary spherocytosis is incorrect, the disorder can arise as a new mutation; well-documented cases of hereditary spherocytosis occur without a positive family history.

The uniform success of splenectomy in abolishing hemolysis is in itself a diagnostic clinical feature of hereditary spherocytosis. If significant hemolysis persists after splenectomy in a patient presumed to have hereditary spherocytosis, the presumptive diagnosis is incorrect. Elliptocytes are readily identified on the stained blood film (Figure 8–1). Because this generally represents a benign anomaly, hereditary elliptocytosis should only be considered the cause of anemia when evidence for hemolysis, such as an elevated reticulocyte count, is found.

Evaluation of a patient presumed to have hereditary spherocytosis includes the following:

1. Hematologic evaluation, with attention to red cell morphology, the mean corpuscular hemoglobin concentration (MCHC), and the reticulocyte count.

2. An osmotic fragility test to confirm the presence of spherocytosis.

3. An antiglobulin test (see chapter 6) to rule out an autoimmune hemolytic anemia as a cause for spherocytosis.

4. An autohemolysis test, which may be of some value when the diagnosis is in doubt in atypical cases.

5. If the diagnosis is in doubt, estimation of red cell enzyme activities.

Hematologic Findings

Blood Cell Measurements. Hemoglobin levels in patients with hereditary spherocytosis and hemolytic ovalocytosis frequently range between 90 and 120 g/L (9 and 12 g/dl), and the mean corpuscular volume (MCV) is usually in the normal range but may be elevated in the presence of prominent reticulocytosis. The MCHC characteristically is elevated to levels as high as 370 g/L (37 g/dl) (normal, 260 to 340 g/L, or 26 to 34 g/dl). The reticulocyte count usually ranges between .05 and .15 (5% and 15%). The degree of reticulocytosis is characteristically greater than in other hemolytic anemias when there is a similar hemoglobin level.

Peripheral Blood Smear Morphology. The central morphologic finding in hereditary spherocytosis is the presence of spherocytes on the peripheral blood film. Ovalocytosis is diagnosed when most or all of the cells on the smear have an oval shape with a long diameter that is 2 or more times the short diameter. Spherocytes appear as slightly smaller than normal, densely staining red cells with diminished or absent central pallor (Figure 8–2). The increased intensity of staining is caused in part by the fact that the spherical cell is thicker. In addition, the MCHC is generally somewhat increased. In mild forms of the disease, these cells may not be present in large numbers. Moreover, the appearance of red cells varies greatly in different parts of the blood film, even when it is well prepared. Improper technique in preparing the smear may result in the appearance of artifactual spherocytes to an inexperienced observer. Prominent macrocytosis and polychromasia may be present with very high reticulocyte counts.

Bone Marrow Examination. The bone marrow characteristically shows erythroid hyperplasia, except during aplastic crises, when erythroid activity is diminished.

Other Laboratory Tests

8.1   Osmotic Fragility Test

Purpose. The osmotic fragility test is necessary to confirm the morphologic findings of spherocytosis.

Principle. The osmotic fragility of red cells is basically a measurement of the extent of redundancy of the red cell membrane. In a hypotonic medium, red cells fill with water until the osmotic pressure inside the cell is reduced to that outside the cell. The red cell membrane is normally sufficiently redundant so that the volume of the cell can increase to about 1.8 times the resting volume before becoming a perfect sphere. Once a cell reaches this volume (the critical hemolytic volume), further entry of water produces lysis. A cell that is spherocytic in the resting state has less membrane redundancy than a cell that is normally biconcave. For this reason, less water can enter before the cell lyses.

Specimen. Blood freshly drawn into heparin or EDTA is used.

Procedure. The osmotic fragility test is performed by adding

Table 8–1   Normal Values for Osmotic Fragility Tests

NaCl (%)	Lysis (%)	
	Fresh	Incubated
0.20		95–100
0.30	97–100	85–100
0.35	90–99	75–100
0.40	50–95	65–100
0.45	5–45	55–95
0.50	0–6	40–85
0.55	0	15–70
0.60	0	0–40
0.65	0	0–10
0.70	0	0–5
0.75	0	0

small volumes of blood to a series of tubes containing buffered salt solutions with an osmolarity equivalent to those of 0.20% to 0.9% NaCl solution. A control tube contains distilled water. After standing at room temperature for 1 hour, the tubes are centrifuged, and the percentage of hemolyzed cells is estimated by measuring the amount of hemoglobin released into the supernatant solution. The tests should be carried out on freshly drawn blood and on blood that has been incubated for 24 hours.

Interpretation.   The normal range of values for the osmotic fragility test is presented in Table 8–1 and Figure 8–3. Increased osmotic fragility of the erythrocytes is the basic diagnostic feature of hereditary spherocytosis; unless abnormal osmotic fragility is demonstrated, the diagnosis cannot be considered to be established. It is not uncommon, however, in mild forms of the disease to find a minimal increase in osmotic fragility on freshly drawn blood. In such cases, the incubated fragility may be of some help. Because an increased osmotic fragility merely reflects the presence of spherocytes, this finding does not distinguish hereditary spherocytosis from autoimmune hemolytic disease with spherocytosis, in which the osmotic fragility of red cells is also increased. In the latter disorder, however, the increase of fragility that occurs with incubation is much less. Increased resistance to hemolysis is characteristic of thalassemia, in which an increase of the surface-to-volume ratio of the red cell is present.

Figure 8–3 Osmotic fragility of normal erythrocytes and those from a patient with hereditary spherocytosis. The osmotic fragility is normal in fresh cells from some patients with hereditary spherocytosis, although usually it is increased. The osmotic fragility of normal cells is increased by autoincubation, but that of cells from patients with hereditary spherocytosis is increased to a greater extent than normal.

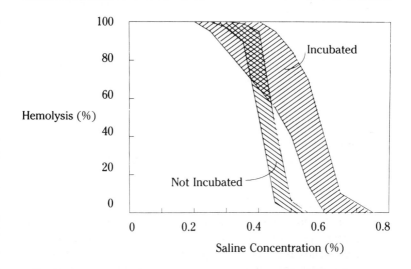

(Reprinted with permission from Beutler E: Osmotic fragility, in Williams WJ, Beutler E, Erslev A, et al (eds): *Hematology,* ed 3. New York, McGraw-Hill International Book Co, 1983, p 1627.)

Notes and Precautions. Reporting osmotic fragility as percent saline concentrations for beginning and completion of hemolysis is an inadequate representation of test results. Osmotic fragility is best appreciated when reported graphically (Figure 8–1).

8.2 Autohemolysis Test

Purpose. The primary usefulness of the autohemolysis test is to assist in the diagnosis of atypical cases of hereditary spherocytosis. While it has also been used in the differential diagnosis of hereditary nonspherocytic hemolytic anemia, the availability of specific enzymatic assays has made the autohemolysis test obsolete for this purpose.

Principle. When red cells are incubated in their own serum, hemolysis occurs gradually. Although the exact mechanism of lysis is probably quite complex, it seems likely that the inability to maintain cation gradients plays an important role, especially in hereditary spherocytosis.

Specimen. Defibrinated whole blood or whole blood anticoagulated with heparin or EDTA is used as a specimen.

Procedure. The autohemolysis test is carried out by incubating sterile blood with and without the addition of glucose for 48 hours and measuring the amount of hemoglobin released into the plasma.

Interpretation. Autohemolysis is normally less than 3.5% at the end of 48 hours without added glucose and less than 0.6% with added glucose. Autohemolysis in the absence of added glucose is generally greatly increased in hereditary spherocytosis; this increase is prevented to a large extent by the addition of glucose. This pattern has been designated type I autohemolysis.

Notes and Precautions. The autohemolysis test is very non-specific. Type I tests may sometimes also be found in non-spherocytic hemolytic anemia. A high blood sugar level caused by concurrent diabetes mellitus may cause a false-negative test result.

Course and Treatment

Both hereditary spherocytosis and elliptocytosis are essentially benign disorders. Complications that may occur include the development of cholelithiasis and cholecystitis and the occurrence of aplastic crises, particularly after infections. Although splenectomy was once recommended quite universally for patients with hereditary spherocytosis and hemolytic elliptocytosis, it is not clear that it is necessary to perform these operations in all patients.

References

1. Godal HC, Gjonnes G, Ruyter R: Does preincubation of the red blood cells contribute to the capability of the osmotic fragility test to detect very mild forms of hereditary spherocytosis? *Scand J Haematol* 1982; 29:89–93.

2. Jandl JH, Cooper RA: Hereditary spherocytosis, in Williams WJ, Beutler

E, Erslev A, et al (eds): *Hematology,* ed 3. New York, McGraw-Hill International Book Co, 1983, pp 547–552.

3. Mohler DN, Thorup OA Jr: Hereditary hemolytic disorders, in Thorup OA Jr (ed): *Fundamentals of Clinical Hematology,* ed 5. Philadelphia, WB Saunders Co, 1987, pp 258–264.

4. Zail S: Clinical disorders of the red cell membrane skeleton. *CRC Crit Rev Oncol Hematol* 1986; 5:397–453.

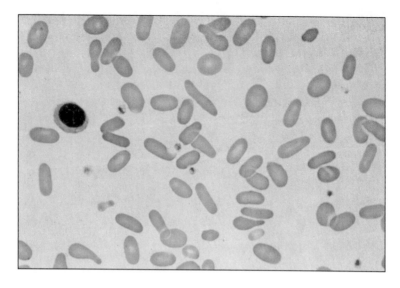

Figure 8–1   Elliptocytes.

Figure 8–2   Spherocytes.

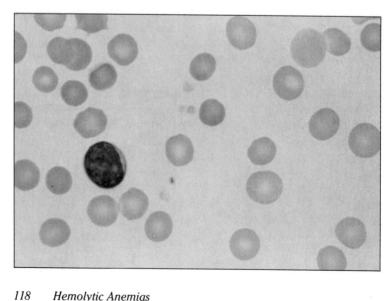

9

Hereditary Erythrocyte Disorders Due to Deficiencies of Enzymes Other than Those of the Hexose Monophosphate Shunt Pathway

Red cells contain the enzymatic machinery to carry out a number of enzymatic processes. The metabolism of glucose to lactate requires 13 enzymes, and several dozen other enzymes have been identified in erythrocytes. Hereditary deficiencies of many red cell enzymes have been documented, and a number of these cause hereditary nonspherocytic hemolytic anemia. Disorders of the hexose monophosphate pathway (HMP) are described in Chapter 10; this chapter addresses all of the other red cell enzyme deficiencies.

Pathophysiology

Because the mature erythrocyte does not contain mitochondria, it must depend entirely on glycolysis for the energy needed for such vital functions as maintenance of membrane integrity and operation of the cation pump. About 90% of glycolysis occurs by way of the main glycolytic pathway, in which glucose is broken down to lactate in a series of enzyme-catalyzed reactions (Figure 9–1). The important products of this pathway are adenosine triphosphate (ATP), the major high-energy compound in erythrocytes, and reduced nicotinamide-adenine dinucleotide (NADH), an essential coenzyme for the reduction of methemoglobin. There is a net yield of 2 moles of ATP for each mole of glucose that is metabolized. 2,3-Diphosphoglycerate (2,3-DPG), which alters the affinity of hemoglobin for oxygen

Figure 9–1 Glucose metabolism of erythrocytes. Enyzmes catalyzing the various metabolic steps are underlined. Abbreviations: Hx = hexokinase; GPI = glucose phosphate isomerase; PFK = phosphofructokinase; TPI = triosephosphate isomerase; GAP = D-glyceraldehyde-3-P; DHAP = dihydroxyacetone-P; GAPD = glyceraldehyde phosphate dehydrogenase; 1,3-DPG = 1,3-diphosphoglyceric acid; DPGM = diphosphoglyceromutase; 2,3-DPG = 2,3-diphosphoglyceric acid; PGK = phosphoglycerate kinase; DPGP = diphosphoglycerophosphatase; 3-PGA = 3-phosphoglyceric acid; MPGM = monosphosphoglyceromutase; 2-PGA = 2-phosphoglyceric acid; PEP = phosph(enol)pyruvate; PK = pyruvate kinase; LDH = lactic dehydrogenase; Glu-6-P = glucose-6-phosphate; F-6-P = fructose-6-phosphate; F-1,6-DP = fructose-1, 6-diphosphate.

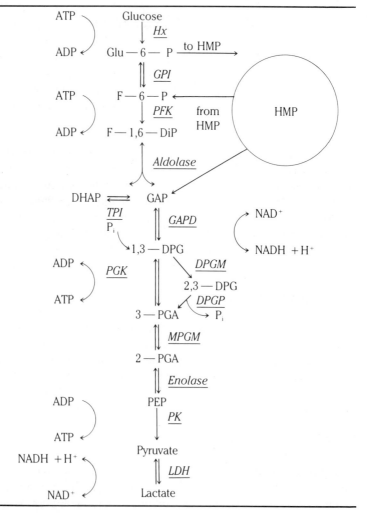

Table 9-1 Main Glycolytic Pathway Deficiencies that Cause Hemolytic Anemia

Hexokinase
Glucose-phosphate isomerase
Phosphofructokinase
Aldolase
Triosephosphate isomerase
Diphosphoglycerate mutase
Phosphoglycerate kinase
Pyruvate kinase

and plays an essential role as a regulator of oxygen delivery to tissues, is a phosphorylated intermediate in this pathway.

About 10% of glycolysis occurs via the HMP shunt, which bypasses the early steps of the main glycolytic pathway, a route that generates reduced nicotinamide-adenine dinucleotide phosphate (NADPH). NADPH is required for reduction of glutathione, which is essential for the protection of hemoglobin and red cell enzymes from oxidative damage (see Figure 10–1).

Hereditary spherocytosis was described fully as a clinical entity at around the turn of the century. In subsequent years, cases were recorded that were characterized by a hereditary hemolytic state first observed during infancy or childhood. In these cases, spherocytes were not present in significant numbers in the peripheral blood film and the osmotic fragility of the red cells of such patients was normal. This group of concurrent disorders is designated as "hereditary nonspherocytic hemolytic anemia" (HNSHA).

One prominent cause of HNSHA is pyruvate kinase deficiency, a defect of the main glycolytic pathway (Table 9–1). HNSHA, however, is known to be a heterogeneous group of disorders. Included in this group, along with deficiencies of the main pathway, are the unstable hemoglobins and disorders of the enzymes of the HMP shunt and glutathione metabolism (Table 9–2).

Clinical Findings

Most patients with HNSHA manifest only an uncomplicated hemolytic state, often associated with splenomegaly. Patients with triosephosphate isomerase deficiency, phosphoglycerate kinase

Table 9–2   Red Cell Disorders Associated with Hereditary Nonspherocytic Hemolytic Anemia

Disorder	Example	Comments
Deficiencies of the main glycolytic pathway	PK deficiency	Relatively common cause
Unstable hemoglobins	Hemoglobin Zürich	
Deficiencies of the HMP shunt pathway	Exceptional G6PD variants	See chapter 10
Deficiencies of glutathione metabolism	Some cases of hereditary glutathione deficiency	See chapter 10

ABBREVIATIONS: PK = pyruvate kinase; HMP = hexose monophosphate; G6PD = glucose-6-phosphate dehydrogenase.

(PGK) deficiency, or glutathione synthetase deficiency may manifest neurologic disorders as well.

Pyruvate kinase deficiency is the most prevalent of the red cell enzyme deficiencies involving the main glycolytic pathway and can serve as the prototype for the others, which are quite rare. Like almost all disorders of the main glycolytic pathway, pyruvate kinase deficiency shows an autosomal recessive mode of inheritance; the exception is PGK deficiency, which is inherited as a sex-linked disorder.

Pyruvate kinase deficiency is usually first detected in infancy or later in childhood because of anemia or jaundice and slight-to-moderate splenomegaly. The severity of the anemia and of the clinical manifestations varies widely from case to case. Any of the characteristic features of chronic hemolytic anemia may be found, including jaundice, splenomegaly, and an increased incidence of gallstones; in patients with severe anemia, aplastic crises have been observed. In severe forms of pyruvate kinase deficiency, splenectomy appears to be beneficial.

Approach to Diagnosis

HNSHA is a conceptually useful classification in the diagnostic evaluation of the red cell enzyme deficiencies. In the autosomal recessive forms of HNSHA, the family history is usually negative unless siblings are affected. Biochemical studies of family members, however, reveal the hereditary nature of the disorder. Routine laboratory studies must ascertain the presence of a nonspherocytic hemolytic anemia. The diagnosis of a specific red cell enzyme deficiency must ultimately be established by a biochemical screen test or assay. Evaluation of these disorders proceeds with the following:

1. Hematologic evaluation, with a search for spherocytes on the blood film.

2. An osmotic fragility test to help rule out hereditary spherocytosis.

3. Hemoglobin electrophoresis to rule out the hemoglobinopathies (see Test 11.1) and an isopropanol stability test to identify unstable hemoglobins.

4. Screening tests for glucose-6-phosphate dehydrogenase (G6PD) deficiency (see Tests 10.1 and 10.2) and for pyruvate kinase deficiency.

5. Appropriate quantitative red cell enzyme assays.

6. Ancillary tests that are part of the diagnostic evaluation of any chronic hemolytic anemia, including Coombs' test to rule out an autoimmune hemolytic process and a sucrose hemolysis test to rule out paroxysmal nocturnal hemoglobinuria.

Hematologic Findings

No pathognomonic hematologic findings are present in pyruvate kinase deficiency or in any of the other glycolytic red cell enzyme deficiency states. Hematologic findings are compatible with chronic hemolytic anemia, and their prominence is proportional to the severity of the anemia. The single most important morphologic criterion for this group of disorders is a negative one, ie, the absence of significant spherocytosis.

Blood Cell Measurements.   In pyruvate kinase deficiency, hemoglobin levels range from 50 to 120 g/L (5 to 12 g/dl) and MCV may be moderately increased. Reticulocytosis is proportional to the severity of the anemia (up to 25%) but may be more markedly increased (to over 50%) after splenectomy.

Peripheral Blood Smear Morphology.   Cells are normocytic, normochromic, or, when in association with reticulocytosis, macrocytic with polychromatophilia; poikilocytosis may be seen. Rare, irregularly contracted, densely staining red cells may be present. Stippling of red cells is prominent in pyrimidine-5′-nucleotidase deficiency.

Other Laboratory Tests

9.1 Fluorescent Screening Test for Pyruvate Kinase Deficiency

Purpose. A series of fluorescent biochemical screening tests is useful for the detection of red cell enzyme deficiencies. In practice, it is often enough to know whether the activity of the enzyme in question is markedly deficient. Slight deviations from normal are not likely to be of clinical importance.

Principle. Instead of measuring the rate of oxidation or reduction of pyridine nucleotide by spectrophotometer, fluorescence visible to the naked eye is used as an indicator. Reduced pyridine nucleotides fluoresce when illuminated with long-wave ultraviolet light, while no such fluorescence occurs with oxidized pyridine nucleotides. In addition to the screening procedure for pyruvate kinase described previously, screening tests are available for glucose-phosphate isomerase, NADH diaphorase triosephosphate isomerase, and G6PD (chapter 10).

Pyruvate kinase catalyzes the phosphorylation of ADP to ATP by phospho(enol)pyruvate (PEP):

$$\text{PEP} + \text{ADP} + \text{Mg}^{++} \xrightarrow{\text{PK}} \text{Pyruvate} + \text{ATP}$$

This reaction is coupled with the NADH-dependent conversion of pyruvate to lactate:

$$\text{Pyruvate} + \text{NADH} + \text{H}^+ \xrightleftharpoons{\text{LDH}} \text{Lactate} + \text{NAD}^+$$

The loss of fluorescence of NADH as it is oxidized to NAD is observed under ultraviolet light.

Specimen. Whole blood collected in heparin or EDTA is suitable for several days at 4° C and for about one day at room temperature.

Procedure. The blood sample is centrifuged, the plasma and buffy coat are aspirated, and a suspension of the red cells is added to a buffered hypotonic screening mixture that lyses the red cells but not the white cells. The screening mixture provides PEP, ADP, NADH, and $MgCl_2$. It is spotted on filter paper immediately after mixing and every 15 minutes thereafter. After the spots are thoroughly dry, the paper is examined under illumination with long-wave ultraviolet light. The patient's sample is compared with that of a healthy control subject.

Interpretation. The first spot should fluoresce brightly. With the normal sample, fluorescence disappears after 15 minutes' incubation. In contrast, in pyruvate kinase–deficient samples, fluorescence fails to disappear even at the end of 45 or 60 minutes' incubation.

Notes and Precautions. False-negative results may be observed if the patient has received a transfusion recently enough that large numbers of transfused cells are still circulating.

9.2   Red Cell Enzyme Assays

Purpose. Assays for red cell enzymes provide quantitative information about their activity and are useful for definitive confirmation of the results of screening tests (see below) and for the detection of heterozygotes when genetic counseling is required.

Principle. Most of the quantitative assays of red cell enzyme activity use spectrophotometric techniques that depend on the absorption of light of the reduced pyridine nucleotide, NADPH, or NADH at 340 nm. The reactions involved in these procedures are linked to the pyridine nucleotide, and the rate of oxidation or reduction of the pyridine nucleotide is measured with the spectrophotometer. Reduction results in the formation NADPH or NADH, with an increase in optical density at 340 nm; oxidation results in formation of NADP or NAD with a decrease in optical density at 340 nm.

Specimen. Blood is collected in EDTA, heparin, or acid-citrate-dextrose. Most red cell enzymes are stable for several days at 4° C under these conditions. The blood should not be allowed to freeze, since washed red cells are used for the enzyme assays and the stability of red cell enzymes is usually less in hemolysates than in intact red cells.

Procedure. The procedure for each enzyme measurement is different. See the references for specific methods.

Interpretation. Interpretation differs for each enzyme. In general, only very severe enzyme deficiencies cause hemolytic anemia.

Even relatively severe deficiencies of enzymes, such as lactate dehydrogenase, glutathione peroxidase, and inosine triphosphatase, are without known clinical effect.

Notes and Precautions.   Quantitative enzyme assays require sufficient time and skill. They are probably best carried out in specialized reference laboratories that are familiar with details of these procedures.

Ancillary Tests

The principal utility of the osmotic fragility test is in the diagnosis of hereditary spherocytosis. Osmotic fragility is clearly increased in hereditary spherocytosis and in autoimmune hemolytic anemia with spherocytosis. Even in such cases, however, osmotic fragility of unincubated blood is occasionally normal, and incubation may be required to demonstrate the abnormality.

The isopropanol stability test is used to screen for the unstable hemoglobins (see Test 11.7).

Course and Treatment

The course of nonspherocytic hemolytic anemia is extremely variable. Pyruvate kinase deficiency may be very severe and require splenectomy early in life. Glucose phosphate isomerase deficiency has even been associated with hydrops fetalis; on the other hand, some patients have a very benign course. Response to splenectomy is variable, but there is no other treatment. Genetic counseling and prenatal diagnosis is possible for most defects.

References

1. Beutler E: *Hemolytic Anemia in Disorders of Red Cell Metabolism.* New York, Plenum Publishing Corp, 1978.
2. Beutler E: Hereditary nonspherocytic hemolytic anemia: Pyruvate kinase deficiency and other abnormalities, in *Hematology,* ed 3. Williams WJ, Beutler E, Erslev A, et al (eds): New York, pp 574–582. McGraw-Hill International Book Co, 1983.
3. Beutler E: *Red Cell Metabolism: A Manual of Biochemical Methods,* ed 3. New York, Grune & Stratton, 1984.
4. Valentine WN, Tanaka KR, Paglia DE: Hemolytic anemias and erythrocyte enzymopathies. *Ann Intern Med* 1985; 103:245–257.

10

Hereditary Disorders of the Hexose Monophosphate Shunt Pathway: Glucose-6-Phosphate Dehydrogenase Deficiency

Glucose-6-phosphate dehydrogenase (G6PD) catalyzes the first step in the hexose monophosphate (HMP) oxidative shunt pathway, resulting in the reduction of (nicotinamide-adenine dinucleotide phosphate (NADP) to NADPH (Figure 10–1). Deficiency of this enzyme is an X-linked genetic abnormality that principally affects the circulating erythrocytes. It is an important cause of hemolytic anemia.

Pathophysiology

NADPH is required as a cofactor for red cell glutathione reductase (GR) to maintain glutathione in the reduced state (GSH). The important functions of GSH in the red cell appear to include the detoxification of low levels of hydrogen peroxide that may form spontaneously or as a result of drug administration, and maintenance of the integrity of the red cell by reducing oxidized sulfhydryl groups of hemoglobin, membrane proteins, and enzymes that may become oxidized. Because G6PD-deficient red cells are unable to maintain glutathione in its reduced state, the ability of the red cell to deal with toxic insults is impaired, and hemolytic anemia results.

G6PD deficiency results from the inheritance of any one of a large number of abnormalities of the structural gene that codes for the amino acid sequence of the enzyme G6PD. Normal G6PD, des-

Figure 10–1 The hexose monophosphate pathway of the erythrocyte: (1) glucose-6-phosphate dehydrogenase, (2) glutathione reductase, (3) phosphogluconate dehydrogenase, (4) ribulose phosphate epimerase, (5) ribose phosphate isomerase, (6) transketolase, and (7) transaldolase.

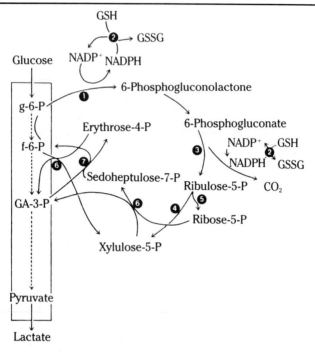

(Reprinted with permission from Beutler E: Energy metabolism and maintenance of erythrocytes. In Williams WJ, Beutler E, Erslev AJ, et al (eds): *Hematology*, ed 3, New York, McGraw-Hill, 1983, p 334).

ignated as B, represents the most common type of enzyme encountered in all population groups that have been studied. G6PD A migrates more rapidly on electrophoresis than the normal B enzyme but has normal enzymatic activity. Approximately 20% of American black males carry this variant. About 11% of American black males have a G6PD variant that has the same electrophoretic mobility as G6PD A but is unstable and results in enzyme deficiency as the red cell ages. This variant, G6PD A−, is the most common clinically significant type of abnormal G6PD among the American black population; red cells from individuals with this variant contain only 5% to 15% of the normal amount of enzyme activity. Among white populations, by far the most common variant is G6PD Mediterranean, which is found frequently in Sicilians, Greeks, Sephardic Jews, and Arabs. Several other variants are common in Asian populations.

Table 10–1   Red Cell Enzyme Deficiencies of the Hexose Monophosphate Shunt Pathway and of Glutathione Metabolism Clearly Associated with Hemolytic Anemia

G6PD
γ-glutamyl cysteine synthetase, GSH synthetase
Glutathione reductase (only total deficiency)

ABBREVIATIONS: G6PD = glucose-6-phosphate dehydrogenase; GSH = reduced glutathione.

Because the gene determining the structure of G6PD is carried on the X chromosome, inheritance of G6PD deficiency is sex-linked. For this reason, the effect is fully expressed in affected males and is never transmitted from father to son but only from mother to son. In females, only one of the two X chromosomes in each cell is active. Consequently, females who are heterozygous for G6PD deficiency have 2 populations of red cells, deficient and normal cells. The ratio of deficient to normal cells may vary greatly. Some heterozygous females appear to be entirely healthy, whereas others are fully affected. The variability of expression of G6PD deficiency in heterozygotes is the result of the variability that is intrinsic to the X-chromosome inactivation process.

Deficiencies of other enzymes in the HMP shunt and glutathione metabolism are comparatively rare (Table 10–1). Hereditary GSH deficiency of the red cell results from a deficiency of either of the two enzymes of GSH synthesis, gamma-glutamyl cysteine synthetase, or GSH synthetase. In some cases, the clinical manifestation of these deficiencies is similar to that of G6PD deficiency; others present with a chronic hemolytic anemia. Some patients with GSH synthetase deficiency also lack GSH synthetase tissues other than red cells. Patients with this condition excrete large amounts of 5-oxoproline (pyroglutamic acid) in the urine and suffer from a progressive neurologic disorder.

Partial deficiency of GR is a "nondisease." Low levels of GR are found in patients with dietary riboflavin deficiency. GR is a flavin enzyme that requires the cofactor flavin-adenine dinucleotide (FAD); GR activity is impaired with FAD deficiency. Near total absence of GR has been reported only once, and this severe deficiency produced a single hemolytic episode in an otherwise hematologically healthy person.

Glutathione peroxidase deficiency does not appear to cause hemolytic anemia. Many hematologically healthy people have

Table 10–2   Drugs and Chemicals Causing Clinically Significant Hemolytic Anemia in Glucose-6-Phosphate Dehydrogenase Deficiency

---

Acetanilid

Methylene blue

Nalidixic acid (NegGram)

Naphthalene

Niridazole (Ambilhar)

Nitrofurantoin (Furadantin)

Primaquine

Sulfacetamide

Sulfanilamide

Sulfapyridine

Sulfamethoxazole (Gantanol)

Thiazolesulfone

Trinitrotoluene (TNT)

---

levels of this enzyme as low as or lower than those found in persons in whom hemolysis was attributed to a deficiency of the enzyme.

Clinical Findings

The most common clinical manifestation of G6PD deficiency is a self-limited episode of drug-induced hemolysis or infection in an otherwise apparently healthy person, beginning 1 to 3 days after administration of an oxidant drug is initiated (Table 10–2). Heinz bodies appear in the red cells, and the hemoglobin concentration begins to decline rapidly. As hemolysis progresses, Heinz bodies disappear from the circulation, presumably as the erythrocytes that contain them are removed by the spleen or the Heinz bodies are "pitted" from the red cells. In severe cases, abdominal or back pain may occur. The urine may turn dark or even black. Within 4 to 6 days, the reticulocyte count is generally increased, except in instances in which the patient has received a drug for treatment of an active infection. In the A− type of G6PD deficiency, the hemolytic anemia is self-limited because the young red cells produced in response to hemolysis have nearly normal G6PD levels and are relatively resistant to hemolysis.

Table 10–3   Clinical Features of Glucose-6-Phosphate Dehydrogenase Variants

G6PD Variant	Clinical Features
Episodic hemolytic anemia with drug administration or infection	Usual manifestation in A− and Mediterranean variants
Favism	Occurs especially in Mediterranean children, not seen in A− type of deficiency
Neonatal icterus	Observed in infants with Mediterranean and Chinese variants, rare in newborn blacks
Hereditary nonspherocytic hemolytic anemia	Seen with rare variants, occasionally seen in Mediterranean type or defect

ABBREVIATIONS: G6PD = glucose-6-phosphate dehydrogenase.

Other stresses that may result in acute hemolytic anemia in people who are severely G6PD deficient are the neonatal state and exposure to fava beans. Rare cases presenting as hereditary nonspherocytic hemolytic anemia are also associated with G6PD deficiency (Table 10–3).

Approach to Diagnosis

The occurrence of episodic hemolysis raises the suspicion that a patient may be suffering from hereditary deficiency of one of the enzymes of the HMP.

Patients with the most common type of G6PD deficiency present with acute hemolytic anemia. In such cases, a careful history regarding ingestion of drugs is important. Other causes of episodic anemia include paroxysmal nocturnal hemoglobinuria (see chapter 12) and some of the unstable hemoglobins (see chapter 11). When the hemolytic nature of the episodes is less apparent, and particularly in cases associated with infection, differential diagnosis includes an aregenerative crisis that may occur in any of the severe hereditary anemias. The rare variants that present as hereditary nonspherocytic hemolytic anemia are discussed in chapter 9. In patients who present with neonatal icterus, fetal-maternal Rh or ABO incompatibility must be ruled out.

Hematologic Findings

The severity of the anemia is extremely variable. The hemoglobin concentration in the blood may be near normal or as low as 50 g/L (5 g/dl). At the beginning of the hemolytic episode, the reticulocyte count may be normal, but if the hemolytic episode has been under way for several days, the reticulocyte count may be elevated in a manner appropriate to the degree of anemia. Indices will be slightly macrocytic if reticulocytosis is present; otherwise, they are normocytic and normochromic. The white count may be low, normal, or elevated because of granulocytosis. The red cell morphology is not usually distinctive. Although "bite" cells have been documented occasionally in patients with drug-induced hemolytic anemia, these patients have not been enzyme deficient. Heinz bodies, particles of denatured hemoglobin and membrane proteins that tend to adhere to the membrane, may be seen on preparations stained supervitally for the enumeration of reticulocytes or those stained supervitally with crystal violet; they are not seen on Wright's- or Giemsa-stained smears.

Other Laboratory Tests

10.1 Fluorescent Screening Test for G6PD

Purpose. The fluorescent screening test is highly reliable for the detection of both severe and mild types of G6PD deficiency in males not undergoing hemolysis.

Principle. In the presence of G6PD and NADP, G6PD is oxidized through 6-phosphogluconate in the following reaction:

$$G6PD + NADP^+ \xrightarrow{\text{G6PD}} \text{6-Phosphogluconate} + NADPH + H^+$$

Since phosphogluconate dehydrogenase (6-PGD) is present in virtually all hemolysates, further reduction of NADP occurs in the following reaction:

$$\text{6-Phosphogluconate} + NADP^+ \xrightarrow{\text{G6PD}} \text{Ribulose-5-P} + NADPH + H^+$$

When mildly G6PD deficient hemolysates are incubated with G6PD and NADP, a small amount of NADPH is formed. In the presence of oxidized glutathione (GSSG), provided in the screening mixture, NADPH is reoxidized in the glutathione reductase reaction:

$$GSSG + NADPH + H^+ \xrightarrow{\text{GR}} 2\ GSH + NADP^+$$

Thus, the screening test measures, in effect, the difference between approximately twice the G6PD activity and the glutathione reductase activity.

Specimen. Blood collected in heparin EDTA or acid citrate dextrose (ACD) solution is satisfactory. Blood that is several weeks old, and even spots of blood collected on filter paper and dried, may be used.

Procedure. Whole blood is added to a buffered screening solution containing saponin, G6PD, NAPD$^+$, and GSSG. After incubation for 5 to 10 minutes at room temperature, the mixture is spotted on filter paper, allowed to dry, and observed for fluorescence.

In patients with the A$-$ variant of G6PD who have recently undergone hemolysis, the test may be modified by centrifuging the blood sample in a microhematocrit tube and using the bottom 10% of the red cell column the reticulocyte-poor, enzyme-deficient cell fraction for the test.

Interpretation. With normal blood, the dried spot is brightly fluorescent; deficient samples show little or no fluorescence. No false-positive or false-negative test results are observed. In patients with the A$-$ variant of G6PD with ongoing or acute hemolysis, however, the remaining young cells and reticulocytes have normal or near-normal G6PD activity, most of the enzyme-deficient cells having been removed from the circulation. Diagnosis of G6PD deficiency under these circumstances can be accomplished either by repeating the screening test in 2 or 3 weeks or by means of modifying the screening test, as noted above. In severe G6PD deficiency of the Mediterranean or similar types in which even very young cells have very low levels of G6PD, a screening test suffices for diagnosis, even in the presence of a severe hemolytic reaction, provided that the patient has not been transfused.

Notes and Precautions. Because G6PD is sex-linked, heterozygotes for G6PD deficiency have 2 red cell populations; some of the red cells are grossly deficient, and others are normal. Although the deficient cells are susceptible to hemolysis, the enzyme activity, as measured on hemolysates, may be only moderately reduced, the extent of deficiency being a function of the proportion of normal and deficient cells in that particular heterozygote. Special methods for the detection of individual cell G6PD may be used to help detect heterozygotes.

10.2   Quantitative G6PD Assay

Purpose. In males not undergoing hemolysis, the G6PD fluorescent screening test is generally adequate for diagnosis, but quantitative enzyme assays may be useful in detecting patients who have undergone hemolysis and in female heterozygotes. The rate of increase of optical density that occurs with the formation of NADPH from NADP is measured at 340 nm in a spectrophotometer.

Specimen. Blood collected in EDTA or ACD solution is satisfactory. The G6PD activity is stable for several weeks at 4° C and for several days at room temperature. The blood should not be allowed to freeze, since enzyme activity is rapidly lost when red cells are lysed.

Procedure. The final assay mixture contains 100 mM TRIS-0.5 mM EDTA buffer (pH 8.0) 10 mM $MgCl_2$; 0.2 mM NADP, and 0.6 mM G6P. The reaction is started by the addition of the G6P, with water being substituted for G6P in the blank cuvette.

Interpretation. Quantitative assay for G6PD activity may reveal the presence of G6PD deficiency in a person who has recently undergone hemolysis. Since G6PD is normally an age-dependent enzyme, activity should be increased in a patient with reticulocytosis. Normal or slightly lower than normal G6PD activity in such a patient implies that G6PD deficiency is present. Enzyme activity in heterozygous females may be below the normal range.

Notes and Precautions. The usual assay for G6PD measures the activity of both G6PD and 6-phosphogluconic dehydrogenase, because the product of the G6PD reaction, 6-phosphogluconolactone, is converted rapidly to the substrate for the 6-phosphogluconate dehydrogenase reaction. In practice, this causes no difficulty. Note the precaution in the diagnosis of heterozygotes discussed under Test 10.1 above.

10.3   Glutathione Reductase Assay

Purpose. The purpose is to determine whether severe glutathione reductase deficiency, a very rare cause of drug-induced hemolytic anemia, is present and to assess the adequacy of riboflavin nutrition.

Principle. Glutathione reductase catalyzes the reduction of oxidized glutathione (GSSG) to reduced glutathione (GSH) by NADPH, which is oxidized to NAD in the process. Flavine adenine dinucleotide (FAD) serves as a cofactor for glutathione reductase. The addition of FAD to the system provides information regarding the extent to which the glutathione reductase apoenzyme is saturated with FAD in the red cell. This, in turn, reflects the state of riboflavin nutriture, since riboflavin is a precursor of FAD.

Specimen. Blood should be collected in EDTA, heparin, or ACD. It can be stored for up to 3 weeks at 4° C or up to 5 days at 22° C.

Procedure. The following reaction mixture is used: 100 mM TRIS-0.5 mM EDTA buffer, pH 8.0; 3.3 mM GSSG; 0.1 mM NADH with or without 1 μM FAD. The rate of increase in optical density at 340 nm is read against a blank from which GSSG has been omitted.

Interpretation. Severe enzyme deficiency (<5% of normal) may be a cause of drug-induced hemolytic anemia or favism. Stimulation of glutathione reductase activity by riboflavin by more than 50% indicates suboptimal riboflavin intake.

Notes and Precautions. Modest glutathione reductase deficiency occurs commonly as a result of inadequate riboflavin intake and probably as a result of genetic polymorphisms. It should not be considered a cause of hemolytic anemia.

10.4   Reduced Glutathione (GSH) Determination

Purpose. Determination of red cell GSH levels is useful in the examination of the red cells of patients with anemia. (See Interpretation below)

Principle. The dithiol compound, dithio-bis-nitrobenzoic acid (DTNB), is reduced by GSH to form a yellow anion, the optical density of which is measured readily at 412 nm.

Specimen. Whole blood collected in heparin, EDTA, or ACD preservative may be used. GSH levels remain unaltered for 3 weeks in ACD solution or for 1 week in EDTA or heparin solutions at

4° C. At room temperature, the assay should be carried out within a few hours.

Procedure. In this procedure, 0.2 mL of whole blood is added to 2.0 mL of distilled water. After removal of 0.2 mL of the lysate for hemoglobin determination, 3 mL of a metaphosphoric acid-EDTA-sodium chloride precipitating solution is added, and the mixture is filtered. Then, 2 mL of the filtrate is added to 8 mL of 0.3 M Na_2HPO_4 solution, 1 mL of DTNB reagent is added, and the optical density is read at 412 nm.

Interpretation. The normal red cell glutathione concentration is 4.5 to 8.7 μmol/g of hemoglobin. A severe deficiency of glutathione results from a genetic defect in one of the two enzymes of glutathione synthesis, viz, gamma-glutamylcysteine synthetase or glutathione synthetase deficiency. Modest reductions of GSH levels and marked instability to challenge by oxidative agents is found in G6PD-deficient red cells. Elevated levels of red cell glutathione are found in patients with myeloproliferative disorders and those with pyrimidine-5-nucleotidase deficiency.

Notes and Precautions. Virtually all of the protein-free DTNB-reducing activity in red cells is due to glutathione. DTNB is reduced readily by other sulfhydryl compounds, however, such as cysteine, and thus the degree of specificity will vary from tissue to tissue.

Ancillary Tests

In patients with severe glutathione deficiency, it is desirable to measure the activities of gamma-glutamylcysteine synthetase and glutathione synthetase. Assay of these enzymes is a relatively difficult radiometric procedure that is best performed by specialized laboratories.

Course and Treatment

Infants with G6PD deficiency and neonatal icterus may require exchange transfusions. Patients with G6PD deficiency should avoid the ingestion of fava beans and the drugs listed in Table 8–1. Splenectomy is not usually useful in the more rare functionally severe types of G6PD deficiency that are associated with nonspherocytic hemolytic anemia.

References

1. Beutler E: *Red Cell Metabolism: A Manual of Biochemical Methods,* ed 3. New York, Grune & Stratton Inc, 1984.

2. Beutler E: Glucose-6-phosphate dehydrogenase deficiency, in Stanbury JB, Wyngaarden JB, Fredrickson DS, et al: (eds): *The Metabolic Basis of Inherited Disease.* New York, McGraw-Hill International Book Co, 1983, p 1629.

11

Disorders of Hemoglobin
Synthesis

Hemoglobin is a tetrameric protein composed of globin and 4 heme groups. The globin is composed of 2 pairs of polypeptides, and each of the 4 polypeptides is associated with 1 heme group. In the hemoglobinopathies, abnormal globin chains are formed at a normal or near-normal rate. The thalassemias or hypochromic anemias are caused by defects in the effective rate of hemoglobin synthesis.

Pathophysiology

Hemoglobin A (HbA) is the major normal adult hemoglobin. It is composed of 2 alpha (α) and 2 beta (β) chains. HbA is therefore depicted structurally as $\alpha_2\beta_2$. The two minor adult hemoglobins are HbA_2 and HbF. The beta chain is replaced by a delta (δ) chain in HbA_2 and by a gamma (γ) chain in HbF. Hemoglobin A_2 is depicted as $\alpha_2\delta_2$ and HbF as a $\alpha_2\gamma_2$. The alpha chain has 141 amino acids; beta, gamma, and delta chains each have 147 amino acids. At birth, HbF is the predominant hemoglobin, but within the first year of life, it is largely replaced. Hemoglobins are then present in the adult proportion of approximately 97% HbA, 2% HbA_2, and 1% HbF. HbA_{1c} is a minor hemoglobin that is formed by posttranslational modification of HbA. This hemoglobin, formed by the addition of glucose to the N terminal of the HbA beta chains, is found in increased amounts in patients with diabetes mellitus. Each globin chain, ie,

Table 11–1 Chemical Differences in Hemoglobin Variants
Caused by Beta-Chain Mutations

Hb	Position	Amino Acid Residue in HbA	Amino Acid Residue in Abnormal Hb
S	6	Glutamic acid	Valine
C	6	Glutamic acid	Lysine
D$_{Punjab}$	121	Glutamic acid	Glutamine
E	26	Glutamic acid	Lysine

alpha, beta, gamma, and delta, has its own autosomal genetic locus. Most hemoglobin variants result from substitutions of a single amino acid. The most common variants, HbS, HbC, and HbE, are beta-chain mutations (Table 11–1). These variants can appear in the heterozygous or homozygous state.

In the thalassemias, globin chains are usually structurally normal but produced in inadequate amounts. The thalassemias are classified according to the chain affected, the most common being alpha-thalassemia and beta-thalassemia. The beta-thalassemic disorders are classified as minor or major for the heterozygous and homozygous states, respectively. Heterozygous beta-thalassemia minor is a common disorder. Combined disorders involving the structural variants and the thalassemias are also seen, the most common of which is sickle beta-thalassemia disease. The alpha-thalassemias are most commonly caused by the deletion of one or more of the four alpha globin genes.

Hemoglobin variants were initially differentiated primarily by their electrophoretic mobility and were assigned letter names. Later, when different hemoglobin variants were discovered with the same mobility, the new variant was distinguished by following the letter previously ascribed to that mobility with the place of discovery of the new variant. Finally, when the exact amino acid structure of a hemoglobin variant was determined, a simple designation was adopted that characterized the amino acid substitution by a superscript to the involved globin chain, eg, for HbS, $\alpha_2\beta_2^{6\ glutamic\ acid \rightarrow valine}$.

Sickle cell anemia refers to the homozygote for HbS, and the sickle cell trait is the heterozygous state. The word "disease" is used for a homozygote with other hemoglobin variants, eg, homozygous HbC disease (HbCC); "trait" refers to the heterozygotes, eg, HbC trait (HbAC). The word "disease" is also applied to the HbS heterozygous state, eg, sickle cell–HbC disease when significant clinical findings are associated with the combination. When letter designations are used for the hemoglobins in the heterozygous hemo-globinopathies, the first letter refers to the preponderant hemoglobin found in the red cell. Thus, HbAS indicates that the concentration of HbA exceeds that of HbS in the red cell of that heterozygous variant.

Clinical Findings

Disorders in hemoglobin synthesis can be divided into those caused by formation of abnormal globin chains, resulting in structural he-moglobin changes (often referred to as the hemoglobinopathies) and the thalassemias, which are associated with a quantitative de-ficiency of effective globin-chain production, ie, decreased quan-tities of normal hemoglobin. Some thalassemias are the result of an abnormal, very unstable globin chain. Combinations of these two types of disorders are also seen (Table 11–2).

Hemoglobin Disorders Caused by Abnormal Globin Chains. Mutations involving the genes that direct formation of globin chains result in amino acid substitutions that may produce pronounced changes in the properties of hemoglobin. A functional classification of the abnormal hemoglobins based on these changes is shown in Table 11–2.

Of the mutant hemoglobins with decreased solubility, the one causing the most common clinically significant hemoglobinopathy is HbS. The heterozygous disorder resulting from this hemoglobin, sickle cell trait, should generally be considered an entirely benign disorder, although on rare occasions it may be responsible for he-maturia. The homozygous disorder is a sickle cell disease, sickle cell anemia, characterized by moderately severe hemolysis and painful crises resulting from microinfarction of blood vessels. When the gene for HbS is inherited together with the gene for certain other abnormal hemoglobins, particularly for HbC (SC disease) or beta-thalassemia (S-thalassemia), sickle cell diseases very similar to sickle cell anemia result. Since the sickle cell gene occurs in approximately 9%, the gene for HbC in 3%, and the gene for beta-thalassemia in 1% of black Americans, these disorders are collectively quite common, affecting approximately 1 in 260 black Americans. Two other hemoglobins in this category are not rare, particularly in the heterozygous state: HbD, which is seen in blacks, and HbE, which is a common mutation in Asian populations. Both of these result in a mild hemolytic anemia, even in the homozygous state. In HbE disease, the anemia is hypochromic and associated with splenomegaly. Hypochromia is also found uniformly in the trait.

The remaining hemoglobinopathies are much less common. Those caused by formation of unstable hemoglobins are inherited as autosomal dominant disorders and are characteristically associated with chronic hemolysis. The anemia is often hypochromic. Some unstable hemoglobins are associated with increased oxygen affinity. In such cases, reticulocytosis may be greater than usually observed for the degree of anemia seen. Hemoglobins in which the essential functional change is increased oxygen affinity result in erythrocytosis. Hemoglobins that have decreased oxygen affinity are very rare and produce anemia with cyanosis.

A mutant hemoglobin that is unable to maintain heme iron in the reduced state and to bind oxygen, designated as HbM, results in hereditary methemoglobinemia. Methemoglobin is brownish, and patients who inherit this hemoglobin have a cyanotic appearance. Like the unstable hemoglobins, those with increased oxygen affinity and the HbMs are inherited as autosomal dominant disorders.

Thalassemias.   Alpha-thalassemia is a common disorder in many parts of the world. Severe forms of alpha-thalassemia are particularly common in Southeast Asia, but mild forms are very prevalent among persons of African ancestry. Because the locus directing synthesis of the alpha chain is duplicated, most persons have four alpha-chain genes, two for each chromosome. Alpha-thalassemia results from the absence or a defect of one or more of these genes. The characteristics of the alpha-thalassemias are summarized in Table 11-3. The most serious clinical consequences result from absence of activity of all four alpha-chain genes, a state that is incompatible with life. The chains synthesized in fetal red cells form gamma$_4$ tetramers designated as hemoglobin Barts. Hemoglobin Barts is unstable, and its oxygen dissociation curve is shifted far to the left. When it is the only hemoglobin formed, fetal death results from a disorder known as hydrops fetalis. If one alpha-chain gene is functional, a less severe disorder occurs. At birth, fetal hemoglobin as well as hemoglobin Barts is present. In later infancy, childhood, and adulthood, the beta chains form beta$_4$ tetramers designated as hemoglobin H. The resulting disorder, HbH disease, is a moderately severe, chronic hemolytic anemia. If 2 normal alpha-chain genes are present, a mild microcytic anemia designated as alpha-thalassemia minor is observed. The presence of 3 normal alpha chains does not result in a clinically detectable abnormality.

Beta-thalassemia is a common disorder, particularly among persons of Mediterranean descent. It is the Mediterranean anemia first described by Thomas Benton Cooley and sometimes known by his name. When only one beta-thalassemic gene has been inherited,

Table 11–2 Functional Classification of Abnormal Hemoglobins

Type of Abnormality	Functional Abnormality	Clinical Disorder[a]
Qualitative (structural) abnormalities	None	No physiologic or clinical disorders
	Aggregation of hemoglobin molecules	Hemolytic anemia
	Unstable hemoglobins[b] with increased susceptibility to oxidative denaturation and formation of inclusion bodies	Hemolytic anemia
	Methemoglobinemia caused by mutations that prevent reduction of heme iron	Cyanosis
Abnormal[b] oxygen affinity	Increased oxygen affinity	Erythrocytosis
	Decreased oxygen affinity	Cyanosis/anemia
Quantitative abnormalities—thalassemias	Alpha-thalassemias with decreased alpha-chain production	Range from mild anemia microcytic to hydrops fetalis
	Beta-thalassemias with decreased beta-chain production	Mild hypochromic anemia to severe hemolytic anemia
	Delta-beta-thalassemias with decrease of both delta- and beta-chain production	Thalassemia-type syndromes

Delta-thalassemias with decreased delta-chain production		No significant clinical or hematologic abnormality
Combined structural disorders with thalassemias	Aggregation of hemoglobin molecule and suppression of normal hemoglobin chain	Disorder usually resembles that seen with structural variant alone but is often milder
Thalassemia-like syndrome	Lepore syndromes resulting from delta-beta fusion chain caused by abnormal crossing over of genes for delta and beta HPFH[c] results from failure to switch from gamma- to beta- and delta-chain production after birth	Clinical syndromes similar to those seen with beta-thalassemia No clinical or hematologic abnormality or mild anemia

ABBREVIATIONS: HPFH = hereditary persistence of fetal hemoglobin.

[a]Homozygous states generally associated with more severe disorder than heterozygotes

[b]Abnormal oxygen affinity frequently seen with unstable hemoglobins

[c]Can be seen in combination with HbS, thalassemia, or HbC

Table 11–3   Alpha-Thalassemias

Genotype	Phenotype	Hematologic Findings
$\alpha\alpha\alpha\alpha$	Normal	Normal
$\alpha\alpha\alpha\alpha^{Th}$	Silent carrier	Normal
$\alpha\alpha\alpha^{Th}\alpha^{Th}$	alpha-thalassemia trait	Mild hypochromic anemia In newborn, HbBarts; in adults, sometimes are HbH inclusions in red cells after BCB incubation
$\alpha\alpha^{Th}\alpha^{Th}\alpha^{Th}$	HbH disease	Hemolytic disease In newborn, increased Hb-Barts; in adult, HbH present; many positive red cells after BCB incubation
$\alpha^{Th}\alpha^{Th}\alpha^{Th}\alpha^{Th}$	Hydrops fetalis	Stillborn, anemic, macerated fetus Cord blood 100% HbBarts

ABBREVIATIONS: BCB = brilliant cresyl blue.

the clinical disorder designated beta-thalassemia minor results. This is a benign, hypochromic microcytic anemia in which the concentration of hemoglobin in the blood may be diminished to 100 or 110 g/L (10 or 11 g/dl) but the red cell count is normal or, very frequently, elevated. In beta-thalassemia minor, the amount of HbA$_2$ is usually increased, because alpha chains that cannot find beta chains with which to combine may combine with delta chains. Slightly elevated levels of HbF are present in about 30% of patients with beta-thalassemia minor. Often, patients with thalassemia minor are mistakenly diagnosed as being iron deficient, because they have a hypochromic microcytic anemia (see chapter 3).

When two beta-thalassemic genes have been inherited, a very serious disorder of infancy and early childhood, thalassemia major, results. It is characterized by massive splenomegaly, extreme erythroid hyperplasia in the bone marrow, severe hemolytic anemia, and failure to thrive. In beta-thalassemia major, prominent elevation of the HbF level ranging from 30% to 100% is found. With HbF values at lower levels in this range, the hemoglobin is distributed heterogeneously among the cell population, helping to distinguish the disorder from the benign condition designated as hereditary persistence of fetal hemoglobin (HPFH), in which a homogeneous distribution is seen.

Beta-thalassemia genes are not all the same. Some result in complete suppression of beta-chain synthesis and are designated a β° genes. Others, which permit some formation of normal beta chains, are designated as β⁺ genes and may result in milder clinical syndromes than the β° variants.

Often classified as beta-thalassemias, delta-beta-thalassemias are associated with suppression of both delta and beta chains and are clinically similar to the beta-thalassemias. Heterozygotes present as thalassemia minor, often with prominent elevation of the HbF level. The homozygotes, however, present as a clinically milder disease than is usually seen with beta-thalassemia major. The Lepore syndromes, which are often classified in this category, are caused by a mutant hemoglobin, Hb Lepore. This hemoglobin results from a cross-over mutation; the hybrid globin chain consists partly of delta chains and partly of beta chains. Hemoglobin Lepore can be detected by electrophoresis.

Approach to Diagnosis

The development of practical procedures using readily available equipment and reagents has enabled the general laboratory clinician to perform a reasonably complete evaluation of most of the more common hemoglobin disorders. However, clinical evaluation and family studies play a particularly important role in evaluating laboratory data in these disorders.

Evaluation of the hemoglobin disorders proceeds with the following:

1. Hematologic evaluation, with attention to red cell morphology and use of supravital stains to detect inclusion bodies.

2. Hemoglobin electrophoresis for the detection of globin-chain variants with altered electrophoretic mobility and measurement of HbA₂ levels; the latter may also be determined chromatographically.

3. If a hemoglobin with an S-like mobility is encountered, tests of hemoglobin solubility as a means of distinguishing HbS from the electrophoretically similar HbD and less frequent variants; solubility tests and the sickling test to screen for sickle cell trait.

4. In some cases, alkali denaturation test for fetal hemoglobin.

5. In some cases, the acid elution test (method of Kleihauer and Betke) to evaluate the distribution of HbF in red cells for the diagnosis of HPFH.

6. The isopropanol stability test for detecting unstable hemoglobins.

7. The test for HbH inclusion bodies.

The following tests may be performed in specialized laboratories:

8. When indicated, spectrophotometric determinations for methemoglobinemia seen with HbMs and measurement of oxyhemoglobin dissociation or $P_{50}O_2$ for detecting hemoglobins with altered oxygen affinity (see chapter 13).

9. Globin-chain synthetic studies when thalassemia is suspected but cannot be confirmed by simpler methods; Southern blotting of alpha globin genes when additional genetic data are needed.

10. Detailed structural analysis of globin chains using "fingerprinting" of tryptic digests by means of electrophoresis, chromatography, and amino acid sequencing.

Hematologic Findings

Hematologic abnormalities associated with the hemoglobin disorders can be classified into (1) those associated with chronic hemolysis, (2) changes characteristic of a particular disorder, (3) findings seen after splenectomy or (in the case of sickle cell disease) findings related to splenic atrophy, and (4) changes seen with aplastic crises, which may accompany infections. The most severe anemia and most striking morphologic changes are seen in the homozygous disorders. The heterozygous states may be normal or may show minimal hematologic abnormalities.

Blood Cell Measurements.   Anemia may be severe, with characteristic ranges for hemoglobin of 50 to 90 g/L (5 to 9 g/dl) in sickle cell anemia and 25 to 65 g/L (2.5 to 6.5 g/dl) in thalassemia major. The heterozygotes may be hematologically normal, as in sickle cell trait, or they may show mild anemia, as in beta-thalassemia minor.

Peripheral Blood Smear Morphology.   See Table 11–4 and Figures 11–1 through 11–4.

Bone Marrow Examination.   Erythroid hyperplasia is proportional to the severity of the hemolysis. A prominent increase in iron deposition is often seen.

Table 11-4   Red Cell Morphology in Disorders of
Hemoglobin Synthesis

Type of Change	Morphology
Changes secondary to hemolysis	Polychromatophilia, fine stippling, macrocytosis—all associated with reticulocytosis; nucleated red cells
Changes associated with splenectomy or splenic atrophy	Basophilic stippling, Howell-Jolly bodies, target cells, Pappenheimer bodies, abnormal poikilocytes
Changes characteristic of specific disorders	
Sickle cell disorders	Sickle cells
HbC disorders	Target cells; hemoglobin crystals may be seen in splenectomized patients
Disorders caused by unstable Hb	Red cell inclusions with supravital stains—Heinz bodies, HbH inclusions
Thalassemia	Microcytosis, target cells, basophilic stippling

Other Laboratory Tests

11.1   Hemoglobin Electrophoresis

Purpose.   Hemoglobin electrophoresis is the principal procedure used to detect and identify abnormal hemoglobins.

Principle.   Electrophoresis is the movement of charged molecules in an electric field. Hemoglobins, like all proteins, are amphoteric; they are charged positively or negatively, depending on the pH of the suspending medium. In a basic solution with a pH of about 8, hemoglobins have a negative charge and migrate toward the positive pole or anode. The relative speeds with which different hemoglobins migrate toward the anode are proportional to their net negative charges. Because HbS contains valine in place of the glutamic acid of HbA, it has a smaller negative charge and a slower anodal mobility than HbA in an alkaline medium. At an acid pH, hemoglobins are positively charged, and their relative mobilities in relation to the anode are the reverse of that seen in an alkaline medium.

Specimen.   Anticoagulated whole blood or washed red cells are used.

Procedure.   Electrophoresis on cellulose acetate at a pH 8.4 to 8.8 is the method of choice for initial electrophoretic testing in the general clinical laboratory. Although use of starch gel as a support medium gives excellent separation of hemoglobins, starch gel electrophoresis is a relatively slow, tedious procedure that is now used primarily by specialized laboratories.

Red cells are hemolyzed and subjected to electrophoresis on cellulose acetate for 15 to 30 minutes. A control hemolysate is run concurrently with the patient sample. Hemoglobins A, A_2, F, S, and C are most often included in controls. After electrophoresis is completed, the membrane is stained, and hemoglobins are identified by their positions. The hemoglobins can then be quantitated by elution and spectrophotometric assay or by scanning the membrane with a densitometer. Electrophoresis in citrate agar at pH 6.2 can be used to complement conventional cellulose acetate electrophoresis (see Interpretation below). The procedure is basically the same as that described for cellulose acetate but requires electrophoresis for 45 to 90 minutes.

Interpretation.   The electrophoretic patterns of some hemoglobin variants are shown in Figure 11–5. Hemoglobins are often divided on the basis of their anodal electrophoretic mobility at an alkaline pH. Slow-moving hemoglobins include C, E, A_2, and O. Intermediate hemoglobins include D, G, S, and Lepore; hemoglobins A and F are more anodal. Among the fast-moving hemoglobins are H, I, and Barts (Figure 11–6). When a prominent band is found in the HbS region on cellulose acetate electrophoresis at pH 8.6, its identity can be confirmed by electrophoresis on citrate agar at pH 6.2; the latter separates HbS from HbD and HbG. Citrate agar also differentiates HbC from HbS, O, E, and A_2 and provides sharp separation of hemoglobins F and A.

Notes and Precautions.   The main limitation of hemoglobin electrophoresis is its inability to detect amino acid substitutions that do not affect charge. Such variants are seen in particular among the unstable hemoglobins and with hemoglobins associated with altered oxygen affinity. Furthermore, as noted previously, different amino acid substitutions may lead to the same change in electrophoretic mobility.

Figure 11–5   Comparison of various hemoglobin samples on cellulose acetate and citrate agar.

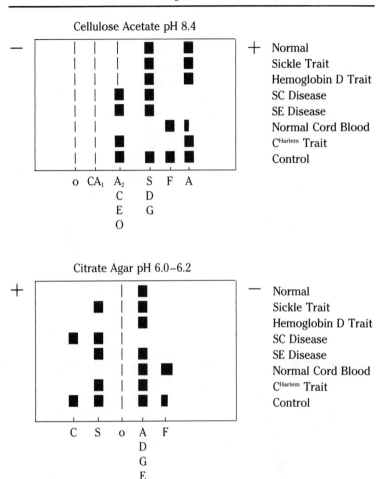

ABBREVIATIONS: o = origin

(Modified with permission from Schmidt RM, Brosious BS: *Basic Laboratory Methods of Hemoglobinopathy Detection.* Publication No. (CDC) 77-8266. Atlanta, DHEW, 1976.)

11.2   Sickle Cell Test

Purpose.   In most cases of sickle cell anemia, a few sickled red cells are observed readily on the routinely prepared stained blood smear. Such sickling is also seen with the heterozygous cell disorders, such as SC disease or the S-thalassemias, in which HbS is the major hemoglobin component. In sickle cell

Figure 11–6   Relative mobilities of hemoglobins on cellulose acetate (TEB), pH 8.4.

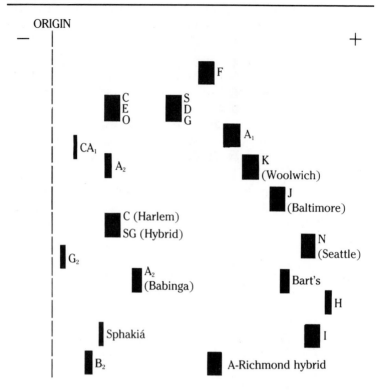

(Modified with permission from Schmidt RM, Brosious BS: *Basic Laboratory Methods of Hemoglobinopathy Detection.* Publication No. (CDC) 77-8266. Atlanta, DHEW, 1976.)

trait and in some sickle cell disorders with a lesser propensity for sickling, however, various maneuvers are required to induce in vitro sickling.

Principle.   When red cells containing HbS are deoxygenated, they sickle. Deoxygenation can be accomplished by mixing a drop of blood with a reducing agent on a slide and covering the preparation with a cover slip.

Specimen.   Venous or capillary blood is used.

Procedure.   The sickle cell test is performed by mixing the amount of blood that adheres to the end of an applicator stick with a drop of freshly prepared 2% sodium metabisulfite solution and covering the suspension with a cover slip. When sickle hemoglobin is present in the red cells, they begin to deform within 10 minutes, assuming crescent and holly-leaf shapes. The preparation is observed on the microscope within 30 minutes by means of the high dry objective.

Interpretation.   The test results are positive for sickle cell traits and for all sickle cell disorders in which HbS is present in a concentration of $\geq 25\%$. Sickling has also been described in other relatively rare variants, such as HbC$_{Harlem}$.

Notes and Precautions.   The most frequently encountered technical problem resulting in a false-negative test result is outdated metabisulfite reagent that has lost its reducing power. With HbS disorders, test results may not become positive until the infant is 1 or 2 months of age because of the relatively high percentage of HbF in the red cells in infancy.

11.3   Solubility Test for HbS

Purpose.   Solubility tests have been used most widely to screen for sickle cell trait, for genetic counseling, and as a means of differentiating HbS from HbD, which are identical on electrophoresis at an alkaline pH.

Principle.   The solubility test is based on the relative insolubility of reduced HbS compared with other hemoglobin variants and HbA in a high-phosphate buffer solution.

Specimen.   Whole blood is used as a specimen.

Procedure.   A solution of 1.24 M KH_2PO_4/1.24 M K_2HPO_4, containing saponin to lyse the red cells and sodium hydrosulfite (dithionite) to reduce the hemoglobin, is used. Blood is added, and the solution is observed for turbidity by noting the patient's ability to read ruled black lines held behind the test tubes. (Commercial kits are available [Sickledex].)

Interpretation.   Positive test results are indicated by a turbid suspension through which the ruled lines behind the test tube cannot be seen. Test results are positive for sickle cell trait and sickle cell disorders; with rare exceptions (eg, HbC$_{Harlem}$) results are negative with all other hemoglobins. The differentiation of sickle cell trait from sickle cell disease may not always be clear since it is based on a quantitative difference in turbidity.

Notes and Precautions.   In the presence of severe anemia, the blood sample usually used may not contain sufficient HbS to yield a turbid solution. With a hemoglobin level less than 70 g/L (7 g/dl), the sample size should be doubled. False-positive results may be seen with lipemic plasma. The solubility test is inadequate as a means of screening for genetic counseling because it fails to detect the important carriers of HbC and beta-thalassemia.

11.4   Alkali Denaturation Test for Fetal Hemoglobin

Purpose.   Measurement of fetal hemoglobin helps to diagnose and differentiate the thalassemias, to diagnose the double heterozygotes with combined thalassemia and a structural hemoglobin variant, and to diagnose the HPFH. Because the mobility of HbF is close to that of HbA on routine electrophoresis, measurement of HbF based on electrophoretic techniques has not been reliable.

Principle.   A rapid and simple method for measuring HbF is based on the fact that it is more resistant to denaturation by a strong alkali than are other hemoglobins.

Specimen.   Anticoagulated whole blood is used.

Procedure.   Alkali is added to a hemolysate. After one minute, denatured hemoglobin is precipitated by the addition of ammonium sulfate. The filtrate contains HbF, which is quantitated spectrophotometrically.

Interpretation.   The normal value for HbF is less than 2% (Table 11–5). Patients with beta-thalassemia minor may have elevated HbF levels of 2% to 5%; those with the less common delta-beta-thalassemia minor may show much higher levels. Patients with homozygous beta-thalassemia show levels of HbF ranging from 30% to 100%. Levels in patients with HPFH range from 15% to 100%. Elevated hemoglobin levels from 2% to 5% have been reported in a large variety of hematologic conditions, including aplastic anemia, pernicious anemia, hereditary spherocytosis, myelofibrosis, leukemia, and metastatic disease with bone marrow involvement.

Notes and Precautions. The alkali denaturation test is very sensitive at low levels of HbF. At levels greater than 10%, however, the method underestimates HbF, and accurate measurement requires special chromatographic techniques.

11.5   Quantitation of HbA$_2$ by Chromatography

Purpose. Levels of HbA$_2$ are elevated in the most common type of thalassemia minor. Quantitation of HbA$_2$ by routine electrophoresis on cellulose acetate has not been uniformly reliable.

Principle. The most accurate and rapid procedure generally available for measuring HbA$_2$ is a chromatographic technique using anion exchange column chromatography to separate HbA$_2$ from HbA.

Specimen. Anticoagulated whole blood is used.

Procedure. HbA$_2$ is separated from HbA by use of a column consisting of diethylaminoethyl(DEAE)-cellulose as the ion exchange resin. The resin is equilibrated with a TRIS(hydroxymethyl)aminomethane phosphate buffer, and the hemoglobin solution is applied. The more strongly charged HbA adheres to the ion exchange resin. HbA$_2$ passes through and is quantitated spectrophotometrically. (Commercial kits with disposable columns are available [HbA$_2$ Quik Column kit, Helena Laboratories, Beaumont, Texas]).

Interpretation. The normal range of values for HbA$_2$ is 1.5% to 3.5% (Table 11–5); in beta-thalassemia, the range is 3.5% to 8%.

Notes and Precautions. A number of hemoglobin variants are eluted from the column under the usual test conditions. These include hemoglobins C, E, O, D, and, to a lesser extent, S. When a value >8% is found, the presence of such a variant is likely. HbA$_2$ may be separated and quantitated in the presence of HbS by eluting the two hemoglobins separately, using buffers with different pH for elution. HbA$_2$ levels may not be elevated in the presence of coexisting iron deficiency.

Table 11–5 Hemoglobin Analysis in Beta-Thalassemic Disorders

Genetic Classification	Clinical	HbA$_2$ (%)
Normal		1.5–3.5
Heterozygotes		
Beta-thalassemia	Thalassemia minor	3.5–8.0
Delta-beta-thalassemia	Thalassemia minor	1.5–3.5
Delta-beta-Lepore	Thalassemia minor	<1.5
Homozygotes		
Beta-thalassemia^0	Thalassemia major	variable
Beta-thalassemia$^+$	Thalassemia major or intermedia	1.5–4.0
Delta-beta-thalassemia	Thalassemia intermedia	0
Delta-beta-Lepore	Thalassemia major	0
Doubly anomolous		
HbS beta-thalassemia$^+$	Sickle cell thalassemia	3.5–8.0
HbS beta-thalassemia^0	Sickle cell thalassemia	3.5–8.0

NOTE: Thalassemia^0 refers to genetic type with no production of beta chains and thalassemia$^+$ refers to genetic type with reduced production of beta chains.

11.6 Acid Elution Test for Fetal Hemoglobin in Red Cells

Purpose. The acid elution test is a staining procedure used to differentiate HPFH from other states associated with high fetal hemoglobin levels.

Principle. When hemoglobin is precipitated inside the red cell and fixed with alcohol, the precipitated HbA and most variants can be solubilized in a buffered solution of citric acid. HbF remains precipitated inside the cell.

Specimen. Whole blood is used.

Procedure. A blood smear is prepared in the usual manner and fixed in 80% ethanol. It is then treated with a citric acid–phosphate buffer (pH 3.3), which elutes HbA from the red cells. The blood film is then stained with eosin, which stains any residual precipitate.

HbF (%)	HbA (%)	Hemoglobin Variant (%)
<2	97	0
<5	>90	0
4–30	remainder	0
2–14	remainder	Hb Lepore ≃ 10
almost 100%	0	0
30–90	remainder	0
100	100	0
75	0	Hb Lepore = 25
8–15	≤20	HbS = 60–70
8–15	0	HbS = 90

Interpretation.   Smears from normal blood show little if any uptake of stain, and cells appear as ghosts. A heterogeneous distribution of fetal hemoglobin is seen in newborn infants, with fetal-maternal transfusion, and in the thalassemias, with elevated HbF levels. HPFH is the only condition in which HbF is evenly distributed among nearly all of the red cells.

Notes and Precautions.   The intensity of the staining often differs markedly from one part of the blood film to another, and considerable experience may be required to interpret this procedure.

11.7   Isopropanol Stability Test

Purpose.   The isopropanol stability test is used to detect unstable hemoglobins.

Principle.   Normal hemoglobin is somewhat unstable in isopropanol. The effect is accentuated with the unstable hemoglobins.

Specimen.   Whole blood is used.

Procedure.   A hemolysate is added to buffered isopropanol and incubated at 37° C. The preparation is observed for precipitation at intervals.

Interpretation.   Unstable hemoglobins generally show turbidity within 5 minutes, while normal hemoglobins do not precipitate until 30 to 40 minutes. False-positive test results may be obtained with sickle hemoglobin, fetal hemoglobin, and methemoglobin.

11.8   Test for HbH Inclusion Bodies

Purpose.   HbH is an unstable hemoglobin that may be difficult to detect on routine electrophoresis. This test is particularly useful for the detection of HbH and may suggest the presence of other unstable hemoglobins.

Principle.   Incubation of whole blood with brilliant cresyl blue causes denaturation of unstable hemoglobin, which precipitates in red cells, resulting in diffuse stippling.

Specimen.   Fresh whole blood is used.

Procedure.   Three to 4 drops of whole blood are incubated with 0.5 mL of a 1% solution of brilliant cresyl blue in citrate-saline solution. Blood films are made at 10 minutes, 1 hour, and 4 hours.

Interpretation.   Positive cells have a diffusely clumped pattern resembling a golf ball with the reticulum staining light blue (Figure 11–7). In HbH disease, ≥50% of the cells on the one-hour slide may be positive. Results with other unstable hemoglobins are variable, and a longer period of incubation is usually required for precipitation. The 10-minute slide is a control that shows the number of reticulocytes present.

Ancillary Tests

Heinz Bodies.   Heinz bodies are particles of denatured hemoglobins that are attached to the cell membrane (Figure 11–4) and are demonstrated with a variety of supravital dyes, such as crystal violet or brilliant cresyl blue. Heinz bodies are found in association with unstable hemoglobin disorders in patients who have undergone splenectomy. They are also seen during acute drug-induced hemolysis.

Incubation of blood with acetylphenylhydrazine and various other reagents that catalyze oxidative damage to hemoglobin results in the formation of Heinz bodies in vitro. The pattern of Heinz body formation when such incubation has been carried out under carefully controlled conditions differs in G6PD deficient and normal cells. This was the basis of one of the early tests for the detection of G6PD deficiency.

Crystal Cells of HbC Disease.   Crystal cells of HbC disease are present in as many as 10% of the circulating cells in patients with this disorder who have undergone splenectomy, but these tetrahedral crystals are rarely seen in blood films of patients who have not undergone splenectomy. In such patients, crystal cells may be produced by hypertonic dehydration of red cells in a 3% NaCl buffer for 4 to 12 hours.

Red Cell Inclusions in HbH Disease.   Red cell inclusions in HbH disease can be produced by incubating whole blood with brilliant cresyl blue (see Test 11.8).

Course and Treatment

The course and treatment of these hemoglobin synthesis disorders varies greatly depending on which mutation is present. Sickling disorders are characterized by disturbances in the microcirculation because sickle cells are rigid and do not pass through capillaries readily. In contrast, the clinical manifestations of HbC disease are minor, being related almost entirely to the moderate anemia that may be present.

References

1. Carrell RW, Lehmann H: The hemoglobinopathies, in Dawson AM, Compston ND, Besser GM (eds): *Recent Advances in Medicine,* ed. 19. London, Churchill Livingston, 1984, pp 223–255.

2. Bunn HF, Forget BG: *Hemoglobin: Molecular, Genetic, and Clinical Aspects.* Philadelphia, W.B. Saunders, 1987.

3. Stamatoyannopoulos G, Nienhuis AW, Leder P, Majerus PW (eds): *The Molecular Basis of Blood Diseases.* Philadelphia, W.B. Saunders, 1987.

4. William WJ, Beutler E, Erslev AJ, et al (eds): *Hematology,* ed 3. New York, McGraw International Book Co, 1983.

5. Wintrobe MM, Lee GR, Boggs DR, et al (eds): *Clinical Hematology,* ed 8. Philadelphia, Lea & Febiger, 1981.

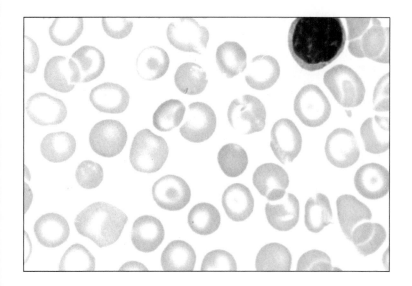

Figure 11–1   Beta-thalassemia minor. Microcytosis and a moderate number of target cells.

Figure 11–2   Hemoglobin C disease. A hemoglobin C crystal in the center and many target cells.

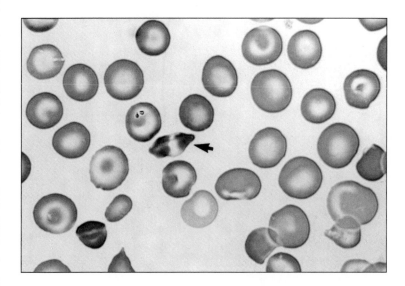

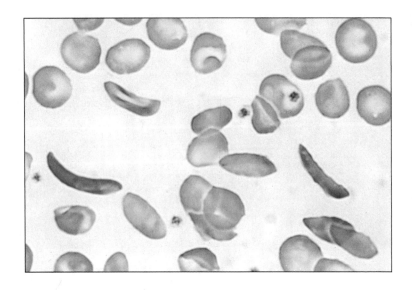

Figure 11–3   Sickle cell anemia. Target cells and several sickled red blood cells.

Figure 11–4   Heinz bodies in red blood cells are seen as coarse dark-staining dots. A few reticulocytes are also present.

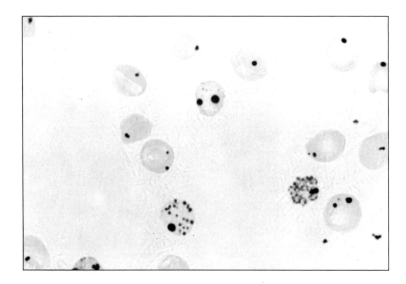

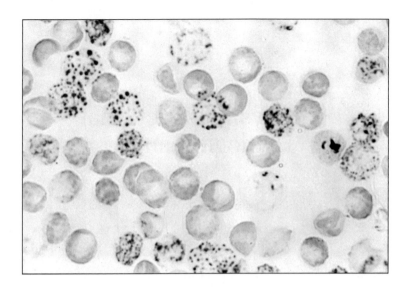

Figure 11–7   Hemoglobin H disease. Many red blood cells contain denatured hemoglobin H granules.

12

Paroxysmal Nocturnal Hemoglobinuria

Paroxysmal nocturnal hemoglobinuria (PNH) is a relatively rare chronic hemolytic disorder in which characteristic abnormalities of the red cell membrane can be demonstrated.

Pathophysiology

The underlying cause of PNH is unknown. It is a clonal disorder of the hematopoietic stem cell that often arises as a sequela of aplastic anemia and is probably caused by an abnormality of the cell membrane. The red cells have a markedly increased sensitivity to lysis by complement, a defect that appears to be shared by other blood cells as well. The complement sensitivity of PNH cells appears to be the result of the loss of "decay accelerating factor" and homologous restriction factor from the membrane. It forms the basis of two of the diagnostic tests of PNH, the sucrose hemolysis test and the acid hemolysis test.

Clinical Findings

The name "paroxysmal nocturnal hemoglobinuria" implies that hemolysis is episodic and that hemoglobinuria is a major feature. The classic presentation of the passage of red urine in the morning on arising, however, usually is not observed. More frequently, chronic hemolysis, often associated with leukopenia and thrombocytopenia, is the predominant feature of the disorder. Hemosiderinuria, not hemoglobinuria, is a constant feature and may cause the development of iron deficiency.

Episodes of abdominal pain may be a prominent symptom. They may be associated with thrombosis of the portal, mesenteric, or hepatic vein. Some patients have severe, refractory headaches that may be caused by small-vessel thrombosis. Thrombophlebitis may occur in the legs or arms and may lead to thromboembolism.

Patients with PNH suffer from irregularly recurring exacerbation in hemolysis, apparently precipitated by events such as infections, operations, and transfusions. The majority of patients with PNH exhibit neutropenia and thrombocytopenia at some stage in their disease. In fact, PNH can rise as a sequela of otherwise typical aplastic anemia.

Approach to Diagnosis

Depending on the predominant features of the presenting illness, PNH may need to be differentiated from other causes of chronic hemolytic anemia, pancytopenia, iron deficiency, and hemoglobinuria and myoglobinuria.

Laboratory evaluation of this disorder proceeds with the following:

1. Hematologic evaluation with complete blood count and study of red cell morphology and bone marrow.

2. Sucrose hemolysis test and test for urine hemosiderin as screening tests for PNH.

3. Acid hemolysis test as a definitive diagnostic test for PNH.

Hematologic Findings

Blood Cell Measurements.   The degree of anemia varies widely, with hemoglobin levels ranging from <60 g/L (6 g/dl) to normal. The mean corpuscular volume (MCV) may be somewhat increased, with prominent reticulocytosis, or indices may be consistent with iron deficiency anemia. The percent of reticulocytes may be markedly elevated; however, the absolute reticulocyte count may be low for the degree of anemia. This discrepancy can be attributed to a bone marrow stem cell defect.

Peripheral Blood Smear Morphology. No characteristic morphologic changes are seen. Macrocytosis and polychromatophilia may accompany prominent reticulocytosis; iron deficiency may result in microcytosis.

Bone Marrow Examination. Normoblastic hyperplasia is the most frequent finding, with adequate numbers of megakaryocytes and myeloid elements. Marrow cellularity, however, may be decreased, or the marrow may be aplastic. Stainable storage iron is often absent, even when obvious iron deficiency is not present.

Other Laboratory Tests

12.1 Sucrose Hemolysis Test

Purpose. The sucrose hemolysis test is the most convenient screening test for PNH.

Principle. An isotonic sucrose solution of low ionic strength appears to enhance the binding of complement to the red cell membrane. When a small amount of serum as a source of complement is added to such a solution, PNH cells are lysed, whereas normal cells are not.

Specimen. Whole defibrinated blood is used.

Procedure. A small amount of fresh, normal, type-compatible serum is added to a buffered sucrose solution. Washed red cells from the patient are added, and the suspension is incubated for 60 minutes at room temperature.

Interpretation. Lysis of >5% is compatible with the diagnosis of PNH. Lysis usually amounting to <5% may be found in the megaloblastic anemias and in autoimmune hemolytic disease. A definitive diagnosis requires performance of the acid hemolysis test (see Test 12.2).

Notes and Precautions. When originally described, it was suggested that the sucrose hemolysis test could be carried out using unbuffered sucrose solutions; however, this may lead to false-negative results.

12.2   Acid Hemolysis Test

Purpose.   The acid hemolysis test is required to make a definitive diagnosis of PNH.

Principle.   A definitive diagnosis of PNH depends on demonstration of the following characteristics of in vitro hemolysis: it occurs with patient cells but not with control cells; it is enhanced by slightly acidifying the serum used; it is abolished by heat inactivating the serum at 56° C; and hemolytic activity is not restored to the heated serum by the addition of guinea pig complement. These characteristics of the hemolytic system can be demonstrated using Ham's acid hemolysis test.

Specimen.   Defibrinated whole blood is used.

Procedure.   The acid hemolysis test is carried out using type-compatible blood from a healthy control subject and blood from a patient with PNH. The following 4 serum preparations should be used from patient and control subject: unaltered serum, serum with a pH adjusted to 6.8 as measured by a pH meter, serum at pH 6.8 that has been heat inactivated to 56° C for 3 minutes, and heated serum to which guinea pig complement has been added. Red cells from patient or control subject are suspended in each of these types of serum.

Interpretation.   Positive test results are those in which hemolysis of the patient's erythrocytes occurs in acidified serum and not in heated serum, either with or without the addition of guinea pig complement. Some hemolysis may be present in the unaltered serum, but this is generally less than that observed in acidified serum. No hemolysis of control cells should occur in any of the tubes.

Notes and Precautions.   Erroneous test results can be obtained by either over- or underacidification of serum. In the test as originally described, the pH of the serum was not verified with a pH meter because such instruments were not available. Careful adjustment of the pH of the serum to 6.8 ± 0.1 is necessary if reliable results are to be obtained.

12.3 Test for Urine Hemosiderin

Purpose. Urine hemosiderin is nearly always present in PNH and may be a valuable aid in making the diagnosis.

Principle. Even in the absence of discernible hemoglobinuria, chronic low-grade intravascular hemolysis is sufficient in PNH to lead to depletion of serum haptoglobin and to result in the presence of hemoglobin in the kidney, which is reabsorbed by the tubules. Tubules become heavily laden with iron, which is excreted in the urine as hemosiderin granules demonstrable with the Prussian-blue stain.

Specimen. A random urine specimen is used for testing urine hemosiderin.

Procedure. The presence of hemosiderin in the urine is demonstrated by adding a drop of a mixture of equal parts of 4% hydrochloric acid and 4% potassium ferrocyanide to the sediment of a centrifuged urine specimen. The mixture is incubated at room temperature for 10 minutes, with frequent agitation.

Interpretation. Hemosiderin appears as blue particles. While considerable emphasis has been placed on the intracellular location of hemosiderin in urine, cells containing hemosiderin may have disintegrated in the urine, and free hemosiderin may be the predominant form. Healthy patients' urine does not contain hemosiderin.

Ancillary Tests

Many other procedures have been described for the detection of PNH. The thrombin activation test, lysis of A cells in the presence of anti-A, and Ham's presumptive tests are all capable of identifying most patients with PNH; however, they are unnecessarily cumbersome and have been superseded by more recently developed procedures, such as the sucrose hemolysis test. Quantitative testing of complement sensitivity may give more precise information regarding the size of the complement-sensitive population; however, it is too complex for routine clinical use. Red cell acetylcholinesterase activity and leukocyte alkaline phosphatase activity are diminished in PNH.

Course and Treatment

The course may be fulminating or chronic. Occasionally, acute leukemia or a myelodysplastic syndrome may supervene. Thrombotic complications, particularly the Budd-Chiari syndrome, may be rapidly fatal. Treatments that have been used include androgenic steroids, corticosteroids, thrombolytic agents, and bone marrow transplantation. The latter may be curative.

References

1. Hartman RC, Jenkins DE Jr: The "Sugar-water" test for paroxysmal nocturnal hemoglobinuria. *N Engl J Med* 1965; 275:155–157.
2. Nicholson-Weller A, Spicer DB, Austen KF: Deficiency of the complement regulatory protein, 'decay-accelerating factor,' on membranes of granulocytes, monocytes, and platelets in paroxysmal nocturnal hemoglobinuria, *N Engl J Med* 1985; 312:1091–1097.
3. Zalman LS, Wood LM, Frank MM, et al: Deficiency of the homologous restriction factor in paroxysmal nocturnal hemoglobinuria. *J Exp Med* 1987; 165:572–577.

13

Acquired Hemolytic Anemia

If the inherited (intrinsic) hemolytic anemias and paroxysmal nocturnal hemoglobinuria (PNH) are excluded, there remains a varied group of hemolytic anemias caused by extrinsic factors such as chemical, physical, and infectious agents, and circulating antibody (Table 13–1). Older terminology grouped the extrinsic hemolytic anemias in the direct Coombs'-positive category; in fact only the antibody-associated anemias are actually in this group. Anemias due to infectious agents or physicochemical damage to the red cell membrane are Coombs'-negative.

If red cell enzyme deficiencies and hemoglobinopathy are excluded, antibody-induced hemolysis becomes the most frequently occurring hemolytic anemia. Antibodies can be produced in response to foreign red cell antigens (alloantibody), to self-antigens (autoantibody), or to drugs bound to the red cell membrane or to plasma proteins. Antibody can also be transfused passively from mother to fetus (erythroblastosis fetalis). In this chapter, we will primarily consider alloantibody following incompatible transfusion; the physicochemical extrinsic causes of increased red cell turnover are much less common and will be discussed in less depth.

Pathophysiology

The mechanism of red cell destruction differs with the underlying cause. Antibodies to red cell antigens foreign to the host result from

Table 13-1   Hemolytic Anemia Caused by Extrinsic Factors

Category	Specific Agent
Infectious	Protozoal—Malaria
	Bacterial—Cholera
	Viral
Physicochemical	Burns
	Chemicals
	Dose-related toxins, eg, benzene,
	phenylhydrazine
	Drugs
	Interaction with red cell enzyme defi-
	ciency
Antibody-induced	Alloantibody
	Incompatible transfusion
	Erythroblastosis fetalis
	Autoantibody
	Warm autoantibodies
	Cold autoantibodies
	PCH
	Drug-induced antibody
	Toxic immune complexes—quinidine,
	quinine
	Haptens—penicillin type/cephalothin
	Alpha methyldopa type
Miscellaneous	PNH

ABBREVIATIONS: PCH = paroxysmal cold hemoglobinuria; PNH = paroxysmal nocturnal hemoglobinuria.

exposure to these antigens through transfusion (IgG, IgM), from previous pregnancy (IgG), spontaneously from unknown causes (IgM), or, rarely, from injection of red cells, an antiquated method of conferring immunity to infectious disease that is occasionally seen in immigrant populations (IgG). Antibody can be present without history of precedent transfusion reaction. The immunoglobulin class of the antibody determines the mode and site of red cell destruction. When IgM antibodies bind to antigen, the classic complement pathway is activated and intravascular hemolysis occurs. When IgG antibody binds to red cell antigens, the sensitized cell membrane is removed piecemeal in the reticuloendothelial system by macrophages with receptors for the Fc portion of the IgG molecule. As portions of the red cell membrane are removed the cell becomes spherocytic and less deformable, so that it is ultimately retained in the splenic cords. In some cases, the IgG antibody activates the classic complement pathway; the reaction usually stops at conversion of complement to C3b and the cell does not lyse. Macrophages in liver and spleen also carry receptors for C3b, which markedly increases the rate of cell destruction when combined with IgG macrophage phagocytosis.

Physicochemical injury to red cells by thermal burn or some chemical agents results in partial loss of red cell membrane. The resultant red cells are smaller and spherocytic, and, therefore, less deformable. They are ultimately removed in the splenic cords. In the case of burns, the injury is full thickness (third-degree), damaging red cells in the underlying microcirculation; as soon as the damaged cells are removed, the hemolysis stops. Infectious agents may disrupt the red cell as they proliferate within it (eg, malaria, babesiosis) or produce enzymes that damage the membrane, as in the case of cholera, which produces neuraminidase.

Clinical Findings

Destruction of red cells produces anemia, malaise, fatigue, pallor, and weakness. Jaundice is seen with rapid red cell destruction, but may be absent in chronic hemolysis. Intravascular hemolysis produces hemoglobinemia and hemoglobinuria often followed by shock and disseminated intravascular coagulation (DIC). Chronic compensated hemolysis gradually causes splenomegaly. Hepatomegaly is seen only in long-standing hemolytic anemia, and may be related to iron deposition in Kupffer cells. Lymphadenopathy is rare unless hemolysis is associated with a hematologic neoplasm.

Approach to Diagnosis

Infectious diseases that produce hemolysis are generally prostrating, eg, bacterial sepsis, so that clinical findings separate them from immune hemolysis. Careful examination of the peripheral smear associated with appropriate history establishes the diagnosis of malaria or other intra-erythrocytic parasites.

The immediate clinical importance of antibody-induced hemolytic anemia depends on whether transfusion has been given in the past 2 or 3 weeks (delayed transfusion reaction) or whether transfusion is being contemplated (preventing transfusion hemolysis). There must be a complete history regarding sources of exposure to red cell products, how recently exposure occurred, and any symptoms associated with the exposure. In immune hemolysis hematologic findings are less important than:

1. Serum antibody screening, which should include several serologic techniques and temperature variations to detect both IgG and IgM antibodies.

2. Antibody identification combined with appropriate antigen typings of the patient's red cells.

3. Direct antiglobulin test if transfusions have been given in the previous 3 to 6 weeks, or if autoimmune hemolysis is suspected.

4. Tests to evaluate acute hemolysis if transfusion reaction is suspected. Such tests include plasma/urine hemoglobin, serum haptoglobin, and serum bilirubin. If intravascular hemolysis has occurred, tests to monitor renal function are also performed.

Hematologic Findings

Hematologic tests are informative only if transfusions are currently being given. An abrupt fall in hemoglobin up to 14 days after transfusion, a failure to maintain hemoglobin levels after transfusion, or the appearance of jaundice suggests incompatible transfusion. Prolonged administration of incompatible blood can result in splenomegaly and lead to the mistaken diagnosis of autoimmune hemolytic anemia. Intravascular hemolysis may result from ABO-incompatible transfusion and with transfusion reactions caused by anti-Kell, anti-Duffy (anti-Fy^a), or anti-Kidd (anti-Jk^a or anti-Jk^b). The latter may cause intravascular hemolysis 10 to 14 days after transfusion. Anti-E, -C, and -S have also caused intravascular hemolysis. Intravascular hemolysis, when followed by disseminated intravascular coagulation, is associated with decreases in F.V, VIII, and platelets.

Blood Cell Measurements.   Variable anemia is present if transfusions are current; otherwise no symptoms occur. One unit of packed red cells should increase the hemoglobin (15 g/L or 1.5 g/dl) or the hematocrit (0.03 or 3%) in an adult of average size. In thermal burns with marked microspherocytosis the mean corpuscular volume (MCV) may be decreased as low as 60 to 70 fL. Histograms produced by newer equipment may show a bimodal distribution of red cell size.

Acute hemolysis may be associated with leukocytosis, sometimes with a left shift.

Peripheral Blood Smear Morphology.   Transfusions that are ABO incompatible are associated with microspherocytes. Disseminated intravascular coagulation can be associated with red cell fragmentation. Thermal burns are associated with transient microspherocytosis lasting 24 to 48 hours. Malarial parasites occasionally enlarge the red cell *(Plasmodium vivax),* but usually produce no specific change. The number of red cells with intracellular parasites parallels the degree of hemolysis.

Bone Marrow Examination. Bone marrow examination is usually not helpful. Prolonged transfusion with incompatible blood results in an increase in marrow iron.

Other Laboratory Tests

13.1 Serum Antibody Screening

Purpose. Serum antibody screening detects the presence of antibody to red cells.

Principle. Antibody to red cell antigens agglutinates or hemolyzes screening cells that have the antigen, provided that the medium of the reaction and the temperature of reaction is appropriate. These tests are widely available, though the reliability of interpretation is variable.

Specimen. Ten milliliters of serum are obtained fresh to conserve complement, since some antibodies are complement-dependent. If blood must be mailed to a reference laboratory, the serum should be separated from the cells to prevent spurious hemolysis. However, red cells must accompany the serum. The serum can be frozen if conditions do not appear optimal—if, for example, it is being mailed to a hot climate, across the continent, or over a holiday.

Procedure. The patient's serum is screened with commercially supplied red cells that have most of the 18 major antigen groups represented. Screening cells and serum are incubated at room temperature to detect IgM antibodies, and at 37° C, followed by the antiglobulin reaction (indirect Coombs' test) to detect IgG antibodies. IgA antibodies are rarely detected in blood group serology. If antibody is strongly suspected, but not detected, laboratories in larger hospitals or reference laboratories automatically perform tests at 4° C or may use enzyme-treated red cells or low ionic saline solution (LISS) as the test medium.

Interpretation. Any degree of hemolysis or agglutination at any stage of the testing is considered positive and graded 0 to 4 + .

The antibody must then be identified to assess transfusion hazard and future availability of blood. Results of antibody screening may be negative despite previous reactions to transfusion or incompatible pregnancies, since antibodies may fade completely with time or are of such low titer that they are detectable only with enzyme-treated red cells or with cells homozygous for the antigen. Suspicious histories should be reported to the laboratory so that technologists can expand their testing beyond the routine screening procedures. Antigen-incompatible transfusions have diminished red cell survival that is sometimes abrupt, as with anti-Jk[a]. Antibody is found in 2% to 3% of the previously transfused population, 2% to 3% of the previously pregnant, and less than 1% of all others, for a combined incidence of 5% to 6%.

13.2   Antibody Identification

Purpose.   Antibody identification assesses current hazard to transfusion, predicts reliability of cross-match procedures, evaluates availability of blood (particularly under emergency circumstances), and detects multiple antibodies.

Principle.   The availability and completeness of identification procedures vary in hospital laboratories, but every area usually has at least one reference laboratory available, and specimens with positive results on screening can be referred by the hospital blood bank. Depending on distance and complexity of the problem, results may require 1 to 5 days.

Specimen.   Serum separated from the clot and a sample of the patient's red cells, either from the clot or from a separate anticoagulated (EDTA) tube, are used as specimens. If serum cannot be tested within 48 hours, it should be stored frozen to conserve complement.

Procedure.   Serum is tested with commercially available panels of 9 or 10 red cell samples for which all antigens are known, as provided on printed protocols. Serum is also tested with the patient's own cells and usually with samples of cord blood as well. Serum and cell samples are incubated at room temperature and at 37° C followed by the antiglobulin reaction. The presence of agglutination or hemolysis is noted and graded. Variability in strength of agglutination, temperature of reaction, or medium of reaction may indicate the presence of more than one antibody. Once antibody specificity is known, the patient's red cells are typed for the appropriate antigen.

Interpretation. Alloantibody agglutinates specific cells of the panel, but not the patient's own. The pattern of reactive cell samples is compared with the protocol sheet to determine specificity. The patient's own cells should be negative for the particular antigen, and if they are not, the antibody specificity is not confirmed and must be re-evaluated.

IgG antibodies act at 37° C by indirect antiglobulin, by enzyme, or by LISS techniques. They usually follow previous transfusion or incompatible pregnancy. Four antibodies are particularly dangerous in transfusion since they cause intravascular hemolysis and/or disseminated intravascular coagulation (DIC): anti-Kell, anti-Fy^a, and anti-Jk^a or anti-Jk^b. The Kidd antibodies may not be found during antibody screening, but rapidly increase their titer with incompatible transfusions, and may cause intravascular hemolysis beginning as long as 10 days after transfusion when the stimulated antibody titer reaches a critical level. The members of the Rh system (anti-D, -c, -E, -e) follow an immunizing stimulus and destroy cells more slowly by splenic sequestration. Rarely anti-E or anti-C have caused abrupt intravascular hemolysis. IgM antibodies bind complement. Although they may follow incompatible transfusion, they more often appear spontaneously and, therefore, unpredictably. They include anti-Lewis^a and anti-Lewis^b, anti-P$_1$, and anti-M. Many believe that alloantibodies reactive at or below room temperature are not clinically significant. However, if the antibody reacts by the antiglobulin phase, the potential for transfusion reactions exists. Transfusion reactions may vary from intravascular hemolysis to unexplained shortened red cell survival. The most lethal IgM antibodies are anti-A and anti-B, involved in major blood group incompatibility. Such incompatibility is almost always caused by errors in patient identification. These antibodies are not detectable by antibody identification techniques, because all the test red cells are group O.

Once identified, antibodies must be permanently recorded, since they may fade with time only to reappear with incompatible transfusions, or be so weak that truly incompatible units appear compatible.

13.3   Direct Antiglobulin (Coombs') Test

Purpose.   The DAT detects globulin coating of circulating red cells, presumably by antibody. It does not distinguish alloantibody from autoantibody. After transfusion, in the absence of autoantibody, the red cells coated are donor cells, as confirmed by testing red cell antigens.

Principle, Specimen, Procedure See Test 7.4.

Procedure. A broad-spectrum reagent should be used to detect any possible reaction. In patients who have received a transfusion in the past 3 months, all tests whose results are positive require elution of the globulin coat and testing to identify the globulin as red cell antibody.

Interpretation. Positive results may vary from $+/-$ to $4+$, depending on the cause. Unlike reactions with autoimmune hemolytic anemia, the DAT tends to be $1+$ or weaker. After massive intravascular hemolysis, the DAT may show negative results since all coated cells are now lysed. The donor cells are a minor population in the patient's circulation, giving a "mixed-field" appearance that is characteristic. Positive test results may be extremely transient. The antibody specificity of the eluate does not match the patient's red cell antigens, although in patients transfused with many units or in those with a DAT of $4+$, the antigens may be difficult to determine. Retesting after 4 to 5 days while withholding further transfusions may clarify the picture.

13.4 Serum Haptoglobin

Purpose, Principle, Specimen, Procedure. See Test 7.3.

Interpretation. The normal range of haptoglobin is 0.4 to 1.8 g/L (40 to 180 mg/dl). Levels less than .25 g/L (25 mg/dl) are consistent with hemolysis. Haptoglobin levels may be transiently decreased after massive transfusion as a result of destruction of senescent red cells without hemolysis.

13.5 Plasma Hemoglobin

Principle. IgM antibodies to red cell antigens activate the classic complement pathway resulting in intravascular hemolysis. IgG antibodies of very high titer may also result in intravascular cell destruction.

Purpose, Procedure, Specimen, and Interpretation.
See Test 7.2.

13.6   Urine Hemoglobin

Purpose.   Free plasma hemoglobin at levels above 1.5 g/L (150 mg/dl) appears in the urine. The test for urine hemoglobin confirms intravascular hemolysis, particularly when venous specimens have been technically difficult to obtain or when obtaining them has been delayed.

Principle.   Plasma proteins, haptoglobin, transferrin, and albumin bind free hemoglobin in normal metabolism. When the renal threshold is exceeded, free hemoglobin is detected in the urine. After incompatible transfusion, this is usually a transient occurrence ending when the incompatible red cells have been lysed.

Specimen.   Random urine is collected within 2 to 3 hours of the clinical episode.

Procedure.   Urine is tested with a dipstick (see chapter 7, Ancillary Tests).

Interpretation.   Normally, no hemoglobin is present in the urine. Significant reactions are 1+ or greater (scale, 0 to 3+). The urine sediment should be examined for red cells (hematuria) not seen with transfusion reactions but accompanying bladder or prostate surgery and catheters. If red cell destruction has been occurring slowly over several days, urine hemosiderin may be present without overt hemoglobinuria.

Course and Treatment

Intravascular hemolysis caused by inadvertant ABO incompatibility activates complement and the coagulation cascade to produce DIC. Hypotension, renal failure, and death may follow. This type of reaction almost always results from improper identification of the patient. The severity of the reaction is dose-related so that treatment requires early recognition of clerical error to stop the transfusion. Patient hydration must be maintained to avoid renal shut down. Twenty percent mannitol has been used as an osmotic diuretic to aid in clearance of hemoglobin. Intravenous steroids have been used, but there is no clinical evidence that they are helpful; although clinical discomfort improves, hemolysis continues unabated. Delayed transfusion reactions produce significant morbidity but less certain mortality. Jaundice and posttransfusion anemia resolve if compatible blood is given. Further transfusion should not be considered until the antibody has been identified and antigen-negative units provided (delayed transfusion reaction) or the patient accurately identified (ABO incompatibility).

If renal failure has occurred, hemodialysis may be necessary to support the patient until renal function returns; in 30% of cases it does not. In delayed or mild hemolytic transfusion reactions, transfusion with compatible blood and time results in resolution of symptoms and an appropriate posttransfusion hemoglobin level. Treatment of catastrophic infectious disease with hemolysis involves prompt and massive treatment of the underlying organism with appropriate intravenous antibiotic therapy. Intravenous or intramuscular steroids are often given, but there is no evidence that the disease course is changed. Such reactions are generally fatal despite supportive therapy. Malaria is treated with chloroquine, primaquin, or other anti-malarials, usually with recovery if treated promptly. Unrecognized falciparum malaria produces severe neurologic and hematologic symptoms and is often fatal.

References

1. Bell CA, Fairbanks VF: Hemolytic disorders, in Fairbanks VF (ed): *Current Hematology.* New York, J Wiley & Sons, 1981, pp 65–122.

2. Issitt PD: *Applied Blood Group Serology,* ed 3. Miami, Montgomery Scientific Publications, 1985, pp 99–111.

3. Kelton JG: Platelet and red cell clearance. *Transfusion Med Rev* 1987; 1:75–84.

4. Mollison PL: The clinical significance of red cell alloantibodies (and autoantibodies) in blood transfusion, in Polesky H, Walker R (eds): *Safety in Transfusion Practices.* Skokie, Ill, College of American Pathologists, 1982, pp 131–150.

5. Mollison PL, Engelfriet CP, Contreras M: *Blood Transfusion in Clinical Medicine,* ed 8. London, Blackwell Scientific, 1987, pp 102–114.

14

Acquired Hemolytic Anemia: Fetomaternal Incompatibility

In fetomaternal incompatibility the fetus receives antibody passively from the mother, who has been exposed to foreign antigens by previous transfusion or has received small infusions of red cells across the placenta during the current or a past pregnancy. Many of the characteristics of incompatible transfusions are similar in fetomaternal incompatibility (hemolytic disease of the newborn).

Pathophysiology

Serologically, in all cases the mother will be negative for the red cell antigen, and her fetus will be positive by virtue of the genetic input of the father. Hemolytic disease of the newborn (HDN) depends on the physicochemical characteristics of the maternal antibody (eg, only IgG antibodies cross the placenta), and they must be avid to bind strongly with the fetal red cell membrane. Evidence suggests that clinical hemolysis correlates with subtype IgG_3; IgG_1 may coat the infant's cells, but is not associated with hemolysis. Coated red cells are sequestered in the spleen and liver and destroyed there, causing enlargement of these organs in the newborn.

The two major types of fetomaternal incompatibility are ABO group incompatibility and Rh incompatibility. The characteristics

Table 14–1   Characteristics of Erythroblastosis Fetalis Caused by ABO and Rh Incompatibility

Findings	ABO	Rh_o
Clinical		
Number of antigen-positive pregnancy	Any, including the first	After the first pregnancy
Clinical severity	Unpredictable	More severe with each antigen-positive pregnancy
Prenatal evaluation	None needed	Anti-Rh_o titer, amniocentesis
Onset of jaundice	3–4 days postdelivery	Immediate
Treatment[a]	None, bilirubin lights, or rare exchange transfusion	None, early delivery, bilirubin lights, exchange transfusion, or intrauterine transfusion
Laboratory		
Direct Coombs' test	± – 1+	2+ –4+
Fetal blood group	A or B	Rh_o positive
Fetal antibody	Anti-A or anti-B	Anti-Rh_o
Maternal blood group	O	Rh negative
Maternal antibody screening	Negative	Positive
Peripheral blood (newborn)	Microspherocytes	Not diagnostic

[a]Treatment options are listed by increasing severity of erythroblastosis

of each are seen in Table 14–1. ABO group incompatibility is very common but usually not clinically severe. The condition is produced by a mother who is blood group O with a fetus who is group A or B. It may occur during any pregnancy, even the first, since it is postulated that secreted A or B substance, not just red cells, cross the placenta to the mother inducing her to produce IgG anti-A or anti-B antibodies in addition to the IgM anti-A and anti-B normally present; the IgG antibody recrosses the placenta to attach to the infant cells. Antibody avidity is usually poor, so disease is slow to appear, usually 3 to 4 days after delivery.

Rh$_o$ (anti-D) incompatibility appears after the first pregnancy as a result of infusion of red cells across the placenta at the first delivery. This is less common with the use of anti-Rh immune globulin. Given at each abortion or delivery, it prevents immune recognition of D antigen and provides immunity to the mother. In 1% of mothers sensitization may occur in the first pregnancy, but clinical disease in the infant does not. Occasionally other antibodies are involved in fetomaternal incompatibility; anti-c, anti-E, and anti-Kell are the most common. The mechanism is the same as for anti-D, but the antibodies are less efficient at causing jaundice in the newborn. Anti-Kell antibodies in a mother almost always indicate past transfusion not incompatible previous pregnancy, since 90% of the population is Kell-negative including mother, father, and their infant.

Clinical Findings

Serologic evidence may exist for HDN without clinical evidence of hemolysis, particularly in ABO group incompatibility. Destruction of red cells is primarily caused by reticuloendothelial sequestration of IgG-sensitized red cells, so that fetal liver and spleen are enlarged, and jaundice is present in the neonatal period. In severe Rh erythroblastosis, red cell destruction occurs in utero; the infant may be born severely anemic with high output congestive heart failure and anasarca (hydrops fetalis), but is not jaundiced until after birth, when placental transport of bilirubin is lost and the neonatal liver must assume bilirubin metabolism. Following delivery the immature infant liver is initially unable to conjugate bilirubin rapidly enough. Jaundice is caused by increased indirect bilirubin, which is lipid soluble and deposited in the lenticulostriate nucleus of the brain (kernicterus). Such deposition can cause mental retardation, motor spasticity, and death.

Approach to Diagnosis

The type of fetomaternal incompatibility producing hemolytic disease of the newborn can be anticipated by transfusion and gestation history, and the following tests:

1. Maternal blood group and antibody screening.

2. Newborn blood group.

3. Direct antiglobulin test of newborn cells and eluate of positive red cells.

4. Peripheral blood smear from cord blood or infant examined for microspherocytes.

5. If serologic evidence is present for erythroblastosis fetalis, serum bilirubin tests are ordered serially.

6. The father's blood is tested with the mother's if serologic evidence of erythroblastosis is not present, yet the newborn is hemolyzing for undetermined causes, and the newborn DAT is positive. This testing is expected to exclude "exotic" incompatibilities between paternal antigens (reflected in the child) and maternal antibody.

7. Although neutralization studies can be performed to classify the maternal antibody as IgG or IgM, knowledge of which helps to estimate likelihood of placental passage, they are rarely necessary or clinically helpful.

Prenatal studies anticipate clinical disease and direct management. These include titration of anti-D in the maternal serum and amniocentesis.

Hematologic Findings

There may be no anemia or severe anemia. The persistent extramedullary hematopoiesis results in increased circulating nucleated red cells (erythroblastosis fetalis). HDN caused by ABO and less common red cell antibodies is usually mild; Rh HDN is progressively severe with each pregnancy, which is reflected in the degree of anemia.

Blood Cell Measurements. Levels of hemoglobin in mild anemia are 140 to 160 g/L (14 to 16 g/dl). In moderate anemia the levels are 100 to 140 g/L (10 to 14 g/dl), and in severe anemia they are 80 to 100 g/L (8 to 10 g/dl). The white count is 10 to 20 × 10^9/L (10 to 20 × 10^3/μl), and the reticulocyte count is greater than 0.10 (10%).

Peripheral Blood Smear Morphology. Morphology shows polychromasia, correlating with the increased reticulocyte count and nucleated red cells greater than 10 per 100 white cells (erythroblastosis). Microspherocytes usually indicate ABO hemolytic disease.

Other Laboratory Tests

14.1   Determination of Blood Group

Purpose.   Testing of the blood group of both the mother and the newborn determines if the mother is negative for antigen and the infant is positive.

Principle.   Maternal red cell antigens and newborn antigens are determined for ABO and Rh_o. Tests can be performed for further antigens if indicated.

Specimen.   Red cells from clots or anticoagulated specimens are washed well with saline before testing. Specimens are stable for at least 7 days. Cord red cells and plasma can be used if the red cells are well washed to remove contaminants. Infant heel-stick specimens can also be used.

Procedure.   Standard typing procedures are direct agglutination of red cells by anti-A, anti-B, and anti-D antibodies. All Rh_o (D) – negative cells are tested for D^u, the partial or gene-suppressed D antigen.

Interpretation.   In ABO hemolytic disease, the mother's blood is group O (ie, negative for A or B antigens) and the infant's blood is group A or B. In Rh hemolytic disease, the mother is Rh negative and the infant is Rh positive. Where the serologic possibility of both ABO and Rh disease is possible, ie, an O-negative mother with an A- or B-positive child, hemolytic disease is more likely caused by ABO incompatibility, since the group incompatibility has usually lysed Rh-incompatible cells throughout the pregnancy. Mothers who are Rh positive are not excluded from having infants with hemolytic disease, since they may be c(hr')-negative, E-negative, and so forth, and their infants positive for these antigens.

14.2   Maternal Antibody Screening and Identification

Purpose.   A positive antibody screening may indicate anti-Rh_o type of hemolytic disease rather than ABO type, where screenings are negative.

Principle. Maternal serum is screened for antibody, usually early in pregnancy and sporadically thereafter to detect IgG or IgM antibodies. The antibody is then identified to assess fetal risk and, if necessary, the father's red cell antigens are tested as a predictive measure of fetal involvement.

Specimen. Serum less than 48 hours old, obtained at the first obstetric visit, is used. A specimen should also be obtained in the third trimester, and more frequently if the early specimen shows positive results, or if the obstetric history warrants it.

Procedure. Serum is incubated with test red cells at room temperature in saline suspension to detect IgM antibodies, and by incubation at 37° C followed by antiglobulin reaction to detect IgG antibodies. All antibodies are identified using the same techniques.

Interpretation. In ABO hemolytic disease only the expected anti-A and anti-B antibodies are found in the group O mother, so the antibody screen is negative. In all other types of hemolytic disease, the antibody screen is positive. The antibody must be identified to determine its significance to the newborn. Only IgG antibodies cross the placenta, and they must coat the infant's red cells to produce symptoms. Common antibodies found in pregnant women are anti-Lewis[a] and anti-Lewis[b]. These antibodies do not produce neonatal disease because they are IgM and cannot cross the placenta, and because all infants are Lewis[a] and Lewis[b] negative. Thus some antibodies are more significant for the mother in a postpartum hemorrhage than for infant HDN.

The current practice of administering Rh immune globulin at 28 weeks gestation to prevent erythroblastosis results in positive maternal antibody screening due to weak anti-D (titer, <4). Unlike antibody produced as a consequence of natural maternal sensitization, these antibodies do not give a "crisp" pattern of identification.

14.3   Direct Antiglobulin (Coombs') Test in the Newborn

Purpose. The DAT detects globulin coating on the newborn's red cells.

Principle. Fetal red cells are coated with passively transmitted IgG antibody specific for antigen.

Specimen. Red cells from specimens of cord blood that is either clotted or anticoagulated can be used. Small capillary specimens from newborn heel-sticks are also adequate. Cord samples are stable for at least 1 week and can be tested when and if clinical findings appear.

Procedure. Broad-spectrum antiglobulin reagent is centrifuged with the newborn's red cells that have been washed with saline to free them of all contaminating substances and serum proteins. Agglutination is graded 0 to 4 +. For all tests producing positive results, adsorbed globulin is eluted and tested for antibody specificity.

Interpretation. Infant DATs are + / − to 1 + for ABO hemolytic disease, 2 to 4 + for Rh hemolytic disease, and 2 to 4 + for hemolytic disease caused by other antibodies. The antibody eluted from the neonatal red cells should match that found in the maternal serum. Antibody found only in cord plasma, but not on cord red cells, is of doubtful significance, indicating poor avidity and, therefore, less likely clinical disease. Antibodies such as anti-c, anti-E, and anti-Kell, adsorbed to fetal red cells produce a strong DAT but usually minimal jaundice. Improved antiglobulin reagents make false-negative tests less common; additional saline wash of the cells diminishes false-negatives resulting from neutralization of the Coombs' reagent. Rarely, elution of an antiglobulin-negative red cell yields antibody because of indetectable numbers of molecules concentrated in the elution process.

Positive DAT results on cord specimens without detectable antibody may indicate adsorption of Wharton's jelly, but the cell control is usually positive. The test should be repeated on blood from a heel-stick or venous sample. If results are still positive, private antibody limited to this family should be considered, and maternal serum or infant's plasma should be tested against paternal red cells for agglutination.

14.4   Acid Elution Stain (Kleihauer-Betke), Postpartum Blood Smear

Purpose. Fetal-maternal hemorrhage (FMH) of even minimal numbers of Rh-positive fetal red cells may sensitize the Rh-negative mother unless she is adequately immunized postpartum with Rh immune globulin. Doses are standardized to compensate for FMH of 15 mL packed red cells or less. The actual volume of FMH can be calculated by staining a postpartum maternal peripheral smear for fetal cells. If the volume of FMH exceeds 15 mL, increased dosage of the Rh immune globulin should be administered. Intrapartum Rh immune globulin is administered at 20 to 28 weeks gestation, but Kleihauer-stained peripheral smears are not useful at this time because the number of potentially positive cells are so minimal.

Principle.   Fetal hemoglobin is resistant to acid elution, whereas adult hemoglobin is not. A postpartum maternal peripheral smear is treated with dilute acid buffer for 10 minutes and then stained. The maternal erythrocyte adult hemoglobin is leached into the buffer leaving ghosted red cells, whereas the fetal red cells remain as dense red erythrocytes.

Specimen.   Very thin peripheral blood smears fixed in 80% alcohol are prepared from postpartum maternal blood collected in EDTA.

Procedure.   Dried smears are placed in McIlvaines buffer (pH, 3.2) for 10 minutes, followed by washing in distilled water to end the reaction. The smear is then stained with erythrosin and counter stained with hematoxylin; 2000 cells are counted. The percentage of densely staining cells with fetal hemoglobin (presumably fetal in origin) is calculated. The percentage can be converted to milliliters by a nomogram, and 300 mg of Rh immune globulin is administered intramuscularly for each 15 mL of packed red cells calculated. Control smears should be made from cord blood specimens (positive) mixed 1 in 10 with adult blood (negative), since occasional marginal cells are seen even with the negative control. Test kits are available using the same principle so that even small laboratories may perform the test.

Interpretation.   Normal adult cells are laked and appear as ghosts. Fetal cells are densely pink and refractile. The volume of FMH is calculated as milliliters of whole blood equal to the percentage of fetal cells × 50. FMH >15 mL packed cell volume requires proportionate additional Rh immune globulin.

Notes.   Adult hemoglobinopathies such as persistent fetal hemoglobin may create a misleading picture. If the volume of FMH suggests significant blood loss in an otherwise well infant with normal hemoglobin, the possibility of hemoglobinopathy in the mother should be considered.

Ancillary Tests

Ancillary tests include ultrasonography, which can demonstrate fetal hydrops. Ultrasound localization of the placenta is also necessary prior to amniocentesis.

Amniocentesis. Measurement of amniotic fluid pigment, probably bilirubin, is helpful in estimating the rate of red cell destruction and expected degree of fetal anemia. The procedure is undertaken when maternal Rh antibody has been identified and has a significant titer (>32). Depending on the titer and the obstetrical history, the first procedure is performed at 28 weeks.

After the placenta has been localized by ultrasound, a fine-gauge needle is introduced percutaneously into the amniotic sac and amniotic fluid is removed for analysis. The fluid is scanned in a spectrophotometer at wavelengths of 350 to 700 nm. Bilirubin has a peak absorbance at 450 nm. If positive findings are present, repeated specimens are obtained every 1 to 2 weeks, or in borderline cases, every few days.

At least 2 specimens are needed to verify an increase in optical density and to determine if the differential absorbtion is increasing, decreasing, or stable. Amniotic fluid (5 to 10 mL) is withdrawn and immediately shielded from light, which degrades bilirubin and causes falsely low results.

With the bladder empty, the placenta is localized by ultrasound. A fine gauge needle is inserted percutaneously under local anesthesia into the amniotic sac, avoiding the placenta and fetal parts. Five to 10 mL of amniotic fluid is withdrawn atraumatically for analysis. The fluid is placed in a container shielded from light, which degrades bilirubin and causes falsely low results. The specimen is centrifuged to separate vernix, and the supernatant is scanned in the ultraviolet spectrum from 350 to 700 nm. The curve is not linear, but has a rise at 450 nm due to bilirubin. A tangent is constructed to create a straight line, and the difference in optical density from the tangent to the peak at 450 nm is the Δ OD. The absorbance is plotted vs wavelength. The optical density rise at 450 nm is common early in pregnancy and decreases after 26 weeks if no red cell sensitization is present. At least 2 specimens are needed to verify an increase in Δ OD and to determine if it is increasing, decreasing, or stable.

Zones have been determined by Liley that correlate with severity of anemia. If the anemia is severe, and fetal lungs are markedly immature, then intrauterine transfusion is considered. If fetal lung maturation is adequate, then early delivery, which permits extra-uterine exchange transfusion, is undertaken. Intrauterine transfusion has a success rate of approximately 85% unless hydrops is present, in which case the success rate is less than 25%.

False elevations in absorbance are seen when hemoglobin or meconium contaminate the specimen, since one of several HbA optical peaks occurs at 450 nm.

Amniocentesis interpretation is based on experience with anti-D antibody. There is no guaranteed extrapolation to other antibodies such as anti-c or anti-E, nor to other causes of hemolysis.

Course and Treatment

Maternal serum is monitored during pregnancy to detect Rh sensitization and follow its course. Rh antibody titers above 32 require amniocentesis to monitor the progression and severity of anemia. Rapid progression may require intrauterine transfusion or early delivery. ABO sensitization is only rarely severe after delivery, often in association with anti-B. There may be correlation with the subclass of IgG antibody. No treatment before delivery is necessary, which is also true for HDN caused by other antibodies such as anti-c, anti-E, anti-Jr^a or other antibodies. Although serologically striking, clinical symptoms are few, and more clinical damage is done by unnecessary amniocentesis, which may result in sensitization to more serious antigens.

Mild jaundice is controlled with bilirubin lights, which oxidize bilirubin in the infant's skin.

References

1. Freda VJ: The antepartum management of Rh disease, in Garratty G (ed): *Hemolytic Disease of the Newborn.* Arlington, Va, American Association of Blood Banks, 1984, pp 33–51.

2. Klemperer M: Perinatal and neonatal transfusion, in Petz LD, Swisher SN: *Clinical Practice of Blood Transfusion.* New York, Churchill Livingstone Inc, 1981, pp 697–705.

3. Mollison PL: Some aspects of Rh hemolytic disease and its prevention, in Garratty G (ed): *Hemolytic Disease of the Newborn.* Arlington, Va, American Association of Blood Banks, 1984, pp 1–32.

4. Sebring ES: Fetomaternal hemorrhage: Incidence and methods of detection, in Garratty G (ed): *Hemolytic Disease of the Newborn.* Arlington, Va, American Association of Blood Banks, 1984, pp 87–118.

5. *Technical Manual American Association of Blood Banks.* Arlington, Va, American Association of Blood Banks, 1985, pp 321–322, 482–484.

6. Bowman JM: The prevention of Rh immunization. *Transf Med Rev* 1988; 2:129–150.

15

Acquired Hemolytic Anemia: Drug Related

Drugs produce hemolytic anemia by interacting with red cell enzymes of the glycolytic pathway or by inducing extrinsic antibodies. The degree of hemolysis can vary from acute intravascular hemolysis to compensated hemolysis of splenic sequestration. In most cases, the hemolytic anemia is reversible when the drug is withdrawn.

Pathophysiology

Although more than 80 different deficiencies of red cell enzymes have been reported, only G6PD and pyruvate kinase deficiency are common, and only G6PD deficiency is associated with drug induced hemolysis. G6PD deficiency does not usually result in hemolytic anemia except when certain oxidant drugs are given. The severity of hemolysis depends on the dose of the inducing drug, the chemical structure of the drug, and the specific variant of G6PD deficiency. These G6PD variants include A− of American Blacks, G6PD Mediterranean, and the Mahidol variant common in Southeast Asians. Hemolysis in the latter two variants is more severe, associated with drugs that do not cause hemolysis in A− variant, eg, quinine, quinidine, and procainamide.

The interaction of an oxidant drug with a G6PD deficient red cell leads to depletion of glutathione (GSH) and inadequate production of NADPH. The depletion of GSH is followed by uncontrolled oxidation of hemoglobin. Hemoglobin degradation products polymerize to form Heinz bodies with resultant membrane damage and reticuloendothelial phagocytosis. Young red cells with more NADPH are less susceptible to oxidative damage, so that as reticulocytosis increases, the effect of low doses of the oxidative drug tends to be self-limited. Drugs that induce hemolysis in susceptible G6PD deficient people are listed in Table 15–1. These drugs do not uniformly cause hemolysis in G6PD deficient people, nor does every drug analogue in a specific category cause hemolysis.

Drugs that cause immune hemolysis have a benzene ring activated by hydroxyl (-OH), amine (-NH), or sulfur (-S) groups. The drug must have a firm binding to a protein carrier, serum proteins, or red cell membrane to produce antibody, and the antibody must have sufficient binding capacity to produce hemolysis. Although by these criteria many drugs are potentially candidates to cause hemolysis, most clinical cases are caused by penicillin or alpha methyldopa. Drugs that induce extrinsic antibodies do so by several mechanisms: toxic immune complexes (quinidine, quinine); hapten formation (penicillins); a positive DAT without hemolysis (cephalosporins); or a true, warm autoimmune hemolytic anemia (AIHA) (alpha methyldopa). Except for the last category, the incriminated drug must be present for hemolysis to occur, although the antibodies persist for life. Table 15–2 lists the drugs commonly involved and their mechanism of action.

Drug-induced immune complexes produce intravascular hemolysis by binding complement to the red cell membrane ("innocent bystander" effect) and activating the classic complement pathway. Such cases are rare and usually restricted to single case reports.

Penicillin and its analogues, when given intravenously, bind to the red cell membranes to produce a hapten. The hapten induces IgG antibody to the penicilloyl moiety, common to drugs of this class and to cephalosporins. Drug-coated cells are destroyed usually within the reticuloendothelial system, although intravascular hemolysis can occur.

The mechanism of antibody production by alpha methyldopa is unknown, although alterations of the endoplasmic reticulum of plasma cells has been postulated to explain the persistence of antibody production long after the drug has been discontinued. Clinical hemolysis rarely begins after the drug has been withdrawn, but if hemolysis is already present, it may not subside for several weeks. Other drugs in the alpha methyldopa class produce serologic findings with minimal hemolysis.

Cephalosporins alter the red cell membrane so that there is nonspecific adsorption of globulins to the red cell. A positive DAT may appear after only 5 to 6 days of therapy.

Nonsteroidal anti-inflammatory drugs are frequently associated

Table 15-1   Drugs Associated with Hemolysis in
Glucose-6-Phosphate Dehydrogenase Deficiency

Analgesics

Acetanilid
Acetylsalicylic acid[a]
Phenocetin[a]

Antimalarial drugs

Primaquine
Pamaquine
Chloroquine[b]
Quinine[b]
Quinicrine
Pentaquine

Sulfonamides and sulfones

Sulfacetamide
Sulfamethoxanzole
Sulfanilimide
Diphenyl sulfone
Thiazole sulfone
Sulfa pyridine

Nonsulfonamide antibacterial agents

Nitrofurantoin
Chloramphenicol[b]
Nitrofurazone (Furadantin)
Nalidixic acid (Negram)

Miscellaneous

Procainamide[b]
Quinidine[b]
Phenylhydrazine
Methylene blue
Toluidine blue

ABBREVIATIONS: G6PD = glucose-6-phosphate dehydrogenase.
[a] Rarely in A− deficient
[b] In G6PD Mediterranean not A−

Table 15–2   Drugs Associated with Immune Hemolysis and the Mechanism of Cell Destruction

Drugs	Route of Administration
Toxic immune complex of (drug + drug Ab + C′)	Oral, variable dose
Quinidine, quinine	
Para-amino salicylate	
Phenacetin	
Ethacrynic acid	
Nonsteroidal anti-inflammatory agents	
Hapten formation	IV >20 mU/day
Penicillin	
Methicillin	
Ampicillin	
Oxacillin	
Carbenicillin	
Nonspecific protein absorption	IM or oral, >4 g/day
Cephalothin	
Cephaloridine	
True, warm AIHA	Oral
Alpha methyldopa	
L-dopa	
Mefenamic acid	
Flufenamic acid	
Chlordiazepoxide hydrochloride (Librium)	
Cimetidine (Tagamet®)	
Cefazolin (Ancef®)	

ABBREVIATIONS: IV = intravenous; IM = intramuscular; AIHA = autoimmune hemolytic anemia; DAT = direct antiglobulin test.

Duration of Therapy	Antibody Class	Hemolytic Symptoms
10–14 days	IgG, IgM, C'	Intravascular hemolysis can occur; single case reports of involved drug; infrequent cause of anemia
10–14 days	IgG	Splenic sequestration; intravascular hemolysis rare
4–6 days	Any protein	Common cause of weakly positive DAT; proven hemolysis rare
6 weeks to 3 months	IgG	10% of patients have positive DAT, 1% hemolyze; splenic sequestration; drug not present for hemolysis. Clinical hemolysis rare despite positive DAT

with hemolysis, which may be caused by both immunocomplex and autoantibody in the same patient.

Clinical Findings

Hemolysis caused by drug interaction with G6PD deficiency may be intravascular, usually abrupt, with severe anemia, hemoglobinuria, and jaundice, and may occur 1 to 3 days after beginning treatment with the oxidant drug. As reticulocytosis begins, the enzyme deficiency is compensated, and the hemolysis will appear to stop.

Drug-induced immune hemolysis is usually less clinically severe, although intravascular hemolysis can occur with all categories. Hepatosplenomegaly and lymphadenopathy are not seen in drug-induced hemolytic anemia.

Approach to Diagnosis

Proper diagnostic evaluation requires an awareness of drugs that commonly cause hemolysis and a suspicion of their involvement in a patient who is currently receiving, or has recently received, such drugs and who has unexplained anemia. Without that suspicion and without narrowing investigation to a specific drug class, proper testing will probably be neither timely nor diagnostic. Evaluation proceeds with the following:

1. Hematologic findings, which determine a normochromic anemia that may be actively hemolytic. Bone marrow aspiration is not usually indicated.

2. Tests for Heinz bodies may be positive in G6PD deficiency.

3. Direct antiglobulin test, which must show positive results, although it may be of variable degree depending on the mechanism of drug action. If the DAT results are not positive, immune hemolysis cannot be proved.

4. Serum antibody screening tests, which are usually negative with standard reagent red cells.

5. Special testing of eluates from Coombs'-positive red cells in parallel with serum against specific drug-treated red cells.

Hematologic Findings

The anemia with intravascular hemolysis may be severe or mild to moderate if well compensated, depending on the drug mechanism of action, the dose, and, if immune, the type of antibody evoked. A reactive leukocytosis may appear. In G6PD deficiency, hemolysis begins as Heinz antibodies appear. As the hemolysis persists, Heinz antibodies are removed in the spleen and tend to disappear.

Blood Cell Measurements.   Hemoglobin can be as low as 20 g/L (2 g/dl) in fatal hemolysis. A mean corpuscular volume (MCV) in the range of 105 to 110 fL reflects reticulocytosis, while the mean corpuscular hemoglobin concentration (MCHC) is usually 300 to 340 g/L (30 to 34 g/dl). The WBC count is 10 to 20 $\times$ 10^9/L (10 to 20 $\times$ 10^3/μl) and may be leukemoid in brisk hemolysis, with a left shift to the myelocyte phase.

Peripheral Blood Smear Morphology.   Nucleated red cells and polychromasia are general findings. Spherocytes may be seen with alpha methyldopa. Target cells are present if jaundice occurs. Bite cells may be seen if Heinz bodies have been extracted in the spleen. Heinz bodies are not seen on Wright's-stained smears, but will be seen on reticulocyte preparations.

Bone Marrow Examination.   The bone marrow is hypercellular with normoblastic erythroid hyperplasia and increased marrow iron (4 +).

Other Laboratory Tests

For specimen collection in immune hemolysis, whole blood is obtained fresh and allowed to clot at 37°C before the serum is separated. Freezing serum samples should be avoided since this frequently disrupts immune complexes. The red cells for testing can be obtained from the clot or from a separately collected EDTA specimen, which prevents nonspecific adsorption of complement. Specimens for evaluation in G6PD deficiency may be collected in EDTA.

15.1   Direct Antiglobulin—(Coombs') Test

Purpose.   The DAT must show positive results for drug-induced immune hemolysis to be considered seriously. Absorbed globulin may be IgG, IgM, or complement. The DAT in G6PD drug hemolysis is negative.

Principle.   No matter what the mechanism of action, all antibody types have in common antibody globulin and/or complement

Table 15–3 Serologic Findings in Drug-Immune Hemolytic Anemia

Mechanism of Action	DAT
Toxic immune complexes (quinine, quinidine)	± −3+ anti-C′
Red cell eluate	Complement
Serum antibody	IgG, IgM
Haptens (penicillins)	2–4+ anti-IgG
Red cell eluate	IgG
Serum antibody	IgG
Nonspecific protein absorption (cephalothin)	± −2+ all or any protein
Red cell eluate	No antibody
Serum antibody	Rarely
True, warm AIHA (alpha methyldopa)	± −4+ anti-IgG
Red cell eluate	IgG
Serum antibody	IgG

ABBREVIATIONS: AIHA = autoimmune hemolytic anemia.
[a] Drug is the specific drug suspected
[b] w+, weakly positive
[c] Agglutination is unrelated to drug treatment of red cells and reflects untreated red cells

attached to the red cell detectable by the DAT. Without a positive direct antiglobulin test, drug-immune hemolytic anemia is unlikely. The adsorbed globulin, once detected, is eluted and tested in parallel with the patient's serum against drug-treated red cells and untreated red cells. The effects of neutralization of the eluate with the suspected drug are also studied.

Procedure. The DAT uses a broad-spectrum reagent. If results are positive, the reaction can be characterized further using monospecific antisera for IgG, IgM, and complement. Eluates are made by organic solvent techniques because these methods precipitate red cell stroma and antibody globulin and, therefore, may detect weak antibody, often critical in drug-immune hemolysis. Tests of the eluate drug-treated red cells frequently require supplemental complement to reproduce the effect in vitro.

	Tests Versus	
Drug-Treated Red Cell[a]	Untreated Red Cell	Drug Neutralization
0	0	0
w+[b] with C'	0	0
4+	0	4+
4+	0	4+
Reacts with and neutralized by related drugs		
1+ -4+	0	0- +
1+ -4+	0	0- +
Cross-reactions with penicillins		
1+ -4+[c]	1+ -4+	0
1+ -4+	1+ -4+	0

Interpretation. Findings for each category of drug-immune hemolysis are summarized in Table 15–3.

15.2 Serum Antibody Tests and Tests With Drug-Treated Red Cells

Purpose. Agglutination of drug-treated cells by patient serum is consistent with drug-immune hemolysis, but it is not as diagnostic as identifying the globulin actually adsorbed to the red cell. For alpha methyldopa, reactions are positive with untreated patient red cells, which defines the antibody as autoantibody.

Principle. In general, the organic drug binds with a serum protein or the red cell membrane to produce a hapten. Antibody production, strength, and avidity vary with the drug and with the patient, as well as the duration and route of exposure to the drug. Avidity of the drug or its complexes for the red cell membrane appears to be the final common pathway to cell sequestration or hemolysis. Ease of demonstration of the drug antibody varies with the mechanism of action.

Procedure.   Tests for the following are available in reference laboratories and most sophisticated hospital blood banks:

1. Toxic immune complexes: Drug pretreated red cells + patient serum + fresh complement, or drug + red cells + patient serum + C'. Concentrations of drugs and serum samples are varied to achieve optimum antigen-antibody concentration. Drug neutralization is not demonstrable.

2. Haptens: Red cells pretreated with weak dilutions of penicillin drugs can be stored in the refrigerator for 2 to 3 weeks for future testing. Treated cells incubated with the patient serum are either positive directly (IgM antibody) or after the indirect antiglobulin reaction (IgG antibody). Antibody can be titered against drug-treated cells or neutralized by the appropriate drug.

3. Nonspecific protein absorption: Red cells can be pretreated with phosphate-buffered cephalothin solutions. Treated cells are incubated with patient serum. Drug neutralization studies are usually not successful. Tests must be performed in parallel with penicillinized red cells to evaluate cross-reactions.

4. True, warm AIHA: Serum agglutinates red cells untreated with the drug. Weak autoantibodies may be demonstrated only against enzyme-treated red cells.

Interpretation.

1. Toxic immune complexes (quinine-quinidine): Negative test results do not exclude the diagnosis of hemolysis since many unknown variables exist. However, this is one of the least common causes of hemolytic anemia in general and of drug-associated immune hemolysis in particular. The DAT is usually ±, generally because of C', which can, on rare occasions, provoke intravascular hemolysis not seen in other types of drug-immune hemolytic anemia. If hemolysis occurs, results of the DAT may be negative. Red cell eluates, because they usually contain insignificant amounts of antibody globulin, may not react with drug-treated red cells.

2. Haptens (penicillins): This type of antibody is common and easily demonstrated, but only IgG antibodies have signifi-

cance in producing clinical hemolysis. The antibody may react with one or more penicillin cogeners, varying for each patient. Cross-reactions with cephalothin-treated cells occur as a result of similarities in chemical structure. Titer of antibody does not correlate well with clinical hemolysis. The DAT is 2 to 4+ with anti-IgG reagents. Weakly positive ($\pm$) DAT results are not usually associated with clinical hemolysis. The appearance of a positive DAT is dose- and time-related, requiring intravenous administration, 10 to 20 M units daily, for at least 10 days. Eluates of patients' red cells and the serum react only with penicillinized red cells (or related drugs), and reactivity is neutralized by solutions of the specific drug or any crossreacting drugs, such as methicillin, ampicillin, and oxacillin. Serum antibody alone is not diagnostic because much of the population has IgM antibodies from dietary exposure. Atopic reactions (urticaria, asthma, etc) are unrelated and are caused by IgE antibody.

3. Nonspecific protein adsorption (cephalosporins): Occurring with moderate frequency, cephalothin-induced protein absorption must be separated from the clinically significant hapten type of antibody. Cephalothin most often produces nonspecific protein absorption with no activity with drug-treated red cells. Occasionally an occult antipenicillin antibody reacts with cephalothin-treated cells, which is misleading. To prove true hemolytic anemia for this category, the eluate must react with cephalothin-treated cells after cross reactions with penicillin have been excluded by prior absorption. The DAT varies from $\pm$ to 2+. Eluates do not react with drug-treated red cells in most cases, since the adsorbed globulin is not antibody but may be anything from fibrinogen to albumin to transferrin.

Only 2 rather doubtful cases of hemolysis caused by cephalothin have been reported. The process is dose- and time-related; the DAT results become positive within 4 to 6 days after oral or intramuscular doses of 6 g/d. Second and third generation cephalosporins act similarly except for cefazolin. Cefazolin reacts like methyldopa with warm autoantibody adsorbed to the red cell. Despite these findings clinical hemolysis does not result.

4. True, warm AIHA (alpha methyldopa): This group is very common and, because antibodies may persist after the drug is withdrawn, its presence is unsuspected until blood is cross-matched for transfusion. The DAT results vary from $\pm$ to 4+, appearing in 10% of patients receiving 1 g/d or more for longer than 3 months. Direct antiglobulin becomes

progressively stronger followed by the appearance of serum antibody. Despite the serologic evidence, only 1% of patients taking alpha methyldopa actually hemolyze. These patients should be monitored with a DAT every 3 to 6 months. Withdrawal of the drug reverses the process, with decrease in serum antibody followed by disappearance of the DAT. The presence of antibody and its specificity determines risk with transfusion. Without serum antibody transfusion, risk is negligible. With serum antibody in a patient with active hemolysis, red cell survival is decreased as for any warm hemolytic anemia.

15.3   Red Cell G6PD Assay

Purpose.   A deficiency of G6PD in a patient with acute hemolysis supports a diagnosis of drug-related hemolysis.

Principle, Specimen, Procedure.   See Test 10.2. Screening tests are available using prepared reagents and fluoridometry, and can be followed by quantitative assays.

Interpretation.   The normal range is 2.2 to 5.0 IU/g Hb. Young red cells have proportionately more G6PD so that marked reticulocytosis may spuriously elevate the level. Low normal G6PD levels in the presence of reticulocytosis should be viewed with suspicion and the patient retested in 4 to 6 weeks after likely drugs have been withdrawn. Similarly, if transfusions have been given, retesting must wait 6 to 8 weeks. Hypochromic anemias may appear to have increased G6PD. Screening tests may miss heterozygote G6PD deficient red cells, so that quantitative assays may be necessary before discarding the diagnosis.

15.4   Heinz Body Test

Purpose.   G6PD deficiency as well as other rarer enzyme deficiencies or unstable hemoglobin are associated with increased numbers of Heinz bodies. This finding is supportive of the diagnosis of drug-induced hemolysis. The test is available in most hospital laboratories.

Principle.   The oxidative pathway of glycolytic red cell enzymes maintains hemoglobin stability. In G6PD deficiency as well as deficiencies of glutathione synthetase deficiency, triose isomerase deficiency, etc, hemoglobin is denatured and precipitates, and is seen as Heinz bodies. Normal red cells can be induced to form Heinz bodies, but G6PD deficient cells produce 3 or 4 Heinz bodies per red cell in the presence of oxidant drugs.

Specimen.   Fresh whole blood is collected in EDTA.

Procedure.   Methyl violet or neutral red is added to a few drops of blood. Smears are prepared from the mixture after 15 minutes, 30 minutes, or 1 hour incubation at room temperature. Red cells can also be incubated with phenylhydrazine before preparation of the smears; this procedure exaggerates the deficiency of G6PD.

Interpretation.   Normal cells may produce a single marginal Heinz body. After phenylhydrazine incubation, G6PD deficient cells may have 3 to 4 Heinz bodies in every cell. If abrupt hemolysis has been present, the test may be negative because of loss of Heinz body–positive cells.

Course and Treatment

Drug-induced hemolysis in G6PD deficiency may be self-limited as reticulocytes with greater concentrations of enzyme are produced. However, intravascular hemolysis can be severe and life threatening, whether caused by G6PD deficiency, penicillin, or alpha methyldopa, the most likely drugs involved. All suspicious drugs are immediately discontinued until the cause of hemolysis is determined. If necessary, the patient can be supported with transfusion. In all cases except alpha methyldopa–type, the antibody is dependent on the presence of the drug and transfusion is tolerated. With alpha methyldopa, antibody persists in the absence of drug. If only the DAT is positive and there is no detectable serum antibody, transfused red cells survive normally. However, in the rare instance of acute severe warm AIHA, transfused cells have a markedly decreased survival, and the risk of death from hemolytic anemia must be weighed against hemolytic complications of transfusion.

Future drug therapy necessitates using drugs not chemically similar to the inciting drug since antibody persists for life. Where alpha methyldopa– or procainamide–type drugs are involved it may be difficult to determine if the hemolysis is caused by unrelated autoimmune disease or by the drug. Active hemolysis of the methyldopa type usually responds to steroid therapy in 1 to 2 weeks. Steroids can then be withdrawn without relapse, although the positive DAT may persist for up to 2 years. If clinical hemolysis is not present, the serologic findings should be allowed to reverse without treatment.

References

1. Bell CA, Fairbanks VF: Acquired hemolytic anemias: In Fairbanks VF (ed) *Current Hematology.* New York, John Wiley & Sons 1981, pp 65–122.

2. Beutler E: Glucose-6-phosphate dehydrogenase deficiency, in Williams WJ, Beutler E, Erslev AJ, et al (eds): *Hematology,* ed 3. New York, McGraw-Hill International Book Co, 1983, pp 561–566.

3. Issit PD: *Applied Group Serology,* ed 3. Miami, Montgomery Scientific Publications, 1985, pp 550–560.

4. Miale JB: *Laboratory Medicine: Hematology,* ed 6. St Louis, CV Mosby Co, 1982, pp 566–588.

5. Nelson DA: Erythrocyte disorders, in Henry JB (ed): *Todd-Sanford-Davidson Clinical Diagnosis and Management by Laboratory Methods,* ed 16. Philadelphia, WB Saunders Co, 1983, pp 1025–1026.

6. Petz LD, Garrathy G: Drug-induced immune hemolytic anemia, in *Acquired Immune Hemolytic Anemias.* New York, Churchill Livingstone Inc, 1980, pp 267–304.

16

Autoimmune Hemolytic Anemia

Autoimmune hemolytic anemia (AIHA) is caused by self-induced antibody to one's own red cell antigens.

Autoimmune hemolytic anemia is divided into two major categories by the laboratory characteristics of the autoantibody: autoantibody that is maximally active at 37°C (warm AIHA) and autoantibody that is maximally active at 4°C (cold AIHA). The clinical and laboratory characteristics of each type are summarized in Tables 16–1 and 16–2.

Pathophysiology

The pathogenesis of the antibody is unknown, although some abnormality of the normal immune pathways is suspected. AIHA can appear at any age, including infancy. The mechanism of cell destruction is mediated through red cell coating by IgG or IgM antibodies and complement.

Warm AIHA is associated with IgG antibody, with or without complement. Monocyte macrophage receptors primarily in the spleen attach to the Fc fragment of IgG leading to piecemeal destruction of the coated red cell. Complement alone absorbed to a red cell membrane causes negligible cell destruction, but when combined with IgG_1, IgG_3, or IgM, antibody cell destruction becomes exponential as receptors for C3 also contribute to cell destruction.

Table 16–1 Characteristics of Autoimmune Hemolytic Anemia

Clinical and Laboratory Findings	Warm AIHA	Cold AIHA
Clinical onset	Abrupt	Insidious
Jaundice	Usually present	Often absent
Splenomegaly	Present	Absent
Age	All ages	All ages
Sex	Slightly increased in females	Increased in females
Associated diseases	SLE, CLL, lymphoma	Viral pneumonia Histiocytic lymphoma
Laboratory		
Peripheral blood	Spherocytes, nucleated red cells	Red cell agglutinates

ABBREVIATIONS: AIHA = autoimmune hemolytic anemia; SLE = systemic lupus erythematosus; CLL = chronic lymphocytic leukemia.

Cold AIHA is associated with IgM antibody and complement. When IgM antibody becomes active at a thermal range approaching 37°C, cell destruction begins as the classic complement cascade is activated, through C1, C4, and C2 to the effector, C3b. C3b activates the membrane-attack system C5 through C9, leading to osmotic lysis. The C3 degradation product, C3b, adheres to the cell membrane. Receptors for C3b exist in the liver and spleen. Further degradation of C3b leaves C3d on the red cell membrane. There are no macrophage receptors for C3d and, although coated, red cell survival reaches a steady state without further macrophage destruction. This effect is seen in ^{51}Cr survival studies as an initial abrupt cell destruction followed by a slower second phase, which may approach normal cell survival.

Clinical Findings

The clinical history often suggests the type of AIHA present. Warm AIHA is of abrupt onset, with jaundice and splenomegaly, and anemia may be severe. Cold AIHA may be post infectious with a similar abrupt onset, and in children it may be associated classically with intravascular hemolysis. However, cold AIHA is more often

Table 16–2 Serologic Findings in Autoimmune Hemolytic Anemia

Test	Warm AIHA	Cold AIHA
Direct Coombs' test	2–4 +	2–4 +
Monospecific sera		
Anti-IgG	1 +	0
Anti-IgG + anti-C'	1 +	0
Anti-C' only	Rare	1 +
Serum antibody	IgG	IgM
Specificity	Anti-e, C, c; Rh precursor; LW; U; Wright[b]	Anti-I/i Pr(Sp₁), Iᵀ
Technique	Indirect antiglobulin, enzyme	Saline or enzyme
Cold agglutinin titer	Normal	>256
Serum complement	Normal or decreased	Decreased
Osmotic fragility	Increased	Normal

ABBREVIATIONS: AIHA = autoimmune hemolytic anemia.

insidious and well compensated, detected only when symptoms of fatigue and pallor associated with profound anemia appear. Cold AIHA is usually not associated with jaundice or splenomegaly despite marked anemia.

Approximately 70% of AIHAs are associated with some underlying disease and classified as secondary (Table 16–3). In general warm AIHA is associated with systemic lupus erythematosus (SLE) or other collagen disease, chronic lymphocytic leukemia, or lymphocytic lymphomas. The hemolytic anemia may precede the associated disease by several years, so these conditions should be screened for by physical examination, complete blood count, and testing for antinuclear antibody periodically. The association of warm AIHA with carcinoma is rare and unpredictable. True AIHA secondary to drug use is of the warm antibody type, as is discussed in chapter 15.

Cold AIHA can be divided clinically into acute postviral, chronic idiopathic, and cold agglutinin disease (CAD). Table 16–4 indicates pertinent characteristics seen in patients with cold AIHA as compared with healthy persons, in whom cold agglutinins are found in

Table 16–3 Diseases Associated with Autoimmune Hemolytic Anemia

	Antibody Specificity	
	Warm Ab	Cold Ab
Malignancy		
Lymphocytic leukemia	Anti-Rh, LW, Wright[b]	NA
Lymphocytic lymphoma	Anti-U, En[a]	
Carcinoma (ovary, thymus, gastrointestinal)		
Non-Hodgkins lymphoma Hodgkin's disease	NA	Anti-I, I[T], Pr (Sp₁)
Collagen disease		
SLE, rheumatoid arthritis, ulcerative colitis	Anti-Rh, LW, Wright[b], Anti-U, En[a]	NA
Infection		
Virus, *Mycoplasma*		Anti-I
Infectious mononucleosis		Anti-i
Clostridia, *E. coli*	Anti-T	
Drugs		
Methyldopa (Aldomet)	Anti-Rh	NA
L-dopa		
Indomethacin		

ABBREVIATIONS: AIHA = autoimmune hemolytic anemia; SLE = systemic lupus erythematosus; NA = not applicable.

low titer. Serologically all 3 types of cold AIHA are similar, varying in the titer of the cold agglutinin. Chronic idiopathic disease is usually seen in elderly women while cold agglutinin disease is usually associated with an underlying lymphoproliferative malignancy. As indicated in Table 16–5, cold agglutinins are normally present. They become abnormal as the titer rises above 1:256; the temperature of agglutination rises toward 37°C; and antibody with complement fixes to the patient's red cells as detected by a positive direct Coombs' test.

Cold AIHA is frequently associated with *Mycoplasma* pneumonia, so that roentgenograms of the chest and *Mycoplasma* titers

Table 16–4 Characteristics of Cold Agglutinins

Clinical Parameter	Physiologic	Post-infection	Chronic Idiopathic AIHA	CAD
Age	Any	Young	Older	Older
Onset	Asymp-tomatic	Acute, 10–14 days	Insidious	Insidious
Spleno-megaly	No	Frequent	No	With lym-phoma
Titer	≤1:32	≥1:64	≥1:256[a]	>1:10,000[a]
Specificity	Anti-I	Anti-I, i	Anti-I, i, Pr$_1$	Anti-I
DAT	0	+ (G,M,C3)	+ (C3)	+ (C3)
Intravascular hemolysis	No	40%	No	Rare
Transfuse?	Yes	Avoid	Avoid	Avoid

ABBREVIATIONS: AIHA = autoimmune hemolytic anemia; CAD = cold agglutinin disease; DAT = direct antiglobulin test.

[a]Representative range for titer

should be obtained. Cytomegalovirus (CMV), Epstein-Barr virus (EBV), measles, and mumps can be associated with AIHA, as can infectious mononucleosis. When cold AIHA is seen with lymphoma, the disease is usually large cell type.

Paroxysmal cold hemoglobinuria (PCH) is closely related clinically to cold AIHA, but differs in that the antibody is IgG and has a characteristic biphasic mode of action, first adsorbing to red cells at low temperature, and then causing intravascular hemolysis and hemoglobinuria as the temperature rises to 37°C. This biphasic hemolysin is the Donath-Landsteiner hemolysin. It is important to diagnose PCH since it is usually self-limited and treated by keeping the patient warm.

Hematologic Findings

Blood Cell Measurements. Anemia may be severe (<30g/L or 3g/dl Hb) with normochromic normocytic indices. There is variable reticulocytosis. In acute hemolysis granulocytosis with a left shift, a nonspecific stress reaction may be present. The leukocytosis can reach leukemoid proportions above 50×10^9/L (50×10^3/μl).

Table 16–5   Serologic Characteristics of Cold Agglutinins

Laboratory Finding	Physiologic Cold Agglutinins	Pathologic Cold Agglutinins
Titer	≤16	>256
Thermal range	4°C	Above 16°C
Direct Coombs' test	Negative	Positive

Peripheral Blood Smear Morphology.   Nucleated red cells, marked polychromasia, and anisocytosis are usually seen. In warm AIHA microspherocytes are present, the result of piecemeal ingestion of antibody-coated red cell membrane by macrophage. Cold AIHA may have marked morphologic changes if it is acutely post-infectious. However, clumping of red cells on the smear caused by cold agglutinins is more common.

Bone Marrow Examination.   The marrow is hypercellular, often approaching 80% cellularity as a result of normoblastic erythroid hyperplasia. Marrow iron is usually markedly increased, reflecting the accelerated erythroid turnover. Prolonged severe hemolysis may result in relative deficiencies of folic acid or vitamin B_{12} with a megaloblastic marrow and ultimately hypoplasia.

In idiopathic, cold AIHA, bone marrow aspiration may not indicate the underlying cause, but in cold agglutinin disease, it may reveal underlying lymphoma. In warm AIHA, marrow aspiration is most informative when the peripheral blood smear shows the presence of lymphocytosis or when lymphadenopathy is present. In the elderly, occult retroperitoneal lymphoma may be present, which will not be diagnosed by marrow aspirate.

Other Laboratory Tests

The following procedures require 15 to 20 mL of blood, which should be obtained and kept at 37°C until clotted; the serum is promptly removed from the cells and frozen to preserve complement. An EDTA specimen is also obtained. EDTA blocks nonspecific absorption of C', which allows a more accurate assessment of the DAT.

16.1   Direct Antiglobulin (Coombs') Test

Purpose.   The DAT detects globulin adsorbed to the patient's red cells and identifies immunoglobulin class. Monospecific reagents are used. C3d is believed to be a clinically significant fraction in AIHA, since it indicates prior absorption of C3 to the red cell membrane.

Principle, Procedure.   See Test 7.4.

Interpretation.   A clinically significant DAT is positive (1 to 4 +) with broad-spectrum reagents. Monospecific reagents are used automatically by sophisticated hospital blood banks and by all reference laboratories to identify the adsorbed globulins in an effort to categorize the AIHA as warm or cold type. In warm AIHA monospecific reagents for IgG or IgG and complement are positive. Monospecific reagents in cold AIHA show only complement since IgM antibody quickly separates from red cells collected at 37°C. Very weak complement reactions (+ / −) are not significant and do not indicate AIHA, whereas such reactions with anti-IgG may be clinically significant occasionally.

Very rarely, AIHA is present without a positive DAT. In such cases, ultrasensitive methods of Coombs' consumption or radioisotopes may reveal antibody molecules on the red cells; however, these tests are not generally available.

16.2   Serum Antibody Detection

Purpose.   These tests detect serum antibody, identify its blood group specificity, and characterize the temperature of reactivity.

Principle.   An indirect Coombs' test, which is often ordered, is only one method for screening the serum for antibody. Other techniques include treating cells with enzymes (ficin, papain, bromelin, or trypsin) to detect very low levels of antibody, and direct agglutination of saline-suspended cells. If screening tests show positive results, the antibody is identified (see also Test 13.2).

Procedure.   The patient's serum and red cell mixtures are tested using the previously mentioned techniques at 37°C and at 4°C. In addition to panels of reagent red cells, the patient's own cells are included as well as specimens of cord blood. The presence of agglutination or of hemolysis is significant and is graded 0 to 4 + (see also Test 13.1).

Interpretation.   Warm autoantibodies are IgG and, rarely, IgM, which agglutinate test cells by indirect antiglobulin tests and enzyme techniques strongly at 37°C and with no increase at

4°C. Specific antibody is found in 30% of cases and is Rh related (e, C, D, c), although the appearance of narrow specificity may only reflect differences in titers of antibody components. In the remainder, the antibody is directed at some primitive precursor of the Rh system or of the Wright system, and all cells are agglutinated except very rare test cells used at reference laboratories such as Rh null cells.

Since antibodies may be present from previous transfusions concurrent with autoantibodies, specificity should be determined. Although transfusions should be avoided, antibody specificity may help in selection of blood that is least incompatible if life-saving transfusion is needed. With steroids, serum antibodies may change specificity or disappear although the positive DAT often persists. The presence of serum antibody correlates more with active AIHA.

Cold autoantibodies are IgM, strongly reactive at 4°C and weaker at 37°C. Sometimes this differential is more apparent with diluted serum. Tests use saline suspensions or enzyme-treated cells. The antibodies may be hemolytic in vitro. Specificity is usually anti-I (reactive with all normal adult cells but not with cord red cells). Anti-i specificity (stronger reactions with cord red cells than adult cells) is seen with the rare AIHA occurring in infectious mononucleosis. Cold autoantibodies should be titered. In order to determine whether antibodies are autoantibodies, the patient's red cell antigens must be determined for the Rh and I systems.

16.3   Eluates of Red Cells

Purpose.   Eluates are prepared to determine if the globulin on red cells detected by the DAT is antibody and, if so, to determine blood group specificity.

Principle.   Red cell antibody-antigen bonds are disrupted by heat or by destroying the red cell membrane.

Procedure.   The test is usually performed automatically by the blood bank or reference laboratory. When the DAT is positive, heating the red cells at 56°C or chemically destroying them with cold organic solvents yields (elutes) the adsorbed antibody, which is then tested in parallel with the serum.

Interpretation.   In warm AIHA eluate antibody identity duplicates the serum. After recent incompatible transfusion in the absence of AIHA, the DAT may yield positive results because of the presence of coated donor cells, but the serum antibody is alloantibody. Antigen typing of red cells in such cases often indicates a mixed field of donor red cells and patient cells. After incompatible transfusion in the presence of AIHA, specificity of eluate and serum antibody may not be clarified until transfused cells have been cleared, usually several days. If eluate does not react with red cells, nonspecific globulin absorption as in myeloma or recent cephalothin therapy should be suspected. In cold AIHA antibody material is not elutable, and there is no reaction with red cells.

16.4   Cold Agglutinin Titer

Purpose.   The presence of abnormal cold agglutinins usually establishes that the AIHA is of the cold antibody type. Titer may indicate underlying disease and follows its progress.

Principle.   Cold agglutinins usually have anti-I specificity and agglutinate saline suspensions of adult red cells because of the I antigen present on the membrane. Rare cold agglutinins with anti-i specificity should not be expected to agglutinate adult red cells to the same titer; cord blood specimens are needed for accurate titers.

Procedure.   The patient's serum is titered in small-volume dilutions of 4, 8, 16, 32, and so forth, and incubated 2 hours at 4°C with a standard suspension of red cells, usually of the patient or of a group O donor, to avoid ABO blood group incompatibility. Cell-serum suspensions are read for agglutination. Titer is the highest serum dilution producing $1+$ agglutination.

Interpretation.   As indicated in Table 16–5 cold agglutinins are normally present. They become abnormal as the titer rises above 1:256. With the rise in titer, the temperature of agglutination often rises toward 37°C, and antibody with complement fixes to the patient's red cells as detected by a positive direct Coombs' test. Physiologic cold agglutinins have titers less than or equal to 16. Titers to 64 are seen after recent respiratory viral infections. Titers are 256 and above in cold AIHA of elderly women or, with viral pneumonia, usually 1000 to 8000. In chronic cold agglutinin disease titers are often 50,000 or higher, but may not always be associated with clinical hemolysis, although vascular occlusion may occur at low temperatures.

    Progress of cold AIHA can be followed by repeating titers weekly in viral pneumonia or idiopathic disease, and monthly in cold agglutinin disease, particularly in lymphoma for which the patient is receiving chemotherapy.

16.5 Donath-Landsteiner Test (Biphasic Hemolysin)

Purpose. The Donath-Landsteiner test diagnoses PCH, which may have a clinical history similar to cold AIHA, but is usually a self-limited disease that is treated conservatively by keeping the patient warm.

Principle. The Donath-Landsteiner test reproduces in vitro a reaction that occurs in vivo. The hemolysin, a complement-dependent IgG antibody, agglutinates cells at 4°C and lyses them at warmer temperatures, usually considered as 37°C. Other hemolysins may react at single temperatures, 4°C or 37°C, but are not biphasic. The Donath-Landsteiner hemolysin does not lyse cells with reverse incubations, 37°C to 4°C.

Procedure. The patient's serum is incubated with test red cells at 4°C and then at 37°C, and serum-cell suspension is observed for hemolysis, which is usually marked (3 to 4+). If biphasic hemolysis is present it is tested against panels of reagent red cells to determine blood group specificity, which is often in the P or I system.

Interpretation. A biphasic hemolysin indicates PCH, occasionally seen in patients with a history that suggests cold AIHA. If intravascular hemolysis has recently occurred, the DAT results may be negative. Paroxysmal cold hemoglobinuria is commonly postviral but can be seen with congenital syphilis so that definitive syphilitic serology, that is, the fluorescent treponemal antibody test should be performed.

16.6 Ham's Test for Acid Hemolysis

Purpose. Ham's test is performed to exclude PNH, which is not caused by serum antibody but by an acquired clonal defect of the red cell membrane. Whenever antibody hemolysis is suspected, PNH should be considered and excluded.

Principle. The patient's red cell is supersensitive to human complement lysis activated at a low serum pH. Human complement and its activator, Factor B (previously C_3PA) is present in all normal serums, including the patient's. The patient's serum is shown to have no antibody against the patient's or any other red cell.

Procedure. Normal sera acidified to pH 6.8 are incubated at 37°C with the patient's red cells and observed for hemolysis, which may be faint to 4 +. Controls are established to prove the defect is limited to the patient's red cells.

Interpretation. False-positive hemolysis is seen if the acidified sera contain a cold agglutinin. True-positives are positive only with human, not guinea pig, complement. The test can be confirmed by sucrose lysis.

16.7 Serum Complement Measurement

Purpose. A decrease in serum complement is most often associated with IgM antibody and cold AIHA. It can, however, be decreased in warm AIHA as well and therefore is not absolute in categorizing AIHA as the warm rather than the cold type.

Principle. Sheep red cells are lysed in the presence of antibody to sheep red cells from rabbits (amboceptor) if complement is present. The source of the complement is the patient's fresh serum. The reaction can be used to quantitate complement.

Specimen. Fresh serum, separated from red cells and immediately frozen, is used as a specimen.

Procedure. Lytic complement tests are not easily performed and often require reference laboratories. Serum complement is measured by lysis of 50% of a spectrophotometrically determined red cell suspension in 1 hour. $C'H_{50}$ is 50 to 100 U in most laboratories, but normal ranges must be determined for each.

Interpretation. Serum complement is decreased in cold AIHA since the antibodies are complement binding. Levels are also often decreased in warm AIHA, with serum showing anticomplementary activity.

16.8   Serum Haptoglobin Quantitation

Purpose.   The absence of haptoglobin is seen in hemolysis or in liver failure. The serum haptoglobin test indicates that hemolysis may be present if liver function is normal.

Principle, Procedure, and Specimen.   See Test 7.3.

Interpretation.   Normal values are usually 0.4 to 1.8 g/L (40 to 80 mg/dl), with active hemolysis values of <0.1 g/L (10 mg/dl). In cold AIHA when pneumonia is present, haptoglobin as an acute reactant protein may be markedly increased, obscuring expected low levels seen with hemolysis, and the test is no longer helpful (see Test 7.3).

16.9   Osmotic Fragility Test

Purpose.   This test is of limited usefulness but is positive in the presence of spherocytes.

Principle.   Spherocytes with increased cell volume have little margin remaining for increased cell water imbibed from hypotonic solutions, and they undergo osmotic lysis.

Procedure.   The patient's red cells are suspended in a series of 10 saline solutions that are increasingly hypotonic. The amount of hemolysis is measured by colorimeter or spectrophotometer and converted to a percentage of cells lysed as compared with a totally lysed specimen. Red cells do not normally lyse until saline is .0045 (.45%) or less.

Interpretation.   Hemolysis increases with the presence of spherocytosis, usually seen in warm AIHA. It is quicker and clinically more satsifactory to review the peripheral smear instead.

16.10   Antibody Titers for Myloplasma and Viruses

Purpose.   Testing for mycoplasma and virus antibody titers identifies, usually in retrospect, an infectious etiologic agent in cold AIHA.

Principle. These antibodies require acute- and convalescent-phase sera obtained 7 to 10 days apart to show a rise in titer of antibody for specific viruses.

Procedure. The tests are usually performed at county or state reference laboratories, which require both specimens to be submitted. The agent suspected should be specified; most common is *Mycoplasma,* occasionally Epstein-Barr virus, or cytomegalovirus.

Interpretation. A three-dilution rise in titer is required for the test to be diagnostic, since previous exposure to these viruses is fairly common. The presence of IgM antibody suggests recent infection.

16.11   Antinuclear Antibody Test

Purpose. Antinuclear antibody by indirect immunofluorescence should be ordered when warm AIHA is diagnosed, particularly in young females, to determine if SLE is the underlying disease, for warm AIHA frequently precedes SLE by months or even years.

Principle. The patient's serum contains antibody to nuclear material (shared by many species). If nuclear material is present, the antibody attaches to it.

Procedure. The patient's serum is incubated with a nuclear antigen source (tissue culture cells, rat kidney, human granulocytes, etc). The antigen-antibody combination is detected by antiglobulin reagent that has been tagged with a fluorescent dye. Microscopy with ultraviolet light causes antinuclear antibody combinations to glow, after which the patient's serum can be titered.

Interpretation. Titers above 1:20 in most laboratories are suspicious and titers of 1:80 or greater are considered diagnostic of SLE. Positive tests of low titer are seen in 3% of the elderly; high titers in the elderly suggest drug-induced AIHA of the methyldopa (Aldomet) type (see chapter 15). Supplemental tests for anti-DNA, anti-Sm may confirm the diagnosis of SLE.

16.12　Evaluation of Occult Lymphoma

Purpose.　Warm AIHA may precede lymphoma by years, but AIHA may be the only visible symptom in concomitant unsuspected disease, usually in the elderly patient.

Principle.　Physical examination should include evaluation of all lymph node areas and evaluation of hepatosplenomegaly.

Procedure.　Noninvasive procedures are utilized. These may include computed tomography of the retroperitoneum, pulmonary hilus, radionuclide scans, and intravenous pyelograms for lateral displacement of ureters.

Interpretation.　A biopsy should be performed on positive findings to confirm the diagnosis.

Course and Treatment

Warm AIHA usually responds in 7 to 10 days to high-dose steroid therapy, which suppresses antibody production and inhibits macrophage adherence. In cases that fail to respond to steroids or relapse immediately as steroids are tapered, immunosuppressive medication or splenectomy that reduces the macrophage pool are usually successful. Intravenous gamma globulin has had limited success after splenectomy.

There is little therapy available for cold AIHA; it does not respond to steroid therapy, immunosuppressives, or splenectomy. In CAD associated with a lymphoproliferative disorder, treatment of the underlying disease often results in improvement of cold agglutinin titers. Chronic idiopathic cold AIHA seen in elderly women waxes and wanes, possibly in relation to urinary tract infections or other stresses.

PCH is usually treated by keeping the patient warm. It is self-limited, responding to recovery from the underlying infection. Aggressive therapy should therefore be avoided.

PNH is not an immune hemolytic anemia, although these patients may be identified during serologic evaluation of true immune hemolytic anemias. Hemoglobin levels are maintained by transfusion of saline-washed or frozen red cells, thus removing plasma proteins that may stimulate further hemolysis.

Although as much as 30% of patients may show no reaction to transfusion, it should generally be avoided in both warm and cold

AIHA, since it induces alloantibodies, further complicating cross-matching, and may increase autoantibody titer and avidity for red cells accelerating hemolysis. It is a temporizing measure since red cell survival is less than 1 week in warm AIHA and may be minutes or hours in cold AIHA. If symptoms of impending stroke or myocardial infarction appear, transfusion may be necessary.

References

1. Bell CA, Fairbanks VF: Hemolytic disorders, in Fairbanks VF (ed): *Current Hematology.* New York, John Wiley & Sons Inc, 1981, pp 65–122.
2. Issit PD: *Applied Blood Group Serology,* ed 3. Miami, Montgomery Scientific Publications, 1985, pp 72–104, 664–665.
3. Landl TH: *Blood: Textbook of Hematology.* Boston, Little, Brown and Co, 1987, pp 297–318.
4. Petz LD, Garratty G: Serologic investigation of autoimmune hemolytic anemia, in *Acquired Immune Hemolytic Anemia.* New York, Churchill Livingstone Inc, 1980, pp 139–184.

The Polycythemias

17

Polycythemia: Primary and Secondary

Erythrocytosis (polycythemia) is defined as an elevated red blood cell volume and is associated with increased hemoglobin level, hematocrit value, and red blood cell count. The terms "erythrocytosis" and "polycythemia" are often used interchangeably, although the latter actually implies an increase in multiple hematopoietic cell lines. For simplicity, however, the terms will be used interchangeably in this chapter. Erythrocytosis can result from an intrinsic bone marrow defect, altered erythropoietin regulatory activity, or decreased plasma volume (Table 17–1).

Polycythemia Vera (Primary Erythrocytosis)

Primary erythrocytosis, or polycythemia vera, is a myeloproliferative syndrome that occurs when all hematopoietic cell lines undergo uncontrolled proliferation with intact maturation. The abnormal cells are derived from a single parent cell, and the proliferation is erythropoietin-independent. The disease has an estimated annual incidence of 4 cases per 1 million population, there is a slight male predominance, and most patients are >40 years of age. The diagnostic features of polycythemia vera are separated into major and minor criteria, as shown below.

Table 17-1   Classification of Erythrocytosis

Type	Examples
Primary	Polycythemia vera
Secondary (physiologically appropriate)	Residence at high altitude Chronic pulmonary or cardiac disease High oxygen affinity hemoglobinopathy Increased carboxyhemoglobin[a] and met-hemoglobin Decreased 2,3 diphosphoglycerate
Secondary (physiologically inappropriate)	Tumors producing erythropoietin or anabolic steroids Cystic renal disease Hydronephrosis Adrenal cortical hypersecretion
Relative (stress)	Disorders associated with decreased plasma volume[b] such as certain diarrhea, emesis, and renal diseases

[a] Carboxyhemoglobin increased in people who smoke

[b] Plasma volume often somewhat decreased in patients who smoke

Major Criteria

1. Elevated red blood cell mass

2. Normal arterial oxygen saturation

3. Splenomegaly

Minor Criteria

1. Platelet count $>400 \times 10^9$/L (400×10^3/μl)

2. White blood cell count $>12 \times 10^9$/L (12×10^3/μl)

3. Elevated leukocyte alkaline phosphatase level

4. Elevated vitamin B_{12} level or vitamin B_{12}-binding capacity

   A diagnosis of polycythemia vera can be made when all 3 major criteria are present or when the first 2 major criteria plus 2 minor criteria are identified.

Secondary Erythrocytosis

Patients with secondary erythrocytosis have an erythropoietinmediated increase in red cell volume that may be either physiologically appropriate or inappropriate. Physiologically appropriate erythrocytosis results from a hypoxic stimulus, such as residence at high altitude, chronic pulmonary or cardiac diseases, high oxygen affinity hemoglobinopathies, and increased carboxyhemoglobin levels. Patients with secondary polycythemia that is physiologically inappropriate do not have tissue hypoxia but have excess production of either erythropoietin or anabolic steroids. Disorders associated with this type of secondary erythrocytosis include: various tumors producing erythropoietin or anabolic steroids; renal disorders, such as cystic disease and hydronephrosis; and adrenal cortical hypersecretion.

Relative Erythrocytosis

In patients with relative or stress erythrocytosis, the primary disorder is one of decreased plasma volume rather than true erythrocytosis.

Pathophysiology

Bone marrow production of red blood cells is regulated by erythropoietin, a hormonelike substance that induces committed bone marrow stem cells to mature into red blood cells. The erythropoietin precursor substance is produced in the kidneys in response to tissue hypoxia. Once oxygen delivery to the tissues is increased, erythropoietin production is suppressed.

In patients with primary erythrocytosis (polycythemia vera), a stem cell defect results in unregulated production of all hematopoietic elements. The production of red blood cells in this disorder is not regulated by erythropoietin.

The excess red cell production in secondary erythrocytosis is erythropoietin-mediated. In patients with physiologically appropriate secondary erythrocytosis, the tissue hypoxia responsible for erythropoietin production can result from decreased oxygen in the atmosphere, impaired oxygen-carbon dioxide exchange in the lungs, or decreased delivery of oxygen to tissues (Table 17–1). In all of the disorders associated with secondary erythrocytosis, the erythropoietin production will decrease if the tissue hypoxia is alleviated.

Physiologically inappropriate erythrocytosis occurs when high levels of erythropoietin, erythropoietinlike substances or anabolic steroids drive the bone marrow to produce excessive numbers of red blood cells in the absence of tissue hypoxia. The disorders associated with this type of secondary erythrocytosis are listed in Table 17–2 and include a variety of neoplasms from the kidney, liver, uterus, overy, adrenal gland, and brain. The nonneoplastic

Table 17–2 Disorders Associated with Physiologically Inappropriate Erythrocytosis

Organ	Disorder
Kidney	Renal cystic disease
	Hydronephrosis
	Transplant rejection
	Renal cell carcinoma
Liver	Hepatoma
Uterus	Leiomyoma
Ovary	Ovarian carcinoma
Adrenal	Pheochromocytoma
	Adrenal cortical hyperplasia
	Hemangioblastoma[a]
Brain	Cerebellar hemangioblastoma

[a]Associated with Von Hippel–Lindau disease

disorders associated with physiologically inappropriate erythrocytosis are largely renal diseases.

The relative or stress erythrocytosis seen in patients with decreased plasma volume can be secondary to either dehydration or excess water loss secondary to renal or gastrointestinal abnormalities. Decreased plasma volume is also a contributing factor to the erythrocytosis frequently seen in heavy smokers.

Clinical Findings

Patients with polycythemia vera are generally middle-aged and present with symptoms related to increased blood volume, thromboembolus, or hemorrhagic phenomena. These patients often experience fatigue, malaise, headache, light-headedness, and pruritus. The postulated cause of pruritus is excessive histamine release by basophils, which may also explain the increased frequency of peptic ulcer disease in these patients.

The thromboembolic and hemorrhagic episodes seen both at presentation and during the disease course in patients with polycythemia vera are secondary to thrombocytosis, platelet functional defects, and hyperviscosity. The fibrinogen level is also often increased and can accentuate the patient's hypercoagulable state.

On physical examination, patients with polycythemia vera frequently have splenomegaly and appear plethoric, with conjunctival and retinal venous engorgement.

The clinical findings in patients with secondary erythrocytosis vary greatly depending on the underlying cause, eg, patients with physiologically appropriate secondary erythrocytosis may have manifestations of cardiopulmonary disease, such as cyanosis, clubbing, and increased respiratory rate. Many other patients with secondary erythrocytosis, however, may have no specific clinical findings. Splenomegaly is not a clinical manifestation of either physiologically appropriate or inappropriate erythrocytosis.

In patients with relative erythrocytosis, the underlying cause of the decreased plasma volume is usually apparent and includes such disorders as diarrhea, vomiting, dehydration, and renal disease. The spleen is generally not enlarged in patients with relative erythrocytosis.

Approach to Diagnosis

Patients should be evaluated for possible primary or secondary erythrocytosis when elevated hemoglobin levels and hematocrit values are detected in the absence of an obvious clinical cause. An algorithm that would encompass all possible diagnostic explanations for erythocytosis is very complex and includes tests rarely performed in routine practice. A simplified approach to the diagnosis of erythrocytosis, however, will allow classification of most patients' diseases.

1. Eliminate cases of relative erythrocytosis by careful clinical evaluation for disorders associated with loss of plasma volume and by measurement of red cell mass.

2. If the patient has an established diagnosis of a neoplasm or renal disease that has been associated with erythrocytosis, consider it a possible cause of erythrocytosis.

3. Assess other hematologic features for abnormalities not readily explained by the clinical setting, notably leukocytosis with left shift, basophilia, and thrombocytosis.

4. Proceed to evaluate for diagnostic criteria of polycythemia vera in patients in whom these other unexplained hematologic abnormalities are identified.

5. In patients with no other unexplained hematologic abnormalities, distinguish between physiologic and nonphysiologic secondary erythrocytosis. Most of the physiologically appropriate cases of erythrocytosis will be secondary to obvious pulmonary or cardiovascular disorders or to smoking. Causes such as high oxygen

affinity hemoglobinopathy, however, require more extensive laboratory investigation.

6. In the absence of polycythemia vera or a physiologic cause for the erythrocytosis, a diverse group of disorders, including occult tumors and renal diseases, should be considered (see Table 17–2).

Hematologic Findings

The hematologic findings of polycythemia vera differ from those of secondary and relative erythrocytosis. In primary erythrocytosis (polycythemia vera), abnormalities are detected in all 3 cell lines in the blood, while secondary and relative erythrocytosis are generally associated with only red blood cell changes.

Blood Cell Measurements. In polycythemia vera, the hemoglobin level, hematocrit value, white blood cell count, and platelet count are all characteristically elevated. The red blood cell indices and red cell distribution width (RDW) are generally normal but may be abnormal in patients with concurrent iron deficiency. The percentage of reticulocytes is within normal limits.

Patients with secondary erythrocytosis have an elevated hemoglobin level and hematocrit value with normal white blood cell and platelet counts. The red cell indices and RDW are generally normal. The absolute reticulocyte count is often elevated.

The elevated hematocrit value noted in patients with relative erythrocytosis is almost always <0.60 (60%) and is not associated with an increased reticulocyte count.

Peripheral Blood Smear Morphology. In polycythemia vera, the erythrocytes are generally normocytic and normochromic, except when there is concurrent iron deficiency. Nucleated red cells may be present. The white blood cell differential count generally shows circulating immature cells and basophilia; eosinophilia may also be present. Platelet counts are increased, and the platelets may be enlarged.

The peripheral blood smear morphology in secondary erythrocytosis is normal, except for the increase in normal-appearing red blood cells. Polychromasia may be present.

No specific morphologic abnormalities are present in blood smears from patients with relative erythrocytosis.

Bone Marrow Examination. In polycythemia vera, the bone marrow is characteristically hypercellular with elevated counts in all 3 cell lines. Although an increase in reticulin fibers can be detected at diagnosis, there is generally a progressive increase in the amount of reticulin fibrosis throughout the patient's disease course. As this fibrosis increases, there is an associated progressive decrease in the cellularity that is sometimes referred to as the "spent phase" of polycythemia vera. Storage iron is often markedly decreased because of increased red cell production, bleeding, and the periodic phlebotomy that is often used for treatment.

Bone marrow examination is generally not necessary to establish a diagnosis of secondary erythrocytosis. If bone marrow is obtained, erythroid hyperplasia will be identified. In patients with relative erythrocytosis, bone marrow examination is not indicated.

Other Laboratory Tests

Laboratory tests that can be utilized to distinguish polycythemia vera, secondary polycythemia, and relative polycythemia are shown in Table 17–3.

17.1   Red Blood Cell Volume

Purpose.   Measurement of the red blood cell volume can be used to distinguish true and relative erythrocytosis.

Principle.   Erythrocyte volume is measured by a dilution technique using radiolabeled red blood cells, with the degree of dilution directly proportional to red cell volume.

Specimen.   Anticoagulated venous blood is used.

Procedure.   A fixed number of the patient's erythrocytes are radiolabeled in vitro and intravenously injected back into the patient. After a 10 to 20-minute equilibrium period, a second sample of venous blood is drawn from the opposite arm. A scintillation counter is used to measure the radioactivity of the injected sample and the second venous sample. Red cell volume is calculated using the formula:

$$\text{Red Cell Volume} = \frac{\text{Injected Radioactivity}}{\text{Radioactivity of Erythrocytes After Mixing}}$$

Interpretation.   An elevated erythrocyte volume is seen in primary and secondary erythrocytosis but not in relative erythrocytosis.

Table 17–3 Laboratory Tests Used to Distinguish Types of Erythrocytosis

Laboratory Test	Test Result: Polycythemia Vera	Secondary Erythrocytosis[a]	Relative Erythrocytosis
Red cell volume	Increased	Increased	Normal
Erythropoietin	Usually decreased	Normal to increased	Usually normal
PO_2	Usually normal	Decreased in some cases	Normal
LAP[b]	Increased	Usually normal[c]	Usually normal[c]
Vitamin B_{12}	Increased	Normal	Normal
Vitamin B_{12} Binding proteins	Increased	Normal	Normal
Carboxy-hemoglobin[d]	Usually normal	May be increased	May be increased
Uric acid	Increased	Normal	Normal
Histamine	Increased	Normal	Normal
Serum iron	Decreased	Normal	Normal
Storage iron (BM)	Decreased	Normal	Normal
Hemoglobin-opathy	Absent	Present in some cases	Absent
Platelet function	Abnormal	Normal	Normal
BM chromo-some abnor-malities	May be present	Absent	Absent

ABBREVIATIONS: BM = bone marrow.

[a] Includes both physiologically appropriate and inappropriate causes of secondary erythrocytosis

[b] Leukocyte alkaline phosphatase

[c] Can be elevated if patient is pregnant, on birth control pills, or if patient has inflammatory disorder

[d] Increased in patients who smoke

Notes and Precautions. Because red cell volume is related to lean body mass, spuriously low values can occur in patients with marked obesity. When ^{51}chromium is used to radiolabel the patient's erythrocytes, the patient should not have previously received antibiotics or ascorbic acid because these substances impair the labeling process, yielding spuriously low results.

17.2 Arterial Oxygen Saturation

Purpose. Arterial oxygen saturation is performed to demonstrate the presence of hypoxemia.

Principle, Procedure. The standard nomogram and spectrophotometric techniques used to measure arterial oxygen saturation are detailed in clinical pathology texts.

Specimen. Arterial blood specimens for blood gas determinations are collected with a minimum amount of heparin, maintained under anaerobic conditions, and analyzed promptly.

Interpretation. When the arterial oxygen saturation is less than the established normal range, hypoxia is present.

Notes and Precautions. Proper and prompt specimen handling is necessary to ensure the accuracy of the result. Normal range values are affected by altitude and need to be established for each laboratory.

Ancillary Tests

Other laboratory tests that can be utilized on a selected basis to distinguish the three types of erythrocytosis are listed in Table 17–3. The characteristic test result for each type of erythrocytosis is also included in this table.

Course and Treatment

The increased blood viscosity associated with erythrocytosis can be the cause of significant morbidity and even mortality in these patients. Blood viscosity increases dramatically as the patient's hematocrit value rises from 0.50 to 0.60 (50% to 60%). As viscosity accelerates, the oxygen-carrying ability of erythrocytes actually decreases. In patients with physiologically appropriate secondary erythrocytosis, this decrease in oxygen delivery leads to further eryth-ropoietin release and greater erythrocytosis. In addition to impaired oxygen delivery, patients with increased blood viscosity are at risk for thrombosis, especially in slow flow rate venous channels.

Polycythemia Vera

Polycythemia vera typically follows an indolent, slowly progressive disease course with gradual evolution from a hypercellular bone marrow picture to bone marrow fibrosis, with associated decline in peripheral blood counts (spent phase). Thrombosis and hemor-rhage caused by increased blood viscosity, thrombocytosis, and platelet function abnormalities are causes of increased morbidity and mortality in patients with polycythemia vera. With proper man-agement, risks from these complications can be substantially re-duced. Without treatment, patients with polycythemia vera have a median survival of about 18 months. With treatment, however, the survival can be extended to 8 to 12 years. Treatment modalities that have been utilized successfully in patients with polycythemia vera include periodic phlebotomy to reduce the hematocrit value, and alkylating agent or radioactive phosphorus therapy to reduce bone marrow production of all hematopoietic elements. Patients under-going periodic phlebotomy should be monitored for the develop-ment of iron deficiency, because hypochromic erythrocytes have increased internal viscosity and decreased deformability that en-hances blood viscosity and further compromises tissue oxygen de-livery. Both alkylating agent therapy and radioactive phosphorus therapy have been associated with increased incidence of myelo-dysplasia and acute leukemia.

Secondary Erythrocytosis

The clinical course and proper management of patients with sec-ondary erythrocytosis is dependent on determining the specific cause of the excessive red cell production. While there is no cu-rative treatment for some cases, such as the high oxygen affinity hemoglobinopathies, other causes, such as certain cardiopulmo-nary disorders, can be alleviated by proper treatment. To reduce blood viscosity, periodic phlebotomy may be indicated for some patients with physiologically appropriate secondary erythrocytosis.

Management of the neoplasm is the primary treatment goal in patients with excessive erythropoietin production by tumor. In a small proportion of patients with tumors of the kidney, adrenal gland, liver, or brain, the erythropoietin production is the first sign that the patient has a neoplasm. Identification of these tumors before they are clinically obvious may be associated with improved survival. Management of the nonneoplastic renal disease is necessary to reduce erythropoietin production in this group of patients with physiologically inappropriate erythrocytosis.

Relative Erythrocytosis

In these patients, the primary cause of the decreased plasma volume is often apparent and can usually be properly treated. Other factors that could aggravate the erythrocytosis, such as hypertension and smoking, should be addressed. The patient's course and treatment vary with the underlying cause of the reduced plasma volume.

References

1. Berk PD, Goldberg JD, Donovan PB, et al: Therapeutic recommendations in polycythemia vera based on Polycythemia Vera Study Group Protocols. *Semin Hematol* 1986; 23:132–143.

2. Ellis JT, Peterson P, Geller SA, et al: Studies of the bone marrow in polycythemia vera and the evolution of myelofibrosis and second hematologic malignancies. *Semin Hematol* 1986; 23:144–155.

3. Golde DW, Hocking WG, Koeffler HP, et al: Polycythemia: Mechanisms and management. *Ann Intern Med* 1981; 95:71–87.

4. Murphy S: Polycythemia vera, in Williams WJ, Beutler E, Erslev AJ, et al (eds): *Hematology,* ed 3. New York, McGraw-Hill International Book Co, 1983, pp 185–196.

5. Brodsky I: The differential diagnosis of the polycythemic states. *Ann Clin Lab Sci* 1980; 10:311–319.

PART 4

Reactive Disorders of Granulocytes and Monocytes

18

Neutrophilia

Leukocytosis is an absolute increase in peripheral white cells above $10 \times 10^9/L$ ($10 \times 10^3/\mu l$). Although the term "leukocytosis" can include eosinophils and basophils, it is generally interpreted as an increase in neutrophilic granulocytes. Thus, neutrophilia is defined by an absolute count greater than $8 \times 10^9/L$ ($8 \times 10^3/\mu l$), or by a percentage of segmented neutrophils and band cells in excess of 0.80 (80%).

Pathophysiology

Granulocytes are derived from a pluripotential stem cell in the bone marrow that also gives rise to the monocyte cell line. Granulocytic maturation progresses from stem cells to myeloblasts, promyelocytes and myelocytes in a series of 3 or 4 cell divisions. Metamyelocytes, band forms, and segmented forms are intermediate and mature nondividing cells. Myelocytes are the largest population of dividing cells that, combined with a half-life of 6 to 7 hours, allows rapid increases in mature granulocytes. Granulocyte distribution is divided into 3 compartments: marrow production (7 to 11 days), circulating granulocyte pool (6 hours), and tissue phase (4 to 5 days). The total granulocyte pool is approximately evenly distributed between circulating granulocytes and those temporarily sequestered in the microcirculation, the marginated pool.

The factors controlling neutrophil migration from marrow to circulating pool are unknown, although colony-stimulating factor may be involved. Neutrophils enter the tissue phase in response to various chemotactic factors derived from complement activation, the fibrinolytic system, lymphokines, bacterial endotoxin, and prostaglandins. Once in the tissue compartment, neutrophils do not return to the circulation, but die there.

The number of circulating or countable granulocytes is determined by: marrow production; rate of entry into the peripheral circulating pool; shifts between circulating and marginated pools; and rate of exit into the tissues. The first two factors are the most important in protracted peripheral granulocytosis, the third in physiologic granulocytosis. Granulocytes act as phagocytic cells whose cytotoxic effect is mediated in part by cytoplasmic granules. The immature cells, blasts and promyelocytes contain primary granules, seen as dense azurophilic masses in progranulocytes. Smaller secondary or specific granules first appear at the myelocyte phase. In the intermediate cells, myelocytes and metamyelocytes, both primary and secondary granules are visible with secondary granules predominating in the mature forms, band forms and polymorphonuclear neutrophilic leukocytes (PMNs). The staining characteristics of the secondary granules with Romanovsky dyes (Wright's or Wright-Giemsa) label the leukocytes as neutrophilic, eosinophilic, or basophilic. Both primary and secondary granules contain enzymes; the primary granules contain peroxidase; and the secondary granules contain alkaline phosphatase, lysozyme, and vitamin B_{12} binding protein. Elevation of the granulocyte count above $50 \times 10^9/L$ ($50 \times 10^3/\mu l$) with some immature cells may simulate chronic granulocytic leukemia, and is therefore categorized as a leukemoid reaction.

Clinical Findings

Clinical findings are related to the underlying disorder. A list of the most common causes of neutrophilic granulocytosis is shown in Table 18–1. The most frequent causes are infection, usually from pyogenic bacteria; inflammation caused by tissue or tumor necrosis; hematologic disorders; and physiologic stress of cold, heat, or exercise. Inflammation or infection is commonly associated with fever, localized pain and swelling, and purulent exudates. In the elderly, inflammation or infection may not provoke neutrophilia, although a shift to the left may be present. Although certain drugs that produce neutrophilia are associated with local irritation of tissue (etiocholanolone, histamine, or endotoxin), others produce no such local effect (heparin, digitalis), but have a stimulatory effect on marrow

Table 18-1   Causes of Neutrophilic Granulocytosis

Physiologic stress or physical agents (usual range: 13 to 30 $\times$ 10^9/L or 13 to 30 $\times$ 10^3/μl)
  Excessive cold or heat
  Exercise
  Postprandial
  Pregnancy (3rd trimester)
  Newborn
  Emotional states (excitement, depression)
  Nausea, vomiting

Infection
  Bacterial:
    Gram positive—*Staphylococcus, Streptococcus, Pneumococcus*
    Gram negative—*E. coli, P. aeruginosa, Pasteurella*
  Rickettsial: typhus
  Parasitic: liver fluke
  Fungal: coccidioidomycosis

Inflammation or tissue necrosis
  Myocardial infarction
  Pneumonia
  Peritonitis
  Collagen disorders (vasculitis, myositis)
  Tumor necrosis

Hematologic disorders
  Acute hemorrhage
  Hemolysis (hemolytic anemia, transfusion reaction)
  Myeloproliferative (polycythemia vera, myeloid metaplasia, or
    myelofibrosis)
  CGL

Drugs/Chemicals
  Etiocholanolone
  Epinephrine
  Digitalis
  Steroids
  Heparin
  Histamine
  Endotoxin

Metabolic
  Diabetic acidosis
  Eclampsia
  Gout (with acute inflammation)
  Thyroid Storm

Idiopathic (10,000–15,000/mm^3)

ABBREVIATIONS: CGL = chronic granulocytic leukemia.

Table 18–2   Findings for Leukemoid Reaction and Chronic Granulocytic Leukemia

Test	Leukemoid Reaction	CGL
White cell count (No. × 10⁹/L)	<100	May be 30–500
%PMNs	Up to 95%	May be normal (60%–70%)
Immature granulocytes	To myelocyte	Usually includes occasional progranulocytes or blasts
Eosinophils, basophils	Normal or decreased	Slightly increased
Nucleated red cells	Occasional	Late, may be common
Bone marrow M/E ratio	6–8:1	≥15:1
LAP	>100	<10

ABBREVIATIONS: CGL = chronic granulocytic leukemia; PMN = polymorphonuclear leukocytes; M/E = myeloid:erythroid ratio; LAP = leukocyte alkaline phosphatase.

or affect the distribution between the circulating or marginated pools (eg, steroids).

Approach to Diagnosis

The differential diagnosis of leukocytosis is reactive process (leukemoid) vs chronic granulocytic leukemia (CGL). Laboratory findings that assist in the differential cell count are listed in Table 18–2. A clinical history of acute infection or inflammation is helpful in excluding CGL or other myeloproliferative disorders such as polycythemia vera, myeloid metaplasia, or myelofibrosis.

1. The total white cell count and differential cell count should be repeated at intervals to establish persistence and magnitude of the neutrophilia. The appropriate interval depends on the toxicity apparent in the patient. At least 4 to 5 hours is necessary to allow significant changes as neutrophils shift from the circulating to the marginated compartment. In the asymptomatic patient the granulocytosis should be documented over several days to 1 or 2 weeks. The serial findings help determine prognosis and whether the next step in diagnostic evaluation, bone marrow aspiration, should be undertaken.

2. Bone marrow aspiration is performed when the granulocytosis does not appear to be physiologic or reactive; eg, when the clinical history is not definitive, the granulocytosis persists or is above $20 \times 10^9/L$ $(20 \times 10^3/\mu l)$, increased immature granulocytes are present, or another cell line is also abnormal. An aliquot should be submitted for karyotype analysis since the presence of Philadelphia chromosome (Ph[1]) is diagnostic of CGL.

3. Leukocyte alkaline phosphatase helps distinguish leukemoid reactions from CGL (see Test 18.1).

4. Appropriate bacteriologic studies are performed if the cause of granulocytosis is suspected to be infection.

Hematologic Findings

Acute granulocytosis caused by physiologic stimuli is transient, usually resulting from a shift of marginated granulocytes to the circulating pool; no change in bone marrow cellularity is therefore expected. Chronic granulocytosis is reflected in increased marrow granulopoiesis with as much as a tenfold increase in granulocyte turnover, which is more marked in children than in adults. A hypercellular marrow results. Even preceding an increase in the rate of turnover, cells may be released prematurely from the marrow, producing a left shift. Increased production of granulocytes in benign conditions has no effect on the size of the liver, spleen, or lymph nodes.

The magnitude of granulocytosis and the relative proportion of band cells to segmented neutrophils may indicate the etiology and the ultimate prognosis. When more than 80% of cells are polymorphonuclear neutrophilic leukocytes (PMNs), contained inflammation above the diaphragm (eg, otitis media, pneumonia, abscess) should be considered. When more than 10% of cells are band cell forms, perforated viscus, inflammation below the diaphragm (eg, perforated diverticulum or appendix, ulcer, or carcinoma of the colon with peritonitis) or hemorrhagic pancreatitis should be considered.

A left shift to the myelocyte phase is seen in severe infections. The presence of blasts or more than occasional promyelocytes indicates extreme marrow stress or CGL. Increased numbers of band cells without granulocytosis, clinical symptoms, or other immature forms suggest Pelger-Huët anomaly. A left shift with nucleated red cells (leukoerythroblastosis) indicates severe marrow stress, as in anoxia or myelophthisis from tumor or leukemia involving the bone marrow. Granulocytosis or left shift with concurrent eosinophilia or basophilia or both suggests CGL.

Blood Cell Measurements.   A total white cell count of 10 to 20 × 10⁹/L (10 to 20 × 10³/µl) is consistent with inflammation or physiologic causes. With a count of 20 to 50 × 10⁹/L (20 to 50 × 10³/µl), leukemoid reaction vs CGL should be considered. A white cell count greater than 100 × 10⁹/L (100 × 10³/µl) is consistent with CGL. In the elderly, the total count may be less than 10 × 10⁹/L (10 × 10³/µl), but a left shift indicates inflammation.

Platelet counts above 400 × 10⁹/L (400 × 10³/µl) can be seen with inflammation, but counts greater than 600 × 10⁹/L (600 × 10³/µl) suggest that the granulocytosis is myeloproliferative or CGL.

Peripheral Blood Smear Morphology.   Toxic granulations are primary granules seen in granulocytes that either result from abnormal persistence during maturation or are caused by premature marrow release, a characteristic of inflammation or infection. Abnormally large granules are also seen in Chédiak-Higashi syndrome. Dohle bodies are amorphous, cytoplasmic masses seen in severe inflammation, massive burns, or infections. Similar inclusions are present in May-Hegglin anomaly, although they differ ultrastructurally. Prolonged granulocytosis produces pseudohypersegmented PMNs with 4 or 5 lobes.

Bone Marrow Examination.   In reactive granulocytosis the marrow is hypercellular 0.70 to 0.80 or 70% to 80%, with increased myeloid/erythroid (M/E) ratio as great as 6:1 or 8:1 associated with a left shift to the myelocyte phase. A shift to myeloblasts or promyelocytes suggests CGL or another myeloproliferative disorder. Usually the only cell line that is increased is the granulocytic, although megakaryocytes may be slightly increased. If megakaryocytes are increased profoundly or the erythroid series appears dysplastic, a myeloproliferative disorder should be considered. In prolonged infection or inflammation, plasma cells may be increased. Karyotype analysis that yields Philadelphia chromosome (Ph¹) is consistent with CGL.

Other Laboratory Tests

18.1   Leukocyte Alkaline Phosphatase (LAP)

Purpose.   The LAP test is useful in differentiating CGL from leukemoid reactions (see also Test 33.1).

Principle.   LAP is an enzyme present in the secondary granules, or more likely, membrane-related cytoplasmic microsomes of maturing neutrophils from the myelocyte phase onward. It is not present in lymphocytes, monocytes, or abnormal and immature neutrophils. Stimulated neutrophils contain increased amounts of LAP. Therefore, the test helps distinguish leukemoid reactions (increased LAP) from the abnormally maturing granulocytes of CGL (decreased LAP).

Procedure.   The LAP test is routinely available in most larger hospital laboratories. Although LAP can be determined quantitatively by enzymatic release from freshly lysed granulocytes, it is usually determined semiquantitatively by specific cytochemical staining of peripheral blood smears. The LAP present in the neutrophils hydrolyzes a substrate of naphthol AS-BI phosphate at pH 8.6; the hydrolyzed product couples to a soluble diazonium dye, Fast Blue RR, forming insoluble brown-to-black azo dye particles in the cytoplasm of the cells at the enzyme sites. The smears are then counterstained with hematoxylin, examined microscopically, and 100 segmented or band neutrophils are counted and graded 0 to 4 + by evaluating the number and color of the particles. The LAP score is calculated by addition of the number of cells times the grade, as shown in the following example. The range of normal scores is 13 to 130, although there may be slight variation in each laboratory.

No. Cells × Grade	Score
20 × 0	0
10 × 1 +	10
20 × 2 +	40
40 × 3 +	120
10 × 4 +	40
	210 = LAP score

Specimen.   Freshly prepared patient and control blood smears, obtained from finger stick capillary blood or heparinized venous blood, and less than 4 hours old, are fixed for 30 seconds in 10% formalin in absolute methanol. EDTA anticoagulant inhibits the reaction and must not be used. If not stained immediately, the fixed slides may be stored up to 6 months in a freezer without significant loss of enzyme activity.

Interpretation.   Normal peripheral smears show 0 to 1 + staining PMNs, band cells, metamyelocytes, and myelocytes yielding scores of 13 to 130 (Table 18–3). Leukemoid reactions have

Table 18–3 Leukocyte Alkaline Phosphatase Scores

<10	10 to 100	>100
CGL	Pregnancy	Leukemoid reaction
PNH	Contraceptives	Pyogenic infection
ITP	ACTH therapy	Polycythemia vera
Infectious mono-nucleosis	Myocardial in-farction	
Pernicious anemia		
Congenital hypo-phosphatasia		

ABBREVIATIONS: CGL = chronic granulocytic leukemia; PNH = paroxysmal nocturnal hemoglobinuria; ITP = idiopathic thrombocytopenic purpura; ACTH = adrenocorticotrophic hormone.

granulocytes with increased LAP (3 to 4+) so that scores are above 100. Intermediate degrees of elevation are seen in pregnancy, in women taking oral contraceptives, in myocardial infarction, and with steroid therapy. Pathologic granulocytes (as in CGL) lack normal enzymatic activity and produce scores less than 10. Other causes of low scores are paroxysmal nocturnal hemoglobinuria (PNH), congenital hypophosphatasia, an inborn error of metabolism, and sometimes myelodysplastic syndrome.

Notes and Precautions. Lymphocytes or blast cells of any cell line do not stain, and peripheral smears with marked increases in either cannot be interpreted. Improperly stored smears lose enzymatic activity and give falsely low LAP scores.

Course and Treatment

The course and treatment of neutrophilia depends on the underlying disease process.

References

1. Beutler E: Leukocyte alkaline phosphatase, in Williams WJ, Beutler E, Erslev AJ, et al (eds): *Hematology,* ed 3. New York, McGraw-Hill International Book Co, 1983, pp 1647–1648.

2. Jandl JH: Granulocytes, in *Blood: Textbook of Hematology*. Boston, Little, Brown & Co, 1987, pp 441–471.

3. Marmont AM, Damasio E, Zucker-Franklin D: Neutrophils, in Zucker-Franklin D, Greaves MF, Grossi CE, et al (eds): *Atlas of Blood Cells: Function and Pathology* (ed 2). Philadelphia, Lea & Febiger, 1988, pp 159–190.

4. Stein RB: Granulocytosis and granulocytic leukemoid reactions, in Koepke JA (ed): *Laboratory Hematology,* ed 1. New York, Churchill Livingstone, Inc, 1984, pp 153–188.

19

Eosinophilia

Eosinophilia is defined as an increase in peripheral eosinophils above 3% or an absolute increase above $0.25 \times 10^9/L$ ($0.25 \times 10^3/\mu l$). The stimulus for eosinophilia may be related to substances (lymphokines) produced by T-lymphocytes. Conditions associated with eosinophilia are summarized in Table 19–1. The most common causes are drug association, allergy, or parasites. Parasitic infestations that cause eosinophilia are characterized by a prominent tissue infestation either during migration or during encysting of the parasite, and often have pulmonary involvement. Allergic reactions associated with eosinophilia are often IgE-dependent reactions and immune complex diseases.

Pathophysiology

Eosinophils spend 3 to 6 days in production in the marrow, have a very short circulation time (less than 1 hour), and survive for 8 to 12 days in tissue, where they apparently function in sequestering immune complexes and in limiting chronic inflammatory reactions. They do not have bactericidal activity; the specific eosinophilic granules contain peroxidase and acid phosphatase, but no alkaline phosphatase or lysozyme. The cell membrane has receptors for IgG and complement. They have limited phagocytic activity. Eosinophils are chemotactically attracted to tissue sites of foreign antigen,

Table 19–1   Conditions Associated with Eosinophilia

Drug Therapy

  Allopurinol

  Phenothiazine

  Heparin

  Streptomycin, penicillins, cephalothin

  Digitalis, quinidine, procainamide, propranolol

Parasitic Infestation

  Trichinosis

  Visceral larva migrans *(Toxocara)*

  Filariasis

  Echinococcus

  Clonorchis sinensis (liver fluke)

  Cysticercosis

  Pneumocystosis

Chronic Infections

  Brucellosis

  Fungal infections

  Leprosy

  Tuberculosis

Malignancies

  Carcinoma of lung, ovary, stomach

Hematologic Disorders

  Pernicious anemia

  CGL

  Hodgkin's disease

  T lymphocyte deficiency (eg, graft v host disease)

Collagen Disease

  Periarteritis nodosa

  Rheumatoid arthritis

(Continued.)

Table 19–1 *Continued.*

Dermatitis

    Dermatitis herpetiformis

    Exfoliative dermatitis (drug-induced)

    Pemphigus

    Bullous pemphigoid

Pulmonary disease

    Löffler's syndrome (eosinophilic pneumonia)

    Farmer's lung (moldy grain)

    Bagassosis (cane fiber, insulation material)

Allergy

    Asthma

    Hay fever

    Urticaria

    Angioneurotic edema

Miscellaneous

    Sarcoidosis

ABBREVIATIONS: CGL = chronic granulocytic leukemia.

antigen-antibody complexes, and vasoactive amines. They limit inflammation by counteracting vasoactive amines and kinins.

Response of eosinophils to inflammation involves an immediate transient accumulation in tissues and prolonged tissue accumulation for days, weeks, or months associated with peripheral eosinophilia and increased bone marrow production of eosinophils. Tissue eosinophils are ingested by macrophages, and Charcot-Leyden crystals are found in secretions or tissue in association with disintegration of eosinophils.

Clinical Findings

The cause of eosinophilia is either clinically obvious or obscure. For this reason, when levels of eosinophils are less than 10%, eosinophilia is often ignored in the absence of clinical signs or symptoms, or other hematologic abnormality. With significant eosinophilia, the liver, spleen, and lymph nodes may be enlarged; the skin or the lungs may be involved, and fever may be present depending on the cause. With chronic hypereosinophilic syndrome there may be myocardial endomyofibrosis with congestive heart failure, bronchial asthma, pulmonary fibrosis, and diffuse central nervous system involvement.

Approach to Diagnosis

Eosinophilia is usually a benign process; its evaluation depends heavily on clinical history. Persistent eosinophilia with levels above 10% should be evaluated by the following:

1. Hematologic findings to determine persistence. Bone marrow aspiration is rarely helpful except to exclude chronic granulocytic leukemia (CGL) when the peripheral blood is suggestive of that disease. Absolute eosinophil count is useful to evaluate therapy.

2. Examination of stool and urine sediment for ova or parasites. Infestation by *Strongyloides, Ascaris, Taenia,* or *Schistosoma* parasites frequently causes eosinophilia.

3. Determination of serum IgE, which is frequently elevated in allergic eosinophilia.

4. Roentgenography of the chest to exclude sarcoid, Löffler's syndrome, or infiltrates secondary to parasites.

5. Muscle biopsy if trichinosis is suspected. In fatal trichinosis eosinophilia may be absent.

6. Biopsy of lymph nodes if persistent lymphadenopathy is present to exclude Hodgkin's disease or sarcoid.

7. Serologic tests for parasites. The available serologic techniques vary with the parasite (Table 19–2). Skin test antigens are not generally available and are not reliable.

Hematologic Findings

Blood Cell Measurements. Eosinophilia is present when an absolute increase in eosinophils above 0.25×10^9/L ($0.25 \times 10^3/\mu l$) is present (normal range, 0.05 to 0.15×10^9/L or 0.05 to $0.15 \times 10^3/\mu l$). The highest elevations are seen in trichinosis, in *Clonorchis sinensis* infections, and in dermatitis herpetiformis. In chronic hypereosinophilic syndrome eosinophil levels are persistently above 1.5×10^9/L ($1.5 \times 10^3/\mu l$). Eosinophils have a diurnal variation, highest in the morning, decreasing in the afternoon.

Bone Marrow Examination. Variable eosinophilia is present that is often unrelated to the degree of tissue or blood eosinophilia. Immaturity of the granulocytic series or myeloid/erythroid (M/E) ratio greater than 10:1 suggests the presence of CGL. Granulomas may be seen in sarcoidosis or tuberculosis.

Other Laboratory Tests

19.1 Stool Examination for Ova and Parasites

Purpose. Examination of stool identifies *Strongyloides, Ascaris,* and *Taenia,* which may cause eosinophilia. Urine sediment should be examined for *Schistosoma mansoni.*

Principle. Parasites with strong tissue phases are those most commonly associated with eosinophilia.

Specimen. Fresh stool specimens are examined on at least 3 occasions.

Procedure. Preparation of a slide for microscopic examination is a standard procedure for most hospital laboratories.

Interpretation. Significant parasites for the diagnosis of eosinophilia are *Strongyloides, Ascaris, Taenia,* or *Schistosoma.* Parasites such as *Amoeba, Giardia, Trichiuris,* and *Enterobius vermicularis* (pinworm) are not associated with eosinophilia.

19.2 Serologic Tests for Parasites

Purpose. Serologic tests confirm exposure to antigens of parasites that encapsulate in tissue and are not readily detected in stool.

Principle. Serologic tests detect rising antibody titer to parasitic antigens. Antibodies may vary with each patient's immune response, the antigenicity of the organism, and the stage of the disease. Not all antibodies react by the same method, since some fix complement, some are flocculins or precipitins, and others are agglutinins. In general, a battery of tests is needed to confirm the diagnosis.

Table 19–2 Serologic Tests for Parasites

Parasite	CF	BF	LA	IHA
Ancylostoma	NA	NA	NA	NA
Ascaris	+	+	NA	+
Cysticercus	+	NA	NA	+
Clonorchis	+	NA	NA	+
Echinococcus	+	+	NA	+
Filaria	NA	+	NA	+
Schistosoma	+	NA	NA	+
Taenia	NA	NA	NA	NA
Trichinella	+	+	NA	+
Toxocara (visceral larva migrans)	NA	+	NA	+

ABBREVIATIONS: + = applicable test; NA = not applicable; BF = bentonite flocculation; CF = complement fixation; IHA = indirect hemagglutinin; IIF = indirect immunofluorescence; LA = latex agglutination; P = precipitin; CSF = cerebrospinal fluid.

aSkin antigens are not regularly available but parasites for which they are used are listed

Specimen. Acute and convalescent serum specimens should be obtained at least 10 days apart. Serum samples may be stored frozen.

Procedure. Tests are not generally available except in county, state, or Centers for Disease Control laboratories, Atlanta. Methods of testing vary with each parasite, but usually include com-

IIF	P	Skin[a]	Comment
NA	NA	NA	No reproducible satisfactory tests
+	NA	NA	All methods unreliable and little used
+	NA	NA	IIF test most specific; IHA sensitive although serum and CSF sensitivity may differ
NA	NA	NA	
+	NA	+	90% correlation with active disease if titer above 256, low titer has poor correlation; some cross-reactions with other parasites
+	NA	NA	60% correlation; false positive at low titer; crossreactive
+	NA	NA	
NA	NA	NA	No tests available
+	+	+	CF correlates with active disease cross-reaction with *Schistosoma*
NA	NA	NA	False negatives are a problem; less than 60% are positive

plement fixation (CF), indirect hemagglutination (IHA), indirect immunofluorescence (IIF), or bentonite flocculation. Latex agglutination tests lack sensitivity as a general class. Skin test antigens are not generally available. Commonly used tests are listed in Table 19–2.

Interpretation.   Rises in titer are clinically significant for active disease, although in many cases titers are already maximal at the time of serologic diagnosis. Antibodies usually require 3 weeks to develop, although eosinophilia may precede them. In chronic disease or in inactive disease, titers fade after 1 or 2 years. Significant titers vary with each disease and technique and are reported by the testing agency.

19.3 Serum IgE Measurement

Purpose. Levels of IgE are elevated in eosinophilia caused by parasitism or atopic disease, eg, dermatitis, hay fever, or asthma.

Principle. IgE (reaginic) antibodies result from skin-sensitizing antigens that may be introduced through the skin or through bronchopulmonary or gastrointestinal systems. IgE is present in minute amounts that can be measured only in nanograms, and requires sensitive radioimmunoassays for quantitation.

Specimen. Heparinized plasma or serum, which may be stored frozen, is used as a specimen. Specimens should be shipped frozen.

Procedure. Several radioimmunoassay (RIA) variations are available commercially as test kits. Radioimmunoassay by competitive protein binding is sensitive to 5 ng/mL. Although serum inhibitors can interfere with the test, it is reasonably accurate for elevated levels. Noncompetitive protein-binding RIA uses a double antibody sensitive to picogram levels and is unaffected by serum inhibitors. The most widely available method is radioimmune precipitation assay (RIPA), which also uses a double-antibody technique. Antibody to IgE plus iodine-125–labeled IgE is incubated with the patient's serum. The antibody becomes complexed with radiolabeled IgE and IgE of the patient. The complexes are precipitated with a second IgG antibody and the insoluble immune complexes are counted.

Interpretation. The normal range for serum IgE is 0.4 to 4000 IU/mL. Values are age dependent; they are very low in cord blood and approach adult levels by the time the patient is 12 years old. Serum IgE levels fluctuate with exposure to the inciting allergen, but may rise several times their original levels. T-lymphocytes influence IgE levels so that T-cell malignancies and Hodgkin's disease may be associated with increased IgE levels. Normal levels of IgE make parasitism as the cause of eosinophilia less likely. Eosinophilia with normal levels of IgE suggests nonallergic causes of asthmatic symptoms.

Ancillary Tests

1. Nasal smears or sputum cytology for eosinophils. Sputum eosinophils suggest Löffler's pneumonia. Nasal eosinophilia is common in allergic rhinitis. Charcot-Leyden crystals may be present.
2. A chest roentgenogram is useful to exclude Löffler's pneumonia or sarcoidosis.
3. Biopsy of enlarged lymph nodes to exclude Hodgkin's disease or filariasis in endemic areas.
4. Biopsy of the gastrocnemius muscle, diagnostic in most cases of trichinosis, is used only in severely ill patients in whom the diagnosis is in doubt.

Course and Treatment

Treatment depends on the underlying cause if it can be determined. In chronic hypereosinophilic syndrome, patients often die with congestive heart failure. In some cases this condition may be related to eosinophilic leukemia. Hypereosinophilic syndromes have been treated with antihistamines, glucocorticoids, and, if related to CGL, with hydroxyurea and other chemotherapeutic agents.

References

1. Adkinson NF Jr: Measurement of total serum immunoglobulin E and allergen-specific immunoglobulin E antibody: Tests for immunological drug reactions, in Rose NR, Friedman H (eds): *Manual of Clinical Immunology,* ed 3. Washington, DC, American Society of Microbiology, 1984, pp 664–670.
2. Fanci AS, Harley JB, Roberts WC, et al: The idiopathic hypereosinophilic syndrome: Clinical, pathophysiologic, and therapeutic considerations. *Ann Intern Med* 1982; 97:78–92.
3. Pincus SH, Schooley WR, DiNapoli AM, et al: Metabolic heterogeneity of eosinophils from normal and hypereosinophilic patients. *Blood* 1981; 58:1175–1181.
4. Smith JW, Gutierrez Y: Medical parasitology, in Henry JB (ed): *Todd-Sanford-Davidsohn Clinical Diagnosis and Management by Laboratory Methods,* ed 17. Philadelphia, WB Saunders Co, 1984, pp 1209–1271.

20

Basophilia

Basophilia is a very rare disorder in which the peripheral proportion is greater than 0.01 (1%) or $0.06 \times 10^9/L$ ($0.06 \times 10^3/\mu l$). Disorders in which circulating basophils may be increased are listed in Table 20–1.

Pathophysiology

The precursor cell is a marrow pluripotent stem cell for the granulocytic series. The basophil has a segmented nucleus and deep blue-violet granules that contain heparinlike mucopolysaccharide and histamine. The basophil circulates briefly before ending in tissue, usually at the site of antigen-induced injury. The cell degranulates in response to IgE antibodies that attach to Fc receptors on the cell membrane. Tissue mast cells resemble basophils, although their granules are ultrastructurally and histochemically different, and the nucleus is ovoid rather than segmented. Animal studies suggest that the basophil may be a different morphologic or physiologic phase of the mast cell. Basophils may increase in hypersensitivity of both immediate and delayed type. Mast cells are present in the tissue phase of chronic hypersensitivity reactions; urticaria pigmentosa is the cutaneous form of systemic mastocytosis.

Table 20–1   Disorders with Increased Basophils

Myeloproliferative Disorders

    Chronic granulocytic leukemia

    Myeloid metaplasia

    Polycythemia vera

Hypersensitivity Reactions

Ulcerative Colitis

Viral Pox Diseases

    Smallpox

    Chickenpox

Myxedema

Hodgkin's Disease

Hematologic Disease

    Hemolytic anemia

    Basophilic leukemia

Ionizing Radiation

Clinical Findings

Basophils are known to increase in some hypersensitivity reactions, excessive radiation, myeloproliferative disorders, including polycythemia vera, myelofibrosis with myeloid metaplasia, and chronic granulocytic leukemia (CGL). Because of the association with granulocytic proliferative disorders, clinical findings in basophilia are dependent on the degree of abnormality in the granulocytic series. Hepatosplenomegaly is often present in hematologic disorders. With mild basophilia there are nonspecific symptoms, so that evaluation is not undertaken in the isolated instance. With basophils greater than 0.80 (80%) the diagnosis of basophil leukemia is appropriate.

    Mastocytosis is a rare disease with infiltration of the skin, liver, spleen, and bone by mast cells. The most common form of the disease is urticaria pigmentosa, a benign self-limited disorder, usually subsiding in adolescence. The histaminelike reactions of degranulating mast cells are seen in the skin as urticaria or dermatographia. Adult forms of the systemic disease tend to persist and to be more serious. There is mast cell infiltration of the skin, bone marrow, gastrointestinal wall, and viscera. Fever and weight loss may be present. Symptoms of histamine release provoke intermittent flushing, hay fever, or asthma with bronchospasm, dyspnea, hypotension, palpitations, and diarrhea. Hepatosplenomegaly and lymphadenopathy are present in 50% of patients. Gastrointestinal bleeding is frequent. Bone lesions include osteoporosis and, occasionally, osteosclerosis.

Approach to Diagnosis

Chronic granulocytic leukemia and other myeloproliferative disorders should be excluded (chapter 33), since these are the most important and most likely causes of an increase in circulating basophils. If urticaria pigmentosa is suspected, skin biopsy is more useful than a hematologic workup. Special stains, such as specific esterase, toluidine blue or Giemsa, are required to demonstrate the basophilic granules of mast cells. In the rare patient with systemic mastocytosis, there may be intermittent increases in circulating histamine.

Hematologic Findings

Minor increases in basophils are usually not associated with any specific etiology. Findings are otherwise related to the specific disorder; in hematologic disorders all cell lines may be involved; and in hypothyroidism or ulcerative colitis findings may be limited to normochromic or hypochromic anemia. In mastocytosis there can be anemia, leukocytosis, and eosinophilia, as well as basophilia. Rarely, mastocytosis may end in basophilic leukemia.

Blood Cell Measurements. Basophils are noteworthy when they represent more than 0.03 (3%) of the differential white cell count. Except in myeloproliferative disorders, there are no abnormalities of other cell lines and no specific morphologic findings. When basophils constitute greater than 0.80 (80%) the diagnosis of basophil leukemia is likely.

Bone Marrow Examination. Bone marrow examination is useful in the diagnosis of myeloproliferative disorders and mastocytosis. Differentiation of basophils from mast cells may be difficult on bone marrow examination. Mast cells may be increased in the marrow as a nondiagnostic reaction to many stimuli, including met-

Table 20–2 Metabolic and Histochemical Differences Between Basophils and Mast Cells

	Basophil	Mast Cell
Granules	Peroxidase Heparin Histamine	Heparin precursor Histamine
Acid phosphatase stain	Absent	Present
PAS stain	Strongly positive	Weakly positive

ABBREVIATIONS: PAS = periodic acid–Schiff.

astatic tumor, malignant lymphoma, myelodysplastic syndrome, and marrow hyperplasia. Histochemical differences between basophils and mast cells are listed in Table 20–2. In systemic mastocytosis the bone marrow is usually hypercellular; erythrophagocytosis can be seen. Mast cells often display variable morphology and may be difficult to identify. The specific esterase stain is helpful in identifying mast cells in the biopsy specimen.

Other Laboratory Tests

20.1 Serum and Urine Histamine Quantitation

Purpose. Histamine release correlates with skin tests for reaginic allergy rather than with basophilia. The assay is a research tool that may support the diagnosis of mastocytosis. In systemic mastocytosis there may be intermittent increases in circulating histamine not seen in basophilia. The test is available from some reference laboratories.

Principle. Histamine is extracted from whole blood or urine into butanol at an acid pH. It is coupled with *o*-phthaldehyde in a highly alkaline pH, forming a fluorescent compound measured by either manual or automated fluoridometry. The technique is sensitive to 0.05 ng.

Specimen. Whole blood is collected in a plastic vial containing fluoride and potassium oxalate. If frozen and stored in plastic, the specimen is stable for up to 30 days, but it is usually tested within 2 to 3 hours. An aliquot from a 24-hour urine specimen can also be used. The aliquot should be frozen within 3 hours of the end of collection and stored in plastic.

Procedure.   Histamine is extracted from whole blood or urine by a laborious procedure that removes plasma proteins and competing compounds such as histidine. The extract is coupled with o-phthaldehyde to yield a fluorescent compound measured by a fluoridometer. Another assay technique uses radiometric transferases to shift carbon-14 methyl groups from S-adenosyl methionine to the unlabeled histamine.

Interpretation.   Normal values for whole blood are 3.0 to 9.0 μg/dL and for urine, 17 to 68 μg/24 hours.

Course and Treatment

The clinical course for basophilia is related to the underlying disease, eg, CGL and other myeloproliferative disorders. Mast cell tumors that produce significant histamine flushing and bronchoconstrictive symptoms are treated with antihistamines and cimetidine. Basophilic leukemia is usually resistant to chemotherapy.

References

1. Brunning RD, McKenna RW, Rosai J, et al: Systemic mastocytosis: Extracutaneous manifestations. *Am J Surg Pathol* 1983; 7:425–438.

2. Ferrito MC: Eosinophils and basophils, in Stein JH (ed): *Internal Medicine.* Boston, Little Brown & Co, 1983, pp 1593–1594.

3. Kass L: *Bone Marrow Interpretation,* ed 2. Philadelphia, JB Lippincott, 1985, p 233.

4. Siraganian RP, Hook WA: Histamine release and assay methods for the study of human allergy, in Rose NR, Friedman H, Fahey JL (eds): *Manual of Clinical Laboratory Immunology,* ed 3. Washington, DC, American Society for Microbiology, 1986, pp 675–680.

5. Webb TA, Li CY, Yam LT: Systemic mast cell disease: A clinical and hematopathologic study of 26 cases. *Cancer* 1982; 49:927–938.

6. Zucker-Franklin D: Basophils, in Zucker-Franklin D, Greaves MF, Grossi CE, et al (eds): *Atlas of Blood Cells: Function and Pathology,* ed 2. Philadelphia, Lea & Febiger, 1988, pp 287–320.

21

Monocytosis

Monocytosis exists when there are more than 10% monocytes in the peripheral blood, ie, the absolute monocyte count is >0.50 × 10^9/L (0.50 × 10^3/μl) for adults, >0.80 × 10^9/L (0.80 × 10^3/μl) for children, and >1.2 × 10^9/L (1.2 × 10^3/μl) for newborns.

Pathophysiology

The marrow precursor cell has not been identified, but a stem cell leading to both monocytic and granulocytic cell lines is postulated. Thus many similarities in metabolism and function are seen between the two cell types. Following development in the marrow, monocytes circulate in the peripheral blood for 1 to 3 days before migrating into tissues where they differentiate into macrophages. Tissue macrophages may be seen as histiocytes, multinucleated giant cells, and epithelioid cells in granulomas.

Monocytes function, as does the neutrophil, in bacterial phagocytosis. Monocytes are processors of antigen for T-lymphocytes. They synthesize, secrete and degrade complement components, and produce interleukin-1 (IL-1). Macrophage and monocyte cell membranes have receptors for the Fc fragment of IgG and for complement. Particles, whether bacteria, fungi, tumor cells, or red cells, coated with these globulins are ingested in cytoplasmic vacuoles and destroyed by cytoplasmic hydrolytic enzymes.

Monocytosis is often transient and it correlates poorly with disease states. Of the diseases listed in Table 21–1, monocytosis is associated most commonly with neutropenia of all types (familial, cyclic, and drug-induced), the recovery phase of infection or inflammation, and Hodgkin's disease. Monocytosis may indicate marrow recovery phase in agranulocytosis. In the past, infectious disease with tissue destruction was considered the most important cause of monocytosis, but changes in therapy have altered this. Tissue destruction in chronic infection, such as subacute bacterial endocarditis (SBE), or disseminated candidiasis, is an important factor in monocytosis. In reticuloendothelial hyperplasia (eg, SBE) monocytes may be seen in peripheral blood or tissue with ingested red cells or, rarely, white cells and platelets. Stasis encourages this phenomenon so that specimens from the earlobe are more helpful than finger sticks or venous specimens in demonstrating erythrophagocytosis. The latter phenomenon, however, is rarely helpful in diagnosis.

Clinical Findings

Physical findings depend on the underlying cause. Hepatosplenomegaly is associated with myeloproliferative disorders and lipoidosis. Reticuloendothelial hyperplasia produces splenomegaly.

Approach to Diagnosis

The proportion of monocytes in the peripheral blood should be correlated with clinical history. Monocytosis associated with white cell counts $<1 \times 10^9/L$ $(1 \times 10^3/\mu l)$ is compatible with the compensatory monocytosis of neutropenia. When leukocyte values are $>10 \times 10^9/L$ $(10 \times 10^3/\mu l)$ the increase in monocytes parallels the increase in granulopoiesis.

The most common causes for monocytosis are indolent infections, such as *Mycobacterium tuberculosis* and *Mycobacterium lepra*, SBE, and the recovery phase for neutropenia (Table 21–1). Because destruction of tissue is associated with monocytosis, roentgenograms of the chest and appropriate cultures of blood or tissue may be helpful.

Hematologic Findings

Blood Cell Measurements.   In a healthy person monocytes comprise 0 to 0.09 (0 to 9%) of the white cells with an absolute

Table 21–1 Diseases Associated with Monocytosis

Physiologic
  Normal newborn
Infections
  Bacterial
    Brucellosis
    Tuberculosis
    Leprosy
    Subacute bacterial endocarditis
    Recovery phase of acute infections
  Rickettsial
    Rocky Mountain spotted fever
    Typhus
  Protozoal or parasitic
    Malaria
Hematologic disorders
  Myeloproliferative disorders
  Myelogenous and monocytic leukemias
  Myelodysplastic syndrome
  Malignant histiocytosis
  Hodgkin's disease
  Agranulocytosis
  Cyclic neutropenias
Collagen disorders
  SLE
  RA
  Polyarteritis
Gastrointestinal
  Sprue
  Ulcerative colitis
  Regional enteritis
Miscellaneous
  Postsplenectomy
  Lipidoses (Gaucher's, Niemann-Pick, Hand-Schüller-Christian diseases)

ABBREVIATIONS: SLE = systemic lupus erythematosus; RA = rheumatoid arthritis.

count of 0.3 to 0.5 × 10⁹/L (0.3 to 0.5 × 10³/μl); this count is somewhat higher in children. Monocytosis is normal in the first 2 weeks of life.

Peripheral Blood Smear Morphology. In monocytosis of infection, azurophilic granules are prominent, and there may be cytoplasmic vacuolization. Ingestion of red cells seen in monocytes in blood smears from the earlobe often indicates the presence of SBE.

Bone Marrow Examination. Bone marrow studies are helpful only if hematologic disorders are suspected. Histologic sections may show granulomas in miliary tuberculosis. Bone marrow cultures are not usually helpful since the specimen is too limited; blood cultures should be performed.

Other Laboratory Tests

21.1   Blood Culture

Blood cultures may be considered negative after 3 have yielded no organisms, if anaerobic techniques have been included.

21.2   Rickettsial Serology

Rickettsial serologic tests use febrile agglutination titers. Results are significant only if 1 titer is elevated. Anamnestic elevations of all titers increase with fever of any origin.

Course and Treatment

The clinical course varies with the underlying disorder, as does the treatment. Genetic disorders progress clinically unrelated to peripheral blood morphology. Splenectomy in the storage diseases has limited success and is performed mainly to relieve hypersplenism associated with secondary thrombocytopenia.

References

1. Cassileth PA: Monocytosis, in Williams WJ, Beutler E, Erslev AJ, (eds): *Hematology*, ed 3. New York, McGraw Hill, 1983, pp 861–864.

2. Johnston RB, Zucker-Franklin D: The mononuclear phagocyte system: Monocytes and macrophages, in Zucker-Franklin D, Greaves MF, Grossi CE, et al (eds): *Atlas of Blood Cells: Function and Pathology,* ed 2. Philadelphia, Lea & Febiger, 1988, pp 323–357.

22

Neutropenia

Neutropenia (granulocytopenia), defined as a decrease in neutrophilic granulocytes to less than $1.5 \times 10^9/L$ ($1.5 \times 10^3/\mu l$), is often associated with a relative lymphocytosis. Thus the peripheral white cell differential count may be misinterpreted as a lymphocytic disorder unless the low total white cell count is noted and an absolute granulocyte count is calculated. Granulocytopenia may be caused by decreased production in the marrow, increased utilization (ie, loss to the tissues), or shifts from the circulating to the marginated pool (Table 22–1). The most common causes are related to drugs, collagen disease, viral infection, and hypersplenism, usually secondary to hepatic cirrhosis.

Pathophysiology

Granulocytopenia becomes clinically significant in terms of infection when the total neutrophil count is less than $1 \times 10^9/L$ ($1 \times 10^3/\mu l$). Since granulopoiesis in the marrow requires 4 to 5 days, a time lag may follow toxic insult to the marrow before granulocytopenia is evident, and, similarly, before recovery is noted.

Drug-associated neutropenia may be caused by direct chemical suppression of marrow production, or may be secondary to toxic immune complexes formed by the drug, its antibody, and complement, destroying cells peripherally. These complexes adhere to the

Table 22–1   Causes of Granulocytopenia[a]

Decreased marrow production
  Toxicity caused by drugs, chemicals, or irradiation
    Chemotherapeutic (cytotoxic)
    Noncytotoxic drugs
    X-ray, gamma irradiation
    Chemicals (benzene, CCl_4, DDT)
  Bone marrow replacement (myelophthisis)
    Cancer
    Leukemia or lymphoma
    Myelofibrosis
  Abnormal granulopoiesis, congenital
    Fanconi's anemia (neonatal aplasia)
    Familial cyclic neutropenia—exaggerated oscillation
    Familial benign neutropenia
  Abnormal granulopoiesis, acquired
    PNH
    Immune injury
    Collagen disease
      SLE
      RA with splenomegaly (Felty's syndrome)
  Aplastic anemia
  Nutritional
    Vitamin B_{12}
    Folic acid

Increased destruction or utilization in peripheral blood or tissue
  Hypersplenism
    Splenomegaly with RA (Felty's syndrome)
  Virus
  Immune
    Leukocyte antibody
    Drug antibody—innocent bystander cell
  Surface injury
    Hemodialysis
    Pump-oxygenator in open heart surgery
  Prolonged inflammation

Shift from circulating to marginated pool
  Peritoneal dialysis

ABBREVIATIONS: PNH = paroxysmal nocturnal hemoglobinuria; SLE = systemic lupus erythematosus; RA = rheumatoid arthritis.

[a]May be part of pancytopenia in some categories

Table 22-2 Noncytotoxic Drugs Associated with Neutropenia

Antimicrobial drugs

    Chloramphenicol

    Semisynthetic penicillins (oxacillin, methicillin)

    Sulfonamides (trimethoprim-sulfamethoxazole)

    Clindamycin

    Nitrofurantoin

    Gentamicin

Tranquilizers or psychotropic drugs (phenothiazines, tricyclics)

Antithyroid drugs

    Phenylbutazone

    Indomethacin

Diuretics

    Thiazides

    Ethacrynic acid

Hypoglycemic agents

    Sulfonamide derivatives

Miscellaneous drugs

    Quinidine

    Procainamide

    Allopurinol

    Cimetidine

surface of the target cell (platelet, white cell, or red cell) resulting in cell lysis. Drugs frequently responsible for neutropenia are listed in Table 22-2.

Granulocytopenia seen in systemic lupus erythematosus (SLE) is of moderate degree and unknown cause, possibly antibody. It may be associated with thrombocytopenia and is most often seen in young females. Rarely, rheumatoid arthritis is associated with splenomegaly and hypersplenism (Felty's syndrome), which produces sequestration granulocytopenia.

Cyclic neutropenia is a diagnosis made by excluding all other likely causes. It is frequently familial with slightly increased frequency in black females. The mechanism of disease appears to be periodic pluripotential stem cell failure.

Viral infections appear to induce white cell damage that may increase neutrophil utilization, margination, or sequestration, resulting in transient neutropenia with lymphocytosis.

Clinical Findings

Neutrophil levels below $0.5 \times 10^9/L$ ($0.5 \times 10^3/\mu l$) are associated with a significant risk of bacterial infection, both endogenous and nosocomial. Presenting symptoms are commonly pharyngitis, gingivitis, or proctitis. Cellulitis, pneumonia, and urinary tract infections with septicemia result and, if marrow recovery is not prompt, death ensues. Spiking fevers and chills are seen with the onset of infection. Regional lymphadenopathy is usually present. Hepatosplenomegaly is related to underlying leukemia, lymphoma, or myelofibrosis. There may be mild-to-moderate splenomegaly with hepatic cirrhosis producing hypersplenism with variable neutropenia.

Approach to Diagnosis

Hematologic tests should define whether the disease is caused by lack of production, as in aplasia, myelofibrosis, or granulocytic arrest, or is caused by peripheral destruction by toxic immune complexes, virus, white cell antibody, chemicals, or splenic sequestration. Splenomegaly or hepatomegaly support splenic sequestration as the cause.

Relative lymphocytosis usually indicates peripheral, specific destruction of granulocytes by drugs, viruses, or arrest of maturation of the granulocyte series in the marrow. Decrease in more than one cell line suggests generalized marrow suppression or peripheral splenic sequestration. Where there is major damage to the marrow, the relative distribution of granulocytes and lymphocytes is generally maintained, despite decreases in absolute numbers of each cell type.

Diagnostic evaluation should include an extensive history of current and recent (6 weeks) drug therapy or exposure to toxins. Physical examination should document the size of both the spleen and the liver.

Bone marrow examination is indicated when the white cell count is persistently below $3 \times 10^9/L$ ($3 \times 10^3/\mu l$) or when another cell line is also abnormal, in order to determine marrow cellularity or arrest in cell maturation, ie, defective granulopoiesis due to injury of a precursor stem cell.

Other correlative tests include:

1. Granulocyte antibody detection to determine an immune cause, as in familial, neonatal, or cyclic neutropenia.
2. Screening tests for antinuclear antibodies to document underlying SLE or rheumatoid arthritis, eg, Felty's syndrome.
3. Spleen scans with technetium (Tc 99m) may document splenic enlargement and increased activity.
4. Chromium-51 survival studies of red cells can also demonstrate splenic red cell sequestration. This method is indirect, since studies of granulocyte kinetics are not generally available.

Hematologic Findings

Blood Cell Measurements. The neutrophil count is less than 1.5×10^9/L (1.5×10^3/μl). If hypersplenism is present, there may be moderate normochromic anemia (80 to 100 g/L or 8 to 10 g/dl) and variable thrombocytopenia (30 to 90 $\times$ 10^9/L or 30 to 90 $\times$ 10^3/μl).

Peripheral Blood Smear Morphology. Although the total number is decreased, the morphology of granulocytes is normal. Neutrophil counts below 1×10^9/L (1×10^3/μl) (1000/mm^3) indicate significant risk from infection and toxic granulations or Döhle bodies may be present in neutrophils. A left shift with neutropenia indicates severe infection or inflammation, with increased tissue utilization and destruction of granulocytes. Monocytosis may be present and is partly compensatory. Associated thrombocytopenia indicates severe insult to the marrow or peripheral sequestration.

Bone Marrow Examination. Bone marrow examination is usually necessary when the white cell count is persistently below 3×10^9/L (3×10^3/μl) or when anemia or thrombocytopenia are present. Bone marrow aspirate and biopsy should always be performed for a complete evaluation. Neutropenia associated with a hypocellular (<20%) or aplastic marrow is seen with drug or chemical toxicity, and is usually associated with decreases in megakaryocytes or erythroid precursors resulting in peripheral pancytopenia. Neutropenia associated with a hypercellular marrow (>80%) and a normal maturation sequence suggests splenic sequestration. Normocellular or hypercellular marrow with partial or complete arrest in granulocytic maturation may be seen with drug insults. The effects of marrow arrest on peripheral blood are delayed for 4 days as the available granulocytes are released, circulate, and marginate. Partial arrests are difficult to appreciate unless a careful marrow differential is made; less than 6% stab cells and polymorphonuclear neutrophilic leukocytes (PMNs) is consistent with arrest.

Other Laboratory Tests

22.1   Antinuclear Antibodies

Purpose.   The presence of antinuclear antibodies suggests that the cause of granulocytopenia is collagen disease, probably SLE, and, less frequently, rheumatoid arthritis.

Principle.   Patient serum containing antinuclear antibodies may react with a variety of nuclear constituents. The antibodies are not species specific, so that the reagent nuclear material may be rat kidney, human granulocytes, or tumor cells taken from tissue culture. Various indicator systems, such as latex agglutination, can be used, but indirect immunofluorescence has 98% sensitivity and has the advantage that the pattern of immunofluorescence can be characterized as homogeneous, speckled, or nucleolar.

Specimen.   Serum is stored in a refrigerator or frozen.

Procedure.   The patient's serum is incubated with a source of nuclear antigen. The antibody globulin attaches to the antigen and is detected by anti–human globulin reagent tagged with fluorescein dye. Microscopic evaluation under ultraviolet light causes all positive (antinuclear antibody) attachments to glow. Serum samples can then be titered; the normal value is a titer <10.

Interpretation.   A titer > 80 is consistent with SLE, while a titer of 10 to 80 may indicate either SLE or rheumatoid arthritis, so that this test result should be followed by specific testing to detect rheumatoid factor. Normal titers increase with age so that 3% of the population above age 65 may have a titer of 1:80. Tests for antinuclear antibody are more sensitive and specific than conventional lupus erythematosus (LE) cell preparations. Screening for anti-DNA, anti-Sm, and anti-nRNP antibodies can be performed to assess the disease further, although these tests are not necessary for diagnosis. Anti-histone antibodies are frequently present in procainamide-induced LE.

22.2 Rheumatoid Factor

Purpose. The presence of rheumatoid factor (RF) suggests that rheumatoid arthritis is the cause of granulocytopenia.

Principle. Rheumatoid factor is IgM antibody against IgG. All tests are based on incubating an indicator particle coated with IgG with the patient's serum. If IgM RF is present, it will agglutinate or clump the indicator. The specimen can be titered.

Specimen. Serum is used as a specimen.

Procedure. Tests for RF include latex particles coated with IgG from rabbits or humans, and the sheep cell agglutination (Rose-Waaler) test, which uses enzyme-treated sheep red cells tested in parallel with untreated sheep red cells.

Interpretation. Significant titers for the latex test for RF are 1:80 or above, while the significant titer for the sheep cell test is >1:8. Nonspecific sheep red cell antibodies can be detected and excluded by the parallel testing. False-positive tests correlate with increased fibrinogen levels, and false-negative tests are common in inactive disease.

22.3 Leukoagglutinins

Purpose. Detection of leukoagglutinins implies a direct immune cause for leukopenia. Positive test results only in the presence of specific drugs imply drug-induced immune neutropenia. The test as used for drug antibody has a low sensitivity and poor correlation, and is available on a research basis only. The test for anti-granulocyte antibody in the absence of a drug is available in specialized reference laboratories, but has limited specificity.

Principle. Suspensions of test granulocytes are incubated with the patient's serum. Evidence of cytotoxicity or leukoagglutination is determined by a variety of indicator systems including leukoagglutination, complement fixation, indirect immunofluorescence, and vital dye exclusion. No single technique is satisfactory since the antibodies involved may be direct-reacting IgM or indirect IgG, and not all are complement binding. The tests can be performed in the presence or absence of specific drugs to attempt to correlate neutropenia with drug-dependent antibody.

Specimen.   Fresh serum is stored frozen to preserve complement. The patient's granulocytes are usually not used since collection of adequate numbers is difficult with neutropenia. For drug studies the patient must be free of all suspect drugs for 5 days to allow clearing of the drug from plasma proteins in order to obtain a baseline.

Procedure.   Fresh granulocytes are separated from whole blood collected in EDTA using Ficoll-Isopaque gradient centrifugation. For a wider antigen pool, 3 to 5 donors should be tested. Cell suspensions are incubated briefly with the patient's serum sample at room temperature, and reactions are evaluated by agglutination under phase microscopy, indirect immunofluorescence, or trypan blue dye exclusion. In drug studies dilutions of drug (1:10, 1:40, 1:100) and of patient serum samples are necessary to strike the optimum antigen-antibody concentrations. Supplemental complement may be necessary.

Interpretation.   All results must be 3 to 4 +, since cell damage resulting from the test procedure is a major technical difficulty. Nonspecific aggregation yields false-positive interpretations. Alloantibodies in previously pregnant or previously transfused patients may give agglutination, but are not necessarily significant. False-negative reactions are a major problem, and these tests cannot be used to exclude antibody-induced leukopenia. Cytotoxic antibodies to human leukocyte antigens (HL-A) do not correlate with neutropenia, since these antigens are on lymphocytes.

22.4   Granulocyte Antibodies

Principle.   Granulocyte antibodies can be seen in autoimmune, chronic, or neonatal neutropenia.

Specimen.   Serum is used as the specimen and should be kept refrigerated.

Procedure.   Manual procedures that investigate relatively few cells are being supplanted by flow cytometry combined with indirect immunofluorescence. Serum samples with the potential granulocyte antibody are incubated with neutrophils obtained from normal buffy coat and from the patient's buffy coat. Granulocytes coated with specific antibody are detected by indirect immunofluorescence, and the cell suspension is evaluated cell by cell using a flow cytometer.

Interpretation. Granulocyte antibodies are unrelated to HL-A. Tests for leukoagglutinins are generally directed at detecting cytotoxic HL-A antibodies, and as such they tend to be less specific.

Notes and Precautions. Granulocytes should be treated with paraformaldehyde to remove membrane immunoglobulins that can give falsely positive reactions by indirect immunofluorescence. Manual techniques are associated with low sensitivity.

Ancillary Tests

Other tests to study phases of granulocyte production, circulation, and pool sizes are research tools that are not generally available, and their interpretation is not well established. Such tests include measurement of total granulocyte pool by serum vitamin B_{12} binding capacity, granulocyte survival time measured by chromium-51 half-life as for red cells, and granulopoiesis measured indirectly by serum lysozyme. In the latter test low levels of lysozyme are difficult to measure, and significantly low levels are not established. The normal fragility of granulocytes further limits all three tests.

Course and Treatment

The course of neutropenia is variable depending on the potential for the marrow to recover. In acute neutropenia, if the absolute neutrophil count remains below $0.5 \times 10^9/L$ ($0.5 \times 10^3/\mu l$), death from fulminating sepsis occurs quickly. The sites that are the common source of infection (pharynx, lungs, urinary tract) are cultured for bacteria and fungi, and broad-spectrum antibiotics, such as carbenicillin and aminoglycosides, are administered until the results of cultures are available. The toxic agent or drug, if known or suspected, must be removed from the patient's environment immediately to permit the marrow to recover. Lithium carbonate has been used with limited success to stimulate granulopoiesis when marrow suppression has been caused by a drug. Granulocyte transfusions are effective for the short term, as a temporizing measure until marrow recovery occurs. This procedure is not indicated when there is no such potential, eg, extensive marrow replacement by tumor or in myelofibrosis.

In chronic asymptomatic neutropenia no therapy is indicated, and, in some cases, the condition spontaneously abates with time, eg, cyclic neutropenia. Splenectomy in neutropenia of Felty's syndrome has been helpful in 50% of patients.

References

1. Finch SC: Neutropenia, in Williams JW, Beutler E, Erslev AJ, et al (eds): *Hematology*, ed 3. New York, McGraw-Hill International Book Co, 1983, pp 773–793.
2. Ferrito MC: Abnormalities of phagocytes, in Stein H (ed): *Internal Medicine*. Boston, Little Brown & Co, 1983, pp 1584–1588.
3. Lalezari P: Neutrophil and platelet antibodies in immune neutropenia and thrombocytopenia, in Rose NR, Friedman H, Fahey JL (eds): *Manual of Clinical Laboratory Immunology*, ed 3. Washington, DC, American Society of Microbiology, 1986, pp 630–632.

23

Functional Defects of Granulocytes

Diseases associated with functional defects of granulocytes are summarized in Table 23–1. These diseases are characterized by repeated bacterial or fungal infections beginning early in life, or infections with otherwise low-virulence organisms in patients with normal granulocyte counts. Most of these involve inherited disorders of immune globulins, complement, or the hexose monophosphate shunt.

Pathophysiology

Neutrophil function involves chemotaxis, phagocytosis, and bacterial killing. Chemotaxis and phagocytosis are dependent on external factors involving immune (antibody) globulin and complement opsonins, C3a, C5a, and C567. Bacterial killing requires production of hydrogen peroxide intracellularly by anaerobic glycolysis and the hexose monophosphate shunt, and utilizes the myeloperoxidase in primary granules of granulocytes.

One of the most severe functional disorders is a heritable defect at multiple functional levels seen in chronic granulomatous disease. Chronic granulomatous disease (CGD) is a sex-linked disorder of granulocyte function in males, and rarely, an autosomal recessive disease of females that leads to early death from infection. In some cases CGD has been associated with the absence of red cell antigens

Table 23–1 Conditions Associated with Functional Granulocyte Defects

---

Extrinsic Defects

  Immunoglobulin opsonin defects

    Agammaglobulinemia, congenital or acquired

    Immune suppression

    Pathologic immunoglobulins (myeloma)

  Complement deficiencies

    C_3

    C_5

  Drugs, toxins

    Adrenocorticoids—inhibit chemotaxis

    Cytotoxic drugs

    Diabetes mellitus—inhibits phagocytosis

Intrinsic Defects

  Defective hydrogen peroxide generation

    Chronic granulomatous disease

    Complete G6PD deficiency (whites)

  Myeloperoxidase deficiency

  Unknown mechanism

    Chédiak-Higashi syndrome

ABBREVIATIONS: G6PD = glucose-6-phosphate dehydrogenase.

---

in the Kell system and with bizarre red cell morphology suggesting abnormalities of cell membrane and cytoskeleton. With repeated infections granulomas appear in the liver, spleen, lymph nodes, and lungs. Macrophages in these involved organs and in bone marrow contain a gold-brown pigment, lipochrome.

Myeloperoxidase deficiency is a rare autosomal-recessive disorder of primary granules that results in defective production of myeloperoxidase. The polymorphonuclear leukocytes (PMNs) ingest, but do not kill, catalase-positive organisms, eg, *Staphylococcus aureus,* because a defective oxidase system is not activated when the cell membrane is stimulated. Some patients show repeated infections, yet other patients show no increased incidence of infection.

Acquired transient defects secondary to drugs are poorly understood.

Clinical Findings

Clinical findings in patients with diseases of granulocyte dysfunction are secondary to infection, and can include regional lymphadenopathy, fevers, hepatosplenomegaly, and eczematoid or lupuslike skin eruptions.

Approach to Diagnosis

Neutrophils function as phagocytes by a complex interaction of immunoglobulins, complement, and neutrophil enzymes. Total evaluation of patients who show an inability to handle infections should screen for defects of all phases.

The specific tests of defective granulocyte function as seen in CGD and myeloperoxidase deficiency measure the contribution of peroxidase to phagocytosis by the following tests:

1. The nitroblue tetrazolium (NBT) dye is a test of nonimmune phagocytosis and measures the contribution of peroxidase qualitatively.

2. Myeloperoxidase stain, which identifies the presence of the enzyme in neutrophil cytoplasm, also provides qualitative measurement.

3. Additional tests for CGD include Kell red cell antigen typings, absent in some types of CGD, and G6PD screening tests since the hexose monophosphate shunt works poorly in CGD and myeloperoxidase deficiency, as well as in primary enzyme deficiency.

4. Tests of extrinsic factors indirectly involved in granulocyte function are quantitation of immunoglobulins to diagnose agammaglobulinemia and total lytic complement (CH50) as a screening test of complement function. If CH50 is decreased, specific assays for C3 and C5, the chemotactic complement, can be performed.

Hematologic Findings

Blood Cell Measurements. The presence of granulocytosis reflects infection. Granulocytopenia is seen in Chédiak-Higashi syndrome.

Peripheral Blood Smear Morphology.   In some types of CGD, marked red cell poikilocytosis is seen, even in asymptomatic patients.

Bone Marrow Examination.   Granulocytic hyperplasia in a hypercellular marrow with a left shift reflects infection. Granulomas are seen in marrow histologic sections in CGD, and histiocytes with lipochrome pigment may also be seen.

Other Laboratory Tests

23.1   Nitroblue Tetrazolium Dye Test

Purpose.   The nitroblue tetrazolium (NBT) test is used to evaluate granulocyte phagocytic function. Test results are negative in CGD. Originally devised to differentiate bacterial from nonbacterial infections, it is now used most often to measure opsonin ability.

Principle.   Unstimulated PMNs do not ingest the dye NBT, but PMNs stimulated in vivo by bacterial infection or in vitro by latex particles or endotoxin do ingest the dye. Once ingested, cell peroxidases reduce the dye to blue crystals (formazan) that can be seen microscopically. This does not occur in CGD.

Specimen.   Fresh heparinized whole blood is used as a specimen. EDTA anticoagulated specimens are not satisfactory, since EDTA inactivates C1q, decreasing this complement-dependent reaction.

Procedure.   Heparinized blood samples from patients incubated with and without endotoxin for a brief period are added to NBT dye solutions and incubated further. The colorless dye is reduced by peroxidase to blue-black formazan granules in neutrophils and monocytes. Blood smears are prepared from each reaction mixture and stained with Wright's stain. A control sample is treated similarly. One hundred PMNs are counted and the percentage with formazan granules is reported. If untreated smears are negative, the results of the endotoxin-stimulated smear are reported.

Interpretation.   A positive range for the NBT test is 29% to 47%, while negative results are less than 10%. The normal unstimulated PMN contains less than 10% formazan crystals. Stimulated PMNs can contain up to 90% formazan granules but usually contain less. Each laboratory, of course, determines its own normal range. Negative results on NBT tests are seen in CGD, complement deficiencies, and agammaglobulinemia; stimulation by endotoxin is of no help in these instances. Patients with normal responses may have a negative test result even during infection if antibiotic therapy is being given; however, in this case, the endotoxin-stimulated NBT test gives positive results. True-negative test results remain negative with the endotoxin-stimulated NBT test. NBT dye reduction is low in patients receiving aspirin, steroids, or phenylbutazone. Negative results should be confirmed by demonstrating white cell bactericidal defects.

23.2 Myeloperoxidase Stain

Purpose. Cytochemical staining detects absence of myeloperoxidase in granulocytes. Active myeloperoxidase implies that opsonin function is intact. Myeloperoxidase deficiency produces a clinical picture similar to that of CGD.

Principle. Peroxidase of granulocytic secondary granules reduces azo dyes, producing insoluble complexes at the site of enzyme action.

Specimen. Freshly prepared blood films are used as a specimen. They should be stained within a few hours, since peroxidase is unstable in light. Smears stored in the dark are usable for 2 to 3 weeks.

Procedure. Hydrogen peroxide (H_2O_2) and colorless dye are layered over the peripheral smear. Peroxidase converts H_2O_2 to O_2 and H_2O, which oxidizes the colorless dye, such as benzidine, to blue-black. A methyl-green or safranin counterstain allows easier identification of granulocytic cell series and monocytes.

Interpretation. Normally maturing granulocytes are strongly positive. Absent staining is seen in cells with deficient peroxidase. Myeloperoxidase deficiency is a rare defect of bactericidal activity against *S aureus* and *Candida*. In CGD, peroxidase staining is normal or increased.

Ancillary Tests

In some types of CGD the Kell blood group antigens (Kell, cellano, Js^a, Js^b, Kp^a, Kp^b) are absent, resulting in Kell null red cells. Following transfusion the serum may contain antibodies of all Kell antigens, agglutinating all red cells except the patient's own or those of other patients with CGD and defective Kell antigens.

Other tests that may be useful include biopsy of lymph nodes for granulomas and lipochrome-pigmented histiocytes in CGD and quantitation of immunoglobulins G, A, and M to document agammaglobulinemia.

Course and Treatment

There are repeated infections, often with early death. Treatment with appropriate antibiotics is indicated. The natural course of untreated CGD includes recurrent infections, septic lymphadenitis, diffuse granulomatosis and death within 5 to 7 years. Regular administration of trimethoprim-sulfamethoxazole (TMP-SMX) with penicillin and nystatin profoundly reduces the incidence and severity of infection.

References

1. Curnutte JT (ed): *Phagocytic Defects I: Abnormalities outside of the respiratory burst,* Hematology/Oncology Clinics of North America, vol 2, no 1. Philadelphia, WB Saunders Co, 1988.

2. Curnutte JT (ed): *Phagocytic Defects II: Abnormalities of the Respiratory Burst,* Hematology/Oncology Clinics of North America, vol 2, no 2. Philadelphia, WB Saunders Co, 1988.

3. Hong R: Immunodeficiency, in Rose NR, Friedman H, Fahey JL (eds): *Manual of Clinical Laboratory Immunology.* Washington, DC, American Society for Microbiology, 1984, pp 702–716.

4. Salmon C, Cartron JP, Rouger P: *The Human Blood Groups.* New York, Masson Publishing USA, 1984, pp 361–376.

5. Southwick FS, Stössel TP: Phagocytosis, in Rose NR, Friedman H, Fahey JL (eds): *Manual of Clinical Laboratory Immunology.* Washington, DC, American Society for Microbiology, 1986, pp 326–328.

24

Leukocytic Disorders of Abnormal Morphology

A varied class of hereditary disorders of granulocytic morphology is summarized in Table 24–1. In general, the disorders are of nuclear morphology or characterized by persistence of primary type granules or by abnormal granules. Except for the Pelger-Huët anomaly, all disorders are associated with major clinical abnormalities, such as albinism, Hurler's syndrome, and, with thrombocytopenic hemorrhage, repeated severe infections and early death.

Pathophysiology

These disorders are heritable gene defects. Transient morphologic abnormalities can also be acquired with severe infection or chemotherapy.

Clinical Findings

Clinical findings vary with the anomaly (see Table 24–1). Patients with Pelger-Huët anomaly and the majority of those with May-Hegglin anomaly are asymptomatic. Thrombocytopenia or functional platelet disorders are common to two anomalies, May-Hegglin and Chédiak-Higashi syndrome. The latter may have hepatosplenomegaly with infiltration of these organs by histiocytes and T lymphocytes. The Chédiak-Higashi syndrome may show decreased granulopoiesis and shortened survival of granulocytes. Defective degranulation of neutrophil and natural killer cell granules in Chédiak-Higashi syndrome impairs host resistance to bacterial and viral infections, and to neoplasia.

Approach to Diagnosis

Except in Pelger-Huët anomaly, it is unlikely that the hematologic findings will call attention to the disease. Instead, clinical findings of thrombocytopenic hemorrhage and severe or repeated infection in early life warrant close examination of a peripheral smear for morphologic abnormalities in both the patient and close relatives, eg, siblings, parents, and children. A white cell count and platelet count are also necessary.

Hematologic Findings

Pelger-Huët anomaly, found in 1 in 6000 people, is an autosomal-dominant trait that results in failure of nuclear lobe segmentation in neutrophils and eosinophils. The homozygous defect results in round nuclei, fewer cytoplasmic granules, and enlarged secondary granules. The heterozygous defect results in bilobed or "spectacle" nucleus. The neutrophil is functionally normal. When concurrent infection occurs the bilobed nucleus appears more immature and is round. In pseudo–Pelger-Huët anomaly, seen in leukemia, pre-leukemia, metastatic carcinoma, and with some drugs, cytoplasmic granules are absent or decreased.

Patients with May-Hegglin anomaly are usually in good health, despite a mild leukopenia and thrombocytopenia. Ultrastructural studies show dense fibrils of messenger RNA similar to those seen with infection or chemotherapy. The disorder may be caused by an unknown metabolic disorder, which is transient in the acquired form and permanent in the inherited disorder. Thrombocytopenia may be caused by a maturation defect manifested in the appearance of many large bizarre platelets.

Alder-Reilly granule anomaly reflects abnormal lipid storage of other organs.

Chédiak-Higashi syndrome is a rare autosomal-recessive disorder involving not only blood, but lymph nodes, spleen, liver, and skin. Neutrophil inclusions result from fusion of lysozymes. The neutrophil has poor chemotaxis, degranulation, and bactericidal activity because of the failure of giant granules to fuse with phagocytic vacuoles. Thus, the disorder may be due to abnormal cell

Table 24-1 Granulocytic Disorders of Abnormal Morphology

Disorder	Morphology	Inheritance	Frequency	Associated Clinical Findings
Pelger-Huët anomaly	Bilobed nuclei in mature PMN	Autosomal dominant	1:6000	None
May-Hegglin anomaly	Leukopenia, Döhle bodies bizarre platelets	Autosomal dominant	Rare	Thrombocytopenic bleeding, infection, lymphomas, death in childhood
Alder-Reilly anomaly	Giant granules	Autosomal recessive	Rare	Associated with some forms of mucopolysaccharidosis
Chédiak-Higashi syndrome	Giant granules in PMNs, eosinophils and platelets; leukopenia; occasionally giant granulation in lymphocytes, monocytes	Autosomal recessive	Rare	Thrombocytopenic hemorrhage, repeated infection, atypical lymphocytic, histiocytic proliferation in liver, spleen, lymph nodes, brain; albinism

ABBREVIATIONS: PMN = polymorphonuclear leukocyte.

membrane function; similarly, the associated albinism may be caused by abnormal melanocyte activation. The platelet dysfunction appears to be due to storage pool deficiency.

Blood Cell Measurements.   The granulocyte count is often decreased in Chédiak-Higashi syndrome and May-Hegglin anomaly.

Peripheral Blood Smear Morphology.   Giant cytoplasmic granules are seen in leukocytes in Chédiak-Higashi syndrome or Alder-Reilly anomaly. Döhle bodies are found with the May-Hegglin anomaly or severe infection, and large azurophilic inclusions in lymphocytes accompany the Chédiak-Higashi syndrome. Platelets are large in May-Hegglin and Bernard-Soulier anomalies.

Bone Marrow Examination.   There are no diagnostic morphologic findings. Lipoid histiocytes may be seen in sections of marrow in lipidoses.

Course and Treatment

The course varies with the underlying disorder, eg, no symptoms with Pelger-Huët anomaly and in most patients with May-Hegglin anomaly, to severe symptoms and early death with Hurler's syndrome. Chédiak-Higashi syndrome has been associated with recurrent severe infections and a lymphomalike disease with early death. Ascorbic acid and A-cyclic nucleotides improve neutrophil and platelet function, but have no effect on the final course of the disease.

References

1. Bessis M: *Blood Smears Reinterpreted.* New York, Springer International, 1977, p 122.
2. Brunning RD: Morphologic alterations in nucleated blood and marrow cells in genetic disorders. *Hum Pathol* 1970; 1:99–124.
3. Jandl JH: Leukocyte anomalies, in *Blood: Textbook of Hematology.* Boston, Little, Brown & Co, 1987, pp 571–588.
4. Marmont AM, Damasio E, Zucker-Franklin D: Neutrophils, in Zucker-Franklin D (ed): *Atlas of Blood Cells: Function and Pathology,* ed 2. Philadelphia, Lea & Febiger, 1988, pp 192–200.

Reactive Disorders of Lymphocytes and Lymph Nodes

25

Reactive Disorders of Lymphocytes

Reactive disorders of lymphocytes result in a polyclonal proliferation of T- or B-lymphocytes, which may be seen as lymphocytosis or lymphoid tissue hyperplasia or both. Lymphocytosis is age-dependent and, in the adult, is an absolute increase in lymphocytes above $3.5 \times 10^9/L$ ($3.5 \times 10^3/\mu l$). In the child under 4 years of age, lymphocytosis is the norm, and only lymphocyte counts above $6 \times 10^9/L$ ($6 \times 10^3/\mu l$) are considered significant; in infants absolute lymphocyte counts are occasionally as high as $8 \times 10^9/L$ ($8 \times 10^3/\mu l$). Causes of lymphocytosis are listed in Table 25–1. Leukocytosis secondary to absolute lymphocytosis is uncommon, but may be seen in pertussis, infectious mononucleosis, infectious lymphocytosis, and lymphocytic leukemia. Lymphocytosis without an increase in total white cell count is seen in acute viral exanthems such as measles, roseola infantum, and rubella. The lymphocytosis seen in postperfusion syndrome is believed to result from acute infection by cytomegalovirus (CMV), or, rarely, Epstein-Barr (EB) virus, and is transmitted by the lymphocytes of whole blood transfusion. Lymphocyte leukemoid reactions are associated most often with infectious lymphocytosis (40 to $100 \times 10^9/L$ or 40 to $100 \times 10^3/\mu l$) or pertussis (15 to $50 \times 10^9/L$ or 15 to $50 \times 10^3/\mu l$). Infectious lymphocytosis may be caused by adenovirus, enterovirus, or Coxsackie A virus.

Relative lymphocytosis secondary to granulocytopenia is more frequent than absolute lymphocytosis. The significance of absolute

Table 25-1   Causes of Lymphocytosis

Physiologic (4 months to 4 years)

Acute infections

    Infectious mononucleosis

    Infectious lymphocytosis

    Cytomegalovirus infection (including postperfusion syndrome)

    Pertussis

    Brucellosis

    Typhoid—paratyphoid

    Viral exanthems—measles, rubella, varicella, mumps, roseola infantum

    Toxoplasmosis

    Infectious hepatitis

    Mycoplasma pneumoniae

Chronic infections

    Congenital syphilis

    Tertiary syphilis

Endocrine

    Thyrotoxicosis

    Adrenal insufficiency

Neoplasms

    Acute lymphoblastic leukemia

    Chronic lymphocytic leukemia

    Lymphosarcoma cell leukemia

Drug sensitivity

    Diphenylhydantoin (Dilantin)

    Para-aminosalicylic acid

lymphocytosis, and, therefore, the aggressiveness with which it is evaluated, differs with age. Newborns and children less than 4 years of age are considerd to be "lymphoid organs" and tend to respond to all antigenic stimuli with lymphocytosis. This characteristic fades as the child reaches puberty, at which time reactive lymphocytosis is stimulated by a narrower range of antigens: infectious mononucleosis, respiratory viruses, and toxoplasmosis are less likely to be primary infections, although they still may be suspected.

Pathophysiology

Lymphocytes are derived from stem cells of thymic origin (T-cells) or from bone marrow (B-cells). T-cells are located in the interfollicular and subcapsular areas of lymphoid tissue in lymph nodes, spleen, and gastrointestinal tract. In a complex interdependent relationship with antigen-presenting cells (monocytes, granulocytes, endothelial cells) and the major histocompatibility complex (MHC), lymphocytes recognize and process foreign antigens. B-cells are found in follicles of lymphoid tissues. When processed antigen is presented to B-cells in soluble form, they enlarge (blast transformation) with cell division and production of clones of daughter lymphocytes or plasma cells. The latter produce specific antibody to the antigen. Antibody either destroys the antigen by cell or particle lysis, or coats it so that phagocytic cells, neutrophils, and monocytes can ingest and destroy the particle. T-cells are the primary agents in cellular immunity, as in rashes and skin tests. B-cells are involved in humoral or antibody immunity since they are directly involved in antibody production. T-lymphocytes can be categorized as helper/inducer cells and as suppressor/cytotoxic cells. T-helper cells respond to soluble antigen, induce B-lymphocytes to secrete immunoglobulins, and transform pre-cytotoxic cells to cell-mediated immune responses as mediated by interleukins. Lymphocytes participating in the recognition process, antibody production, and killing process are permanently committed to respond to the particular antigen on every subsequent exposure, but to no other, and are therefore said to have "memory." When the antigenic stimulus is removed, the lymphocytes return to a waiting state. These lymphocyte subpopulations are identifiable by markers on the cell membrane, including receptors for complement, Fc fragment, and surface immunoglobulins.

T-cells comprise 80% to 90% of circulating lymphocytes, B-cells only 10% to 20%. T-helper cells are approximately 60% and T-suppressor cells are approximately 30% of the total T-cell population. T-cells may survive up to 30 years, B-cells for shorter periods of time. The spectrum of antigens that may incite the immune sequence of cell division and antibody production are legion. Antigen reactivity may be reflected in peripheral lymphocytosis and antibody production, or may be reflected in hyperplasia and enlargement of lymphoid tissue, most often in lymph nodes, but occasionally in the spleen.

Clinical Findings

The significance of lymphocytosis varies with age; in children under 4 years of age, mature lymphocytosis is more likely to be a physiologic process. Reactive lymphocytosis caused by infection is usually of short duration, 3 to 6 weeks, and associated with systemic symptoms, fever, exanthems, pharyngitis, or malaise. In benign lymphocytosis, lymphadenopathy is variable but usually involves at least cervical lymph nodes; generalized lymphadenopathy is rare. Splenomegaly is seen more often than hepatomegaly, although both may be found in infectious mononucleosis or CMV infection.

Approach to Diagnosis

The urgency of testing and its sequence depends on clinical history, symptoms, and age of the patient. The differential diagnosis of reactive vs pathologic lymphocytosis begins with the following:

1. Examination of the peripheral blood determines the magnitude and duration of the lymphocytosis, as well as lymphocyte morphology. The bone marrow aspirate is rarely helpful in reactive processes, but the pattern and extent of infiltration on marrow clot sections or biopsy are helpful in persistent, and, therefore, possibly pathologic lymphocytosis.

2. Serologic tests are performed to document the underlying cause if hematologic and clinical findings are of short duration, suggesting a reactive process. These tests include screening for heterophile and differential absorption tests for infectious mononucleosis, screening for hepatitis B surface antigen (HB_sAg) if lymphocytosis is associated with elevated liver enzymes, tests for cytomegalovirus, *Toxoplasma* titers, or Epstein-Barr virus titer.

3. Biopsy of enlarged lymph nodes is performed if serologic testing is not diagnostic, if lymphadenopathy persists or progresses, and if clinical symptoms such as fever or malaise persist beyond 3 to 6 weeks. Lymph nodes are cultured for virus or bacteria and are also examined microscopically. Lymphocyte suspensions made from the fresh tissue are tested immunologically for cell surface markers to determine monoclonal populations as seen in neoplastic lymphocytosis.

4. T- and B-cell surface markers can be serologically characterized to determine if a monoclonal population is present, as in neoplastic lymphocytosis vs the polyclonal population of a reactive

process. Further characterization of neoplastic lymphocytes aids in treatment and prognosis.

Hematologic Findings

Blood Cell Measurements.   Anemia is usually not present. The white cell count may vary from 5 to 30 $\times$ 10^9/L (5 to 30 $\times$ 10^3/μl). The proportion of lymphocytes is greater than 30% of the total, ie, >3 $\times$ 10^9/L (3 $\times$ 10^3/μl). Normal levels vary with age; at birth, 0.30 (30%) lymphocytes are present; at 6 months, 0.60 (60%); at 4 years, 0.50 (50%); at 6 years, 0.40 (40%); and, in adults, 0.30 (30%). The platelet count is usually normal. Rarely, it is less than 100 $\times$ 10^9/L (100 $\times$ 10^3/μl) with acute viral exanthems.

Peripheral Blood Smear Morphology.   Normally both T- and B-lymphocytes appear as small, uniform cells with scanty cytoplasm. Antigenically stimulated, both T- and B-cells are seen on the peripheral smear as large ameboid cells, and they are termed reactive or atypical lymphocytes (Figure 25–1). Atypical lymphocytes comprise more than 20% of the total, most often in infectious mononucleosis, cytomegalovirus (CMV) infection, and infectious hepatitis. Lymphocytes in infectious lymphocytosis generally remain small. Lymphocytes of varied size and shape usually indicate a reactive process, while morphologic monotony suggests neoplastic lymphocytosis. Azurophilic granules may be prominent as may cytoplasmic vacuoles, the site of lysosomes dissolved in the staining process.

Bone Marrow Examination.   Both aspirated particles and histologic sections of the marrow should be examined for distribution of lymphocytosis. Bone marrow biopsy may be of further help. Lymphocytosis may be diffuse, in small aggregates of 3 to 10 cells, or in nodules. Lymphoid nodules that are small and discrete are usually a reactive phenomenon and are often seen in elderly patients. Rarely, reactive lymphoid nodules may show actual follicle development. Confluence of nodules or many nodules with ill-defined borders suggest neoplastic lymphocytosis. Lymphocytes comprise less than 20% of cells in normal marrow, but may appear as sheets if a nodule in a particle has been smeared. Therefore, to avoid distribution errors, more than one slide must be examined.

In hypoplastic marrow, lymphocytes and lymphoid nodules become more prominent, since they and the stromal support cells are the last to disappear. Lymphocytosis is frequently associated with some degree of plasmacytosis. If both lymphocytes and plasma cells appear mature, they are more likely reactive.

Other Laboratory Tests

25.1 Infectious Serology

Purpose. Serologic tests for infectious agents may determine the specific etiology for reactive lymphocytosis, often restrospectively. Cultures are more specific, but are technically difficult so that sensitivity is 60% or less. Culture techniques are not as widely available as serologic tests.

Principle. After individuals have been exposed to infectious agents, specific antibody titer rises. Antibodies may be IgG, IgM, complement fixing, or precipitating, and they vary with each patient. A rise in antibody titers usually occurs slightly after the onset of lymphocytosis. Both IgG and IgM titers should be ordered since IgG titers may persist for years and not be helpful in the diagnosis of acute disease. IgM titers are consistent with current or recent infection.

Specimen. Acute and convalescent serum is taken 10 to 14 days apart during the period of lymphocytosis. Specimens can be stored frozen for comparison testing.

Procedure. Testing is usually available at county or state health department laboratories or regional reference laboratories. Complement fixation, hemagglutination inhibition, direct or indirect immunofluorescence, or radioimmunoassay (RIA) are helpful techniques (Table 25–2). Serum is serially diluted for all except RIA procedures.

Interpretation. Many patients have been exposed to specific agents early in life. Therefore, a single titer is rarely diagnostic. A threefold or fourfold rise in titer in a 10- to 14-day span is considered significant, since laboratory dilution carry-over could not account for the change. Low-antibody titers may persist for years in toxoplasmosis, EBV or CMV infection, or in rubella.

For CMV and *Mycoplasma* infection, titers of 256 or higher suggest acute infection. For toxoplasmosis, a titer of 1:8 is seen in most adults; titers above 64 are suspicious for acute infection. In infants, positive immunofluorescence using IgG conjugates may represent maternal antibody until the newborn reaches 3 months of age. Therefore, positive test results with IgM conju-

Table 25–2   Serologic Tests in Differential Diagnosis
of Lymphocytosis

Disease	Diagnostic Test	Significant Result
Infectious mononucleosis	Heterophile by kit or Davidsohn differential	Positive Titer >224 resistant to guinea pig kidney absorption
	Anti-EB-viral capsid antigen; Anti-Early Antigen by IF; Anti-EB Nuclear Antigen by ACIF	Positive in 20% of cases; anti-EB early antigen positive in 80% of cases
Hepatitis A (infectious)	RIA test for antibody to Hepatitis A	IgM, current infection; IgG, past infection
Hepatitis B (serum)	HBsAg by RIA	Reactive
Cytomegalovirus	CF	Titer >256 for acute infection, Titer >8 for past infection
Toxoplasmosis	IF CF	Titer >64 Titer >128
Rubella	HI	Titer >10 for past infection, Titer >80 for acute infection
Mycoplasma pneumoniae	CF CAT	Titer >256 Titer >64

ABBREVIATIONS: CF = complement fixation; HI = hemagglutination inhibition; IF = immunofluorescence; RIA = radioimmunoassay; ACIF = anticomplement immunofluorescence; HBsAg = hepatitis B surface antigen; CAT = cold agglutinin titer.

gates are considered more significant, but must be correlated with maternal titers.

Hepatitis B is reported as reactive or nonreactive. The presence of HBsAg, its core antigen (HBcAg), DNA polymerase antigen, and HBeAg in the presence of lymphocytosis are consistent with current infection, the latter two with high infectivity. Tests for *antibody* to core antigen are available. Of the many techniques for HBsAg, RIA is the most sensitive. The presence of HBs antibody is not clinically significant unless a baseline nonreactive test result is known, since antibody is found in 10%

Table 25–3 Characteristic Alteration of Lymphocyte Subsets
In Reactive Disorders

Clinical Disorder	Alteration
Acquired immunodeficiency	Absolute progressive CD_4 decrease
CMV mononucleosis	Transient CD_4 decrease; CD_8 increase persisting months to years
EBV mononucleosis	CD_8 increase during acute disease
Sarcoidosis	Decreased CD_4 cells in blood, increased in lung
Tuberculosis	Chronic relative CD_4 decrease
Viral exanthems	Transient CD_4 decrease during acute disease

ABBREVIATIONS: CMV = cytomegalovirus; EBV = Epstein-Barr virus.

of healthy blood donors and may remain detectable for months
or years. Core antibody is consistent with current virus repli-
cation in liver cells, as seen in acute or chronic active hepatitis.
EBV serology is reviewed in chapter 26.

25.2   T- and B-Cell Markers of Lymphocytes

Purpose.   Tests for T- and B-cell membrane antigens (markers)
determine dominant vs pleomorphic populations, monoclonal
vs polyclonal population of lymphocytes, ie, neoplastic vs reactive lymphocytosis. Some membrane markers by their mere
presence identify malignant differentiation, eg, common ALL
antigen (cALLa), or T_1. Patterns of increase or decrease in specific lymphocyte subpopulations may be diagnostic of disease
or correlate with prognosis in nonmalignant lymphocyte disorders, eg, AIDS or other viral infections (Table 25–3).

Principle.   Each subpopulation of lymphocytes has membrane
markers as defined by functional studies or by monoclonal
antibodies. T-lymphocytes have membrane attachment sites for
sheep red cells and will form a rosette with them. B-lymphocytes, which are related to antibody production, have surface
immunoglobulins. In addition they have receptors for the Fc
fragment of IgG, the basis of rosette formation with antibody-
coated sheep cells, and for C3. Lymphocytes that do not show
T- or B-cell markers as presently defined are termed "null lymphocytes."

Table 25-4 Selected Monoclonal Antibody Markers in Human Lymphocytes, Monocytes, and Granulocytes

CD	Common Names	Cells Identified
T Lymphocytes		
CD[a]	OKT[b], Leu[c]	Common thymocytes
CD1	OKT6, Leu6	0% to 5% blood lymphocytes
CD2	OKT11, Leu5	E-Rosette lymphocytes; T-cell leukemia, lymphoma
CD3	OKT3, Leu4	Most peripheral blood T-cells
CD4	OKT4, Leu3	T-helper/inducer cells
CD5	NA, Leu1	All T lymphocytes
CD8	OKT8, Leu2	T-suppressor cells/Cytotoxic
NA	OKT10, Leu17	Activated T- and B-cells and monocytes, thymocytes, NK cells
NA	OK Ia	Anti-HLA-DR B-cells, activated T-cells, B-cell lymphomas and CLL, monocytes
CD10	CALLA	Non-T ALL, CGL blast crisis, T-cell and B-cell lymphomas
B Lymphocytes		
Anti-IgG polyvalent		Surface Ig–bearing cells, B-cells, Fc-receptor bound IgG on lymphocytes, PMNs monocytes
Anti-Kappa/Lambda		B-cell light chain ratio 2:1—Imbalance indicates monoclonality
CD20	B1	B-cells, not plasma cells
CD19	B4	B lymphocytes, some B-cell malignancies
NA	PC A-1	Plasma cells, plasmacytoid lymphocytes
Monocytes, Granulocytes		
NA	OKM1	Monocytes, granulocytes
CD11	Mo1	Monocytes, granulocytes, null cells, some myelomonocytic, monocytic leukemias

(Continued.)

Table 25-4 *Continued.*

CD	Common Names	Cells Identified
NA	Mo2	Monocytes, macrophages, occas myelo-monocytic leukemia
NA	My4, My7, My9	Monocytes, granulocytes, blood and marrow 40% to 80% AML
Other Markers		
NA	TdT	B-cells, T precursors, cortical thymo-cytes

ABBREVIATIONS: CD = cluster designation; NK = natural killer; CLL = chronic lymphocytic leukemia; ALL = acute lymphoblastic leukemia; CGL = chronic granulocytic leukemia; PMN = polymorphonuclear leukocyte; AML = acute myeloblastic leukemia; NA = not applicable.

[a]Cluster designation, 2nd International Workshop on Human Leukocyte Differentiation; not all monoclonal antibody specifities fall within cluster designates

[b]Ortho-Diagnostics, Inc. Raritan N.J. monoclonal antibody

[c]Leu Beckton-Dickinson Immunocytometry Systems, Mountain View, CA monoclonal antibody

These techniques were tedious, incomplete, and have been supplanted by the rise of a multiplicity of monoclonal antibodies labeled with fluorescent conjugates (fluorescein and rhodamine), combined with flow cytometry that allows extensive sampling and categorization of T- and B-cells, and of T subsets (Table 25-4). Both percentage and absolute numbers of each type of cell can be determined. There are antibodies for membrane markers of nonlymphocytes as well. Many large hospital laboratories and numerous reference laboratories now provide the service.

Specimen.   Lymphocytes are harvested on the day of testing from the buffy coat of 10 to 20 mL of whole blood collected in EDTA, heparin, or citrate. Lymphocyte suspensions can be made from biopsied lymph nodes by finely mincing the tissue and scraping the cells from the surface. Tissue can be held overnight in RPMI-1640 tissue culture media.

The lymphocytes are collected by centrifuge gradient through Ficol-isopaque from the patient's heparinized whole

Table 25–5 Human Lymphocyte Subset Distribution
Normal Range

Monoclonal Antibody		Lymphocyte Type	Normal Range[a]	
			%	Numbers
CD3	(OKT3)	Labels most T lympho-cytes	54–83	900–2550
CD4	(OKT4)	Helper/Inducer cells	30–55	520–1600
CD8	(OKT8)	Suppressor/Cytotoxic cells	15–40	360–1075
NA	(OKT10)	Thymocytes, (?) regenera-tive	0–28	0–660
CD2	(OKT11)	E-Rosette receptor	60–90	950–2700
CD10	CALLA	Common ALL antigen	0–8	0–191
NA	(OK 1-1A)	Normal B-cells, B-cell ma-lignancies	0–16	0–314
sIg (polyvalent)		B-cells	6–31	135–710
Kappa/Lambda		B-cells	19–15	50–410

ABBREVIATIONS: CD = cluster designation; ALL = acute lymphoblastic leukemia; CALLA = commmon ALL antigen; NA = not applicable.
[a]Normal range varies with each laboratory

blood. The buffy layer is 90% lymphocytes, but the interface zone with red cells is contaminated with unwanted granulocytes and mononuclear cells.

Procedure.   Lymphocyte suspensions are incubated with a series of fluorescein- or rhodamine-conjugated monoclonal antibodies that react with cell membrane antigens. The flow cytometer permits individual cells to flow through an orifice. Cells are differentiated on the basis of size and nuclear complexity and the amount of fluorescence generated by laser ultraviolet light. Instead of the limited number of cells evaluated by the manual techniques, a greatly improved statistical sampling is possible. The total lymphocyte count is multiplied by the percentage of each T-cell subset to yield an absolute number for each subset. Table 25–5 lists some of the currently more useful antibodies and their relative percentages.

Interpretation.   In lymphocytosis it is important to determine if the cell population has a dominant or monoclonal population of either T- or B-cells that indicate probable neoplasm. Polyclonal populations are associated with reactive processes. Lymphocytes that do not demonstrate markers are defined as null lymphocytes until a marker is found.

Notes and Precautions. There may be variation in specificity of monoclonal antibodies because of differences in the cell line of the hybridoma from which the clone arises. Normal ranges for each cell type must be determined by each reference laboratory. Antisera produced by Becton-Dickinson Immunocytometry Systems (Mountain View, CA) use Leu nomenclature; antisera produced by Ortho-Diagnostics Inc (Raritan, NJ) uses OKT nomenclature. Several other manufacturers produce other monoclonal antibodies that, in some cases, show cross-reacting specificity. Cluster designation (CD) nomenclature represents an international attempt to amalgamate a confusing mixture of developmental terminology and should be used.

Course and Treatment

The clinical course depends on the cause of the lymphocytosis. Many of the infections associated with lymphocytosis are viral, which limits treatment to supportive measures to prevent or control superimposed bacterial complications. Typhoid is treated with appropriate antibiotic therapy, of which norfloxacen is a new class of antibiotic. *Mycoplasma* responds to erythromycin or tetracycline, but not to other antibiotics.

Endocrine disorders are treated with appropriate hormonal supplementation. Discontinuation of diphenylhydantoin therapy reduces lymphocytosis, but may not alter the associated lymphoid hyperplasia. Lymph node hyperplasia, with or without lymphocytosis, may be slow to resolve. Posterior cervical lymphadenopathy in infectious mononucleosis may persist as small shotty lymph nodes for years.

References

1. Andiman WA: Antibody response to Epstein-Barr virus, in Rose NR, Friedman H, Fahey J (eds): *Manual of Clinical Microbiology,* ed 3. Washington, DC, American Society of Microbiology, 1986, pp 509–514.
2. Claman HN: The biology of the immune response. *JAMA* 1987; 258:2834–2840.
3. Giorgi JV: Lymphocyte subset measurements: Significance in clinical medicine, in Rose NR, Friedman H, Fahey JL (eds): *Manual of Clinical*

Laboratory Immunology, ed 3. Washington, DC, American Association of Microbiology, 1986, pp 236–243.

4. Jackson AL, Warner NL: Preparation, staining and analysis by flow cytometry of peripheral blood leukocytes, in Rose NR, Friedman H, Fahey JL (eds): *Manual of Clinical Laboratory Immunology,* ed 3. Washington, DC, American Society of Microbiology, 1986, pp 226–236.

5. Kaufman L, Reiss E: Serodiagnosis of Fungal diseases, in Rose NR, Friedman H, Fahey J (eds): *Manual of Clinical Immunology,* ed 3. Washington, DC, American Society of Microbiology, 1986, pp 446–466.

6. Miale JB: *Laboratory Medicine: Hematology.* St Louis, CV Mosby Co, 1982, pp 666–671.

7. Patten E: Immunohematologic diseases. *JAMA* 1987; 258:2945–2951.

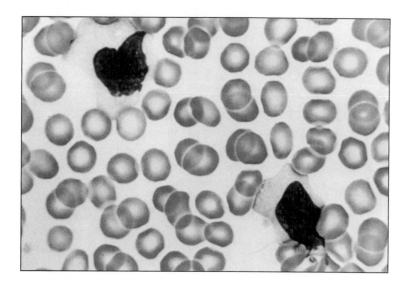

Figure 25–1   Infectious mononucleosis. Peripheral blood with 2 large, reactive lymphocytes.

26

Infectious Mononucleosis

Infectious mononucleosis (IM), a self-limited febrile illness caused by the Epstein-Barr virus (EBV), is a highly specific cause of lymphocytosis. A positive heterophile test is necessary to make the diagnosis.

Pathophysiology

EB virus infects B-lymphocytes that have surface receptors for the virus. Infection results in a morphologic change in the cell, with production of new surface antigens on the cell membrane. These changes activate suppressor T-cells, which undergo morphologic transformation to the atypical cells characteristic of the disease. Activated suppressor T-lymphocytes kill the EBV transformed B-lymphocytes.

Clinical Findings

IM has a prodrome of 3 to 5 weeks followed by the typical clinical findings of fever, malaise, and pharyngitis. IM occurs in all age groups, but most often between the ages of 15 and 25 years. EBV infection without clinical mononucleosis is often inapparent. Young children with EBV infection have a nonspecific febrile illness. The

Table 26–1   Tissues with Heterophile and Forssman Antigens

	IM Heterophile Antigen	Forssman Antigen
Sheep red cell	1+	1+
Horse red cell	2+	0
Ox or beef red cell	1+	0
Guinea pig kidney red cell	0	1+

disease may be epidemic, occurring usually in the spring, or cases may be episodic and isolated.

Nearly all patients have cervical lymphadenopathy with less involvement of other regional lymph nodes. Thirty percent to 50% of the patients have splenomegaly; splenic rupture can occur, but is rarely a cause of death. Ten percent of the patients have hepatomegaly, yet nearly all patients have hepatitis with elevated liver enzymes. In a significant number of patients the pharyngitis is related to *Streptococcus* group A.

Approach to Diagnosis

The diagnosis of IM, unlike other causes of lymphocytosis, requires the presence of heterophile antibodies.

Diagnosis may be difficult when the course is primarily febrile (typhoidal), unless diagnostic tests are repeated over several weeks. IM should be suspected in patients less than 30 years of age who have lymphocytosis. Serologic findings, which appear with the onset of peripheral atypical lymphocytosis include (1) antibody to the causative virus, (2) coincidental antibody-agglutinating sheep red cells (the heterophile antibody), (3) antibody to human red cell antigens (anti-i), and (4) an increase in IgM (Table 26–2). Serologic findings persist into and beyond the convalescent phase, which may be 4 to 6 weeks. The diagnostic approach includes the following:

1. Hematologic evaluation with attention to blood lymphocytosis and lymphocyte morphology. Bone marrow examination is rarely needed unless serologic tests remain nondiagnostic.

2. A positive test for heterophile antibody is required to diagnose IM as the cause of the lymphocytosis. This is usually accomplished by a screening test. If the test is negative in young patients

	Stage of Disease	Diagnostic Test
Heterophile	With lymphocytosis persists 2–3 months	Sheep-cell agglutinins (Davidsohn differential); horse-cell agglutinins (commercial kit tests)
Anti-EBV capsid antigen		
IgG antibody	Persists for years	Immunofluorescence titer 1:80 or 3-dilution rise; IF, complement fixation
IgM antibody	Acute phase	
Anti-i	Rare, during acute phase	Direct antiglobulin test, serum antibody screening; cold agglutinin titer
IgM	Mid-disease and 2–3 months after	Quantitative immunoglobulins

or is positive in a clinical setting inconsistent with IM, it should be followed by a Davidsohn differential absorption test, or EBV serologic tests.

3. The Davidsohn differential absorption test excludes serum sickness or Forssman antibodies from true heterophile antibody, and detects low-titer heterophile antibody seen in young children.

4. Specific viral serologic tests for EBV are rarely needed for diagnosis and do not influence treatment. These tests are useful when clinical symptoms suggest IM, but the heterophile is negative. IgM antibody to EBV capsid antigen (EB-VCA) is positive in 80% of acute infections. IgG antibody and antibody to EB nuclear antigen (EBNA) appear later.

5. Ancillary procedures that indicate the expected rate of recovery include liver function tests.

6. Serologic tests for autoimmune hemolytic anemia are performed if anemia is present. These tests include a direct antiglobulin test, serum antibody screening, and a test for cold agglutinin titer (Table 26–2).

Hematologic Findings

Hematologic findings appear 3 to 4 days after symptoms begin, but may be delayed for 2 or 3 weeks. At the peak of the disease, moderate-to-marked lymphocytosis with hyperplasia of all lymphoid tissue is present. Anemia is uncommon, but autoimmune hemolytic anemia, cold-antibody type, appears in 1% of cases. Antibody specificity is often anti-i but anti-I or anti-Pr have also been reported. The anemia appears 2 or 3 weeks after onset of the disease and is self-limited. Thrombocytopenia is rare, less than 0.1%, and usually moderate, with hemorrhage a very rare event. Thrombocytopenia may be due to direct effects of virus, splenomegaly, or autoantibody.

Blood Cell Measurements. Usually no anemia is present; rarely hemolytic anemia may occur with hemoglobin levels of 90 to 110 g/L (9 to 11 g/dl). MCV is elevated if hemolysis is present, as a result of the increased reticulocyte count. The white cell count is 10 to 20 $\times$ 10^9/L (10 to 20 $\times$ 10^3/μl) with greater than 0.60 (60%) lymphocytes; 0.10 to 0.20 (10% to 20%) lymphocytes are atypical. The platelet count is usually normal, although rarely it may be 80 to 100 $\times$ 10^9/L (80 to 100 $\times$ 10^3/μl).

Peripheral Blood Cell Morphology. The characteristic Downey cell is a transformed (atypical) lymphocyte with an eccentric, oval, often indented, nucleus. The cytoplasm is abundant and pale blue. Downey classified these cells as type I, II, or III, as the cell appeared more and more plasmacytoid with an ovoid nucleus and deeper blue cytoplasm. This classification is of historic interest only and has no clinical significance. If hemolytic anemia is present, spherocytes and nucleated red cells may be seen.

Bone Marrow Examination. Bone marrow aspiration is usually unnecessary. Mild hypercellularity may be present due to reactive granulocytic hyperplasia or to mild diffuse lymphocytosis.

Other Laboratory Tests

26.1   Heterophile Screening Tests

Purpose. Results of the heterophile test must be positive and associated with lymphocytosis to make the diagnosis of IM.

Principle. Subsequent to EBV infection and lymphoid hyperpla-

Table 26–3   Serologic Specificity in Tests to Diagnose Infectious Mononucleosis

Test	Test Antigen
Paul-Bunnell presumptive	2% sheep red cells in saline
Differential absorption	2% sheep red cells in saline
Monosticon[a]	Sheep red cell extract
Diagluto[b]	Horse red cells
Hetrol[c]	Stabilized horse red cells
Monospot[d]	Fresh citrated horse red cells
Mono-Test[e]	Stabilized horse red cells
Mono-Stat[f]	Papain-treated sheep red cells
Confirmikit[g]	Papain-treated horse red cells

ABBREVIATIONS: IM = infectious mononucleosis; FA = Forssman antibody; SS = serum sickness.

[a]Manufactured by Organon Diagnostic Products, West Orange, NJ

[b]Manufactured by Beckman Instruments, Inc., Fullerton, CA

[c]Manufactured by Difco Laboratories, Detroit, MI

[d]Manufactured by Ortho Pharmaceutical Corp., Diagnostic Division, Raritan, NJ

[e]Manufactured by Wampole Laboratories, Cranbury, NJ

[f]Manufactured by Co Lab Industries, Inc.

[g]Manufactured by BBL Microbiology Systems, Cockeysville, MD

sia, IgM antibodies are produced in the human that cross react with antigens found in tissues of other animal species, and are, therefore, heterophilic. Rise in heterophile antibody parallels atypical lymphocytosis and declines with decrease in lymphocytes. Animal tissues that have heterophile antigen are listed in Table 26–3. Heterophile antibody must be distinguished from other cross-reacting, Forssman-type antibodies by absorption tests using animal tissue rich in Forssman antigens that remove Forssman antibodies and leave heterophile antibody. Sheep red cells are the classic source of heterophile antigen, but it is more strongly represented on horse red cells. Both cell types are used in screening test kits, usually stabilized by tanning to allow longer storage (Table 26–4). Sheep red cell suspensions are available commercially for the more classic Paul-Bunnell test.

Differential Absorption	Antibody Specificity
	IM, FA, SS
Guinea pig kidney and beef red cells	IM
	IM, FA, SS
Guinea pig kidney and beef red cells	IM
	IM
Guinea pig kidney and beef red cells	IM, FA
None	IM
None	IM
None	IM

Specimen. Kit tests use serum or plasma. For the Paul-Bunnell test, serum must be complement inactivated at 56° C for 30 minutes, since heterophile antibodies are hemolytic.

Procedure. Commercial test kits for IM screening are widely available. The Paul-Bunnell test requires refrigeration of sheep red cell suspension and is usually available in most reference laboratories and large hospitals.

Screening tests with commercial kits mix a drop of stabilized cell suspension with the patient's serum or serum dilutions on a slide or card. Agglutination indicates a positive test result. Positive and negative serum controls are provided and are run simultaneously. The classic Paul-Bunnell anti-sheep cell titer incubates equal volumes of sheep cell suspension and dilutions

Table 26–4   Representative Patterns in the Davidsohn
Differential Absorption Test

Type of Antibody	Absorption with Guinea Pig Kidney Antigen	Absorption with Beef Red Cell Antigen
Heterophile antibody in infectious mononucleosis	Not removed or less than 3-tube change in titer	Antibody removed
Forssman antibody (normal serum)	Antibody removed	Antibody not removed or incompletely removed
Forssman antibody (serum sickness)	Antibody removed	Antibody removed

of the patient's serum for 30 minutes. The test is read for the
highest serum dilution showing agglutination.

Interpretation.   In Paul-Bunnell tests, titers above 224 are presumptive of IM. Titers of 56 to 224 indicate probable IM but should be confirmed by differential absorption. Diagnosis of IM is not supported by titers less than 28.

Positive agglutination using commercial screening kits suggests IM. Negative agglutination may indicate that the titer is less than 56. The test should be repeated using differential absorption.

Titers for positive agglutination in kit tests are adjusted by formalinization to detect titers of 56 or 112 and above. Fresh horse red cells may detect lower titers. Titers below 56 are frequently found in IM in children under 12 years of age, and kit tests may give false-negative results. False-positive results occur in serum sickness, and approximately 5% of serum samples contain high-titer horse agglutinins unrelated to IM. False-positives are usually excluded by differential absorption tests, since only in IM are Forssman antigens unable to remove the sheep cell agglutination. Low levels of heterophile antibody persist for months and may be recalled anamnestically with other diseases; therefore, all positive results should be correlated with the characteristic lymphocytosis. Seronegative IM is uncommon, usually appearing in young children. The diagnosis of seronegative IM can be substantiated only if EBV antibody titers show a diagnostic rise. If both heterophile and EBV titers are negative, another cause for the lymphocytosis should be found.

26.2 Differential Absorption Tests

Purpose. Absorption tests differentiate heterophile from Forssman antibody.

Principle. IM results in the production of many antibodies directed at antigens shared by humans and other species. The classic diagnosis of IM is defined by the sheep red cell antibody discovered by Paul and Bunnell. The heterophile antigen found on sheep red cells and beef red cells is not found on guinea pig kidney, which has Forssman antigen. Absorption with guinea pig kidney of serum that agglutinates sheep cells and beef cells defines the pattern of heterophile antigen.

Specimen. For the Davidsohn differential absorption test, serum is complement inactivated immediately before testing. For the kit tests, serum or plasma may be used without inactivation.

Procedure. In the Davidsohn differential absorption test, serial dilutions of the patient's serum are incubated with sheep red cells to determine the presumptive titer. Serum aliquots are then absorbed individually with guinea pig kidney or beef cells and retitered against sheep red cells. A three-tube decrease in titer is considered positive absorption. Some kit tests include suspensions of guinea pig kidney or beef cells so that drops of serum can be absorbed with appropriate drops of suspension, and the drop mixtures can then be mixed with stabilized sheep or horse cells to determine patterns of absorption.

Interpretation. Table 26–4 summarizes the diagnostic patterns. Antibody resistant to absorption by guinea pig kidney is characteristic of heterophile antibody. Negative findings for heterophile antibody suggest that the disease is not IM. Titers are a technical means to determine three-tube decrease and do not correspond to activity or severity of disease.

26.3 Anti–EBV Serology

Purpose. Anti–EBV serologic tests are useful in classic, self-limited, acute EBV infection, ie, IM, when the heterophile antibody is negative. The most useful tests in this circumstance

Table 26–5   Characteristic Epstein-Barr Virus Serology

	IM-VCA	IgG-VCA
Acute IM	2+	1+
Convalescing IM	1+	3+
Recurrent IM		
Remote IM	0	1+
Nasopharyngeal Ca	0	2+
Burkitt lymphoma	0	2+

ABBREVIATIONS: IM = infectious mononucleosis; NT = not tested.

[a]EA has 2 components, D and R. Antibodies to R component are frequently seen in children and in recurrent disease. The component usually seen in adults is D

are IgM and IgG antibodies to EBV capsid antigen, (VCA), and IgG antibody to EBV nuclear antigen (EBNA). For persistent fatigue thought to be caused by chronic or recrudescent EBV infection, IgG antibody to VCA and IgG anti–EA (early antigen) are supportive evidence.

Principle.   EBV is the presumed cause of IM. As for many viruses, EBV has a nuclear core and capsule, each with its own antigen. IgM–EB-VCA is positive early in acute IM followed by a decrease in IgM antibody after 1 to 2 months and an increase in IgG-VCA; IgG–VCA fades over several months to a stable low level often maintained for years. Anti-EA rises and falls early in the disease, lasting only a few months. Often the diagnostic rise in titer to the capsid antigens is missed and low levels of anti-EA will be found in only a few patients. Anti–EBNA appears late, persisting for several months before decreasing to low stable levels.

    In chronic EBV infection there is evidence of suppression of T-suppressor lymphocytes with abnormal cellular immunity. Anti IgG–VCA persists at high titer, occasionally with IgM–VCA. Anti–EA also persists whereas anti–EBNA is absent.

Specimen.   Serum can be stored for only 2 to 3 months to preserve complement.

Procedure.   The patient's serum is layered over prepared smears of the EBV infected lymphoblastoid cell line. Reaction of patient antibody to viral capsid antigen is detected by indirect immu-

IgA-VCA	Anti-EA[a]	Anti-EBNA
NT	2 + (D)	Negative
NT	1 +	3 +
	1 + (R)	
NT	0	2 +
2 +	IgA-1 + (D)	
NT	1 +	0

nofluorescence using fluorescein-conjugated anti–human IgG, IgA, or IgM. Similar technique is used for anti–early antigen, except that the lymphoblastoid cell line has been superinfected with virus. Early antigen has 2 components, diffuse (D) and restricted (R), based on the immunofluorescent pattern. Anti–EBNA is detected using anti–complement immunofluorescence. Fresh tissue–cultured Raji cells are layered with patient serum, incubated at 37° C, and rinsed in saline. Fluorescein-conjugated antibody to human C3 is then layered, incubated, and rinsed, and examined by fluorescent microscopy.

Interpretation. Interpretation is summarized in Table 26–5. In acute IM, rising titers of IgM–VCA and IgG–VCA may be seen. Anti–EA is usually not detected, or is detected transiently in the first 3 to 4 weeks. In most children and adults the EA antibody response is to D component, but in children under 4 years of age, antibodies to R component are common. The later rise in titer for anti–EBNA may be helpful; rise in titer should be fourfold to be diagnostic.

In remote IM infection, low unchanging titers of IgG–VCA and anti–EBNA are present.

In chronic EBV infection high titer IgG–anti–VCA exists with persistent low titers of anti–EA. In acute IM, anti–EBNA is absent or very low titer.

In nasopharyngeal cancer, IgA antibodies to VCA and to EA may be present, and are often associated with metastatic disease.

Notes and Precautions. Rheumatoid factor may give a false-positive test result for anti–IgM VCA, so that antibody to at least 1 other antigen should be positive to validate the result.

Course and Treatment

Mononucleosis is a self-limited disease with no specific treatment. The fever usually remits within 10 days. Fatigue and malaise, treated with bed rest, may persist for 6 to 10 months, and severity of symptoms is often related to elevations of liver enzymes. Streptococcal pharyngitis is treated with penicillin. Steroid therapy is occasionally necessary for airway obstruction due to pharyngeal edema, for post-viral Guillain-Barré syndrome (GBS), or for autoimmune hemolytic anemia. Exchange plasmapheresis has had variable success in acute GBS.

Chronic EBV infection is a controversial entity; symptoms of fatigue persist for many months with ambiguous serologic findings. Chronic or previous EBV infection has been described in patients with Burkitt's lymphoma or nasopharyngeal carcinoma. The infection appears related, if not causal, and neoplastic disease appears years later.

References

1. Andiman WA: Antibody response to Epstein-Barr virus, in Rose NR, Friedman H, Fahey J (eds): *Manual of Clinical Microbiology,* ed 3. Washington, DC, American Society of Microbiology, 1986, pp 509–513.

2. Horwitz CA, Henle W, Henle G, et al: Long-term serological follow-up of patients for Epstein-Barr virus after recovery from infectious mononucleosis. *J Infect Dis* 1985; 151:1150–1153.

3. Sumaya CV: Infectious mononucleosis and other EBV infections: Diagnostic factors. *Lab Management* 1986; 17:37–43.

4. Tosato G, Straus S, Henle W, et al: Characteristic T-cell dysfunction in patients with chronic active Epstein-Barr virus infection (chronic infectious mononucleosis). *J Immunol* 1985; 134:3082–3088.

5. Zighelboim EJ: Infectious mononucleosis and other benign disorders of lymphocytes, in Stein JH (ed): *Internal Medicine.* Boston, Little, Brown & Co, 1983, pp 1594–1595.

27

Lymphopenia

Lymphopenia is defined as a total lymphocyte count of $<1.5 \times 10^9/L$ $(1.5 \times 10^3/\mu l)$ in adults, and $<3 \times 10^9/L$ $(3 \times 10^3/\mu l)$ in children. Causes of lymphopenia are listed in Table 27–1.

Pathophysiology

Lymphopenia may be secondary to abnormalities of lymphocyte production (neoplasia, immune deficiency); to loss from mechanical interference with lymphocyte kinetics, as in disorders of the small intestinal lymphatics or thoracic duct that are often associated with the malabsorption syndrome; or to destruction by drugs, viruses, or radiation. Because 80% of circulating lymphocytes are T-cells, disease processes that affect this subpopulation are usually associated with lymphopenia. Specific loss of B-cells is much less evident. Acquired immune deficiency syndrome (AIDS) is caused by infection with the human immunodeficiency virus (HIV), a retrovirus cytopathic for T-helper lymphocytes; the T-helper antigen is the receptor for the virus.

Clinical Findings

T-cells are mediators of cellular immunity, so that lymphopenia is often associated with clinical symptoms of a cellular immune def-

Table 27–1   Causes of Lymphopenia with Diagnostic Methods

Disease	Diagnostic Method
Immunodeficiency syndromes	Quantitative immunoglobulins
Swiss-type agammaglobulinemia	IgG, IgA, and IgM decrease
Agammaglobulinemia with thymoma	IgG, IgA, and IgM decrease
Lymphopenic dysglobulinemia	IgG, IgA decrease; IgM increase
Wiskott-Aldrich syndrome	Platelet count decrease; IgM decrease
Ataxia telangiectasia	IgA decrease; IgE (?) decrease
AIDS	Helper/suppressor ratio < 1.0; biopsies of skin, lymph nodes Cytology (pneumocystis); cultures TB, fungus
Lymphocyte destruction	
Corticosteroids—Cushing's syndrome, iatrogenic	Plasma cortisol
Radiation	History
Alkylating chemotherapy	History
Intestinal lymphocyte loss	
Intestinal lymphangiectasia	Small bowel biopsy; IgA decrease
Whipple's disease	Small bowel biopsy with PAS stain
Right heart failure	EKG, chest x-ray, physical examination
Occlusion of thoracic duct or intestinal lymphatics	Chest x-ray
Neoplasm	
Hodgkin's disease	Biopsy
Terminal carcinoma	Biopsy
Miscellaneous	
Sarcoid	Angiotensin-converting enzyme; lymph node biopsy
Renal failure	Serum creatinine
Miliary tuberculosis	Chest film; sputum culture
SLE	Antinuclear antibody
Aplastic anemia	Bone marrow biopsy

ABBREVIATIONS: PAS = periodic acid–Schiff; SLE = systemic lupus erythematosus; AIDS = acquired immune deficiency syndrome; EKG = electrocardiogram.

icit, such as rashes or eczema and mucocutaneous candidiasis. In AIDS loss of T-helper lymphocytes alters the T-cell helper/suppressor ratio leading to repeated life-threatening infections by opportunistic viral, fungal, and protozoal organisms, malignancies (Kaposi's sarcoma, lymphoma), autoimmune disorders (thrombocytopenia), and neurologic disorders. Opportunistic infections are secondary to *Pneumocystis carinii* (pneumonia), *Mycobacterium avium* (pneumonia or disseminated disease), oral candidiasis, toxoplasmosis, *cryptosporidiosis* (diarrhea), hepatitis B, cytomegalovirus (CMV), and herpes virus infections.

Approach to Diagnosis

Recognition of the most common disorders causing lymphopenia is based on clinical history followed by:

1. Hematologic findings, with attention to leukocyte differential. Bone marrow aspirate differential may lend supportive evidence.

2. Quantitative immunoglobulin determinations, which are needed to classify immunodeficiency syndromes.

3. Ancillary tests that may determine the underlying cause and are easy to perform are those for antinuclear antibodies (in systemic lupus erythematosus), angiotensin-converting enzyme (in sarcoidosis), and serum creatinine (in renal failure).

4. If cellular immunodeficiency is suspected, skin tests, including mumps antigen, are applied. Biopsy of lymphoid tissue or skin may be necessary.

5. T- and B-lymphocyte studies are helpful in defining lymphoproliferative disorders. T-cell helper/suppressor ratios contribute to the diagnosis of AIDS.

6. Appropriate cultures are necessary in immunodeficiency syndromes.

Hematologic Findings

Lymphocytopenia may be associated with thrombocytopenia or anemia in some immunodeficiency syndromes, in aplastic anemia, after irradiation, or with some drugs. Significant lymphopenia occurs at a higher level in children. Depending on the underlying cause, there may be a paucity of palpable lymphoid tissue. Alternatively, enlargement of lymph nodes, spleen, and liver may occur in Hodgkin's disease or sarcoidosis. In the latter condition, hepatomegaly may also be present.

Blood Cell Measurements.　In lymphopenia the lymphocyte count for adults is less than $1.5 \times 10^9/L$ ($1.5 \times 10^3/\mu l$), or less than 10%, and for children it is less than $3 \times 10^9/L$ ($3 \times 10^3/\mu l$). Thrombocytopenia in congenital immunodeficiency is moderate, 30 to $50 \times 10^9/L$ (30 to $50 \times 10^3/\mu l$), but it can be severe in AIDS, 10 to $20 \times 10^9/L$ (10 to $20 \times 10^3/\mu l$). Anemia is mild, normochromic, or absent.

Bone Marrow Examination.　Cellularity varies with underlying disease. It is hypocellular in marrow aplasia, may be hypercellular in Hodgkin's disease, and normocellular in most cases of lymphopenia. Normally, 5% to 20% of cells in bone marrow are lymphocytes. Under 5 months of age, lymphocytes may comprise as much as 40% of cells, but are normally absent. Persistent absence of both lymphocytes and plasma cells after 6 months suggests immunodeficiency. Clot sections or biopsy specimens are necessary to detect sarcoid granulomas or caseating granulomas of *Mycobacterium* infection in AIDS. *Mycobacterium avium-intracellulare* can be detected in marrow histiocytes with PAS stains and may be so numerous that acid-fast stains are not necessary, except to characterize the organism.

Other Laboratory Tests

27.1　Quantitation of Immunoglobulins

Purpose.　Acquired and hereditary immunodeficiency syndromes associated with lymphopenia are often combined with deficient production of immunoglobulins. In AIDS there may be a polyclonal rise in gamma globulin due to stimulation of B-cells by infection.

Principle.　Lymphopenia is usually caused by T-cell deficiency. When a combined deficiency with B-lymphocytes occurs, production of immunoglobulins is altered. This may result in decreases of 1 or more immunoglobulins and elevations of others. Combined deficiencies occur in hereditary disorders, but also in mechanical loss or toxic destruction of the entire lymphocyte pool. Immunoglobulins that are deficient are usually IgG, IgA, or IgM. IgE is rarely involved, and the significance of decreased IgD is unknown.

Procedure, Specimen, and Interpretation.   See Test 38.4.

27.2   Quantitation of T-cells

Purpose.   Quantitation of T-cell subsets may be helpful in diagnosing the underlying cause of lymphopenia and in determining prognosis. The relative percentage and absolute numbers of T-helper and T-suppressor lymphocytes with calculation of the helper/suppressor ratio is the most useful in lymphopenia.

Principle, Specimen, and Procedure.   See Test 25.2.

Interpretation.   Immunophenotyping of lymphocytes with pan–T-cell antibody identifies T-cells, of which 65% are helper cells, and 35% are suppressor cells, in a normal ratio of 1.0 to 2.9. Ratios above 2.9 are usually reactive and caused by decreases in suppressor cells. In almost all cases of AIDS or AIDS–related complex (see lymphadenopathy), ratios are <1.0. Absolute numbers of T4 lymphocytes $<0.4 \times 10^9/L$ ($0.4 \times 10^3/\mu l$) are usually associated with clinical AIDS. In AIDS–related complex (ARC), patients with low T4 lymphocytes frequently progress to clinically overt AIDS. Other infections cause nonspecific elevation of suppressor cells; in these cases, the ratio is also decreased, although usually not <1.0. A low ratio is not diagnostic of AIDS.

Course and Treatment

The clinical course is dependent on the cause of lymphopenia. Congenital immunodeficiency results in significant morbidity and eventually death from infection. Supportive therapy with appropriate antibiotics is helpful. In some disorders transplantation of bone marrow or thymic tissue has reconstituted the lymphocyte population.

HIV infection results in AIDS in at least 50% of patients within 2 to 5 years. AIDS is fatal within 1 to 2 years, death occurring from infection or neoplasm. Current therapy with AZT is palliative and short term, usually producing severe anemia.

Lymphopenia from alkylating agents may recover, but lymphopenia in many diseases does not improve, although it is not life-threatening, eg, in sarcoid, systemic lupus erythematosus, and renal failure.

References

1. Check IJ, Piper M: Quantitation of immunoglobulins, in Rose NR, Friedman H, Fahey JL (eds): *Manual of Clinical Immunology*, ed 3. Washington, DC, American Society of Microbiology, 1986, pp 138–151.

2. Fanci AS, Masur H, Gelman EP, et al: The acquired immunodeficiency syndrome: An update. *Ann Int Med* 1985; 102:800–813.

3. Hong R: Immunodeficiency, in Rose NR, Friedman H, Fahey JL (eds): *Manual of Clinical Immunology,* ed 3. Washington, DC, American Society of Microbiology, 1986, pp 702–719.

28

Lymphadenopathy Without Lymphocytosis

Lymphadenopathy results from neoplastic proliferation of a clone of lymphocytes, or reactive hyperplasia of lymphocytes and histiocytes. Metastatic tumors are an important cause of enlarged lymph nodes. The common causes of reactive lymphadenopathy are toxoplasmosis, viral infection (Epstein-Barr virus or cytomegalovirus infection), venereal infection (syphilis, chancroid, lymphogranuloma inguinale), AIDS or ARC, and less commonly, granulomatous disease (sarcoid, tuberculosis) (Table 28–1).

Pathophysiology

Lymph node enlargement is mechanical, due to a proliferation of lymphocytes, benign or malignant, or infiltration by metastatic carcinoma.

Clinical Findings

Regional lymphadenopathy occurs with metastatic carcinoma, but can be the presenting finding in what will become generalized lymphadenopathy of hematologic neoplasms or immunodeficiency syndrome.

AIDS occurs in certain high-risk populations: homosexual

Table 28–1 Causes of Lymphadenopathy Without Lymphocytosis

Infections

  Parasitic

    Toxoplasmosis

    Lymphogranuloma venereum

    Filaria

  Bacterial

    Plague, tularemia

    Mycobacterium tuberculosis, atypical *Mycobacterium*

    Syphilis, congenital or tertiary

    Chancroid

  Fungal

    Coccidioidomycosis

    Histoplasmosis

  Viral

    Cytomegalovirus

    Infectious mononucleosis

Collagen Disease

  Rheumatoid arthritis

  Systemic lupus erythematosus

Drugs

  Diphenylhydantoin (Dilantin)

  Para-aminosalicylic acid

Neoplastic disorders

  Lymphoma or leukemia

  Metastatic carcinoma

Other

  Sarcoidosis

  Persistent generalized lymphadenopathy

  AIDS or AIDS-related complex

  Cat-scratch hyperplasia

ABBREVIATIONS: AIDS = acquired immune deficiency syndrome.

males, intravenous drug abusers, hemophiliacs, and Haitian immigrants. Vague clinical symptoms of fever, night sweats, malaise, diarrhea, weight loss, and lymphadenopathy may be present for several months before the diagnosis is made. Unexplained opportunistic infection may be the presenting symptom; pneumonia with clinical prostration, dyspnea, and cough caused by *Pneumocystis;* meningitis, or coma, due to toxoplasmosis or cryptococcosis; or diarrhea due to *Cryptosporidiosis,* amebiasis, or giardiasis.

Lymph node hyperplasia also occurs in a variety of infectious diseases or collagen vascular disorders, and symptoms vary with the underlying disease (pulmonary symptoms in sarcoidosis, and renal failure, arthralgia, and arthritis in systemic lupus erythematosus).

Approach to Diagnosis

The logical sequence of diagnostic evaluation involves noninvasive techniques to document the underlying disease before tissue biopsy is performed. Physical examination may determine the extent of lymphadenopathy, but is often supplemented with radiologic examination.

The diagnostic approach includes the following:

1. Chest roentgenogram to document sarcoid hilar adenopathy, tuberculosis, *Pneumocystis* infection, fungal infections, or tumor. CAT scans or magnetic resonance imaging are useful in inaccessible areas such as the chest and retroperitoneum.

2. Serologic tests for infectious agents include RPR, VDRL, or fluorescent treponemal antibody absorption test (FTA-Abs) for syphilis; and HIV antibody testing, if the patient permits, for AIDS.

3. T-cell helper/suppressor ratios in suspected AIDS.

4. Skin tests for tuberculosis, coccidioidomycosis, or histoplasmosis, especially if chest roentgenograms are positive.

5. Biopsy of lymph nodes is often necessary to establish lymph node morphology and to document granulomas or tumors (see chapter 36). If facilities are available some material should be submitted for electron-microscopic examination, which can often detect occult organisms, including viral particles. Persistent, significantly enlarged lymph nodes (>2 cm), in the absence of obvious infection, should always be biopsied.

6. Bone marrow biopsy and liver biopsy are less helpful in the diagnosis of benign lymphadenopathy.

7. All biopsied material should be cultured for routine bacteria, fungus, and *Mycobacterium* tuberculosis. Cultures of bone mar-

row are less successful than those of lymph nodes because of the limited volume of specimen.

8. Ancillary tests include those for angiotensin-converting enzyme in sarcoid, for antinuclear antibodies in collagen disease, and anti-HIV in AIDS or AIDS-related complex.

Hematologic Findings

Lymphocytosis may be transient in many diseases that cause lymphadenopathy and absent at the time of diagnosis. Therefore, hematologic findings may be minimal. Anemia and thrombocytopenia suggest lymphoproliferative malignancy, but may be seen in collagen disease or AIDS. Regional lymphadenopathy may suggest the cause or port of entry of infection: cervical lymphadenopathy, respiratory disease; inguinal, venereal disease; axillary or inguinal, plaque or tularemia; and pulmonary hilus, sarcoid. The location of regional lymphadenopathy draining tumors may suggest the site of the primary tumor: neck, nasopharynx, lung or thyroid; axilla, upper extremity, breast, or, rarely, lung; inguinal, lower extremity, anal, or perineal area; and pulmonary hilus, lung, or, rarely, upper gastrointestinal tract.

Blood Cell Measurements. Findings are variable. If anemia is present, it is normochromic and normocytic. White cell count may be decreased in AIDS or other viral infections ($<4 \times 10^9$/L or 4×10^3/μl), normal, or elevated in lymphoproliferative disorders. Lymphocytosis may be seen in some infectious diseases, neutrophilia, or lymphopenia in others. Platelet counts are normal except in AIDS-related disorders.

Bone Marrow Examination. Bone marrow biopsy or histologic section of aspirate occasionally reveals granulomas in sarcoid, disseminated fungal disease, or miliary tuberculosis. Because of limitation of the specimen, culture is rarely rewarding, except in AIDS where infection can be overwhelming.

Other Laboratory Tests

28.1   Serologic Tests for Infectious Agents

Purpose. High titers for ubiquitous organisms (eg, CMV, *Toxoplasma*), or titers of unusual organisms (as in coccidioidomycosis) are consistent with the causative agent, but are not always present. IgM antibodies are consistent with current disease.

Principle. Infection with various organisms produces specific antibody, as in toxoplasmosis, or nonspecific antibody, such as the reaginic antibodies of syphilis. The presence of antibody may be documented by direct methods using the organism or indirect methods such as complement fixation (Table 28–2).

Specimen. Serum is used as a specimen. In complement fixation tests, specimens from the acute and convalescent phases of disease are required to detect rises in titer.

Procedure. Indirect immunofluorescence (IF) techniques are commonly available. They are performed by incubation of serum dilutions with organisms fixed to prepared glass slides. Specific antibody adheres to the organism. Excess serum is rinsed away and antibody is detected by fluorescein-conjugated antiglobulin reagent. Positive reactions fluoresce using a microscope with ultraviolet light source. Complement fixation techniques are available at state or county health laboratories and other regional reference laboratories. These tests rely on specific antibody (Ab) attaching to antigen (Ag) (*Coccidioides, Histoplasma*, etc) with complement binding (reaction 1). The presence of complement is then determined by lysis of an indicator system, usually a sheep red cell (SRBC) with anti–sheep cell antibody (anti-SRBC) (amboceptor). If complement was not fixed, the indicator system hemolyzes (reaction 2b). If complement fixation has occurred, the indicator system does not hemolyze (reaction 2a). The amount of sheep cell antibody and standardization of the initial amount of complement present in the system must be determined on the day of the test. The test itself is an overnight incubation at 4° C for complement fixation, with addition of the indicator system the following morning. The test is read for hemolysis. Serial dilutions of test serum yield titers.

Reaction 1:
Antigen + Patient Serum Ab +
$$\text{Standardized C}' \rightarrow Ag = Ab = C'$$
$$C' + Ag + Ab$$

Reaction 2a:
$$SRBC + \text{anti-SRBC} + (Ag = Ab = C') \rightarrow \text{No hemolysis}$$

Reaction 2b:

$$SRBC = \text{anti-SRBC} + (C' + Ag + Ab) \rightarrow \text{Hemolysis}$$

Excess of antigen or antibody may be anticomplementary, invalidating the test. Microtiter techniques are available.

Interpretation. Reaginic tests for syphilis serology such as RPR or VDRL are sensitive screening tests, but should be confirmed by the more specific anti-treponemal test, the fluorescent treponemal antibody absorption test (FTA-Abs). Lymphadenopathy appears in congenital and tertiary syphilis. The FTA-Abs IgM test on newborn infants of seropositive mothers cannot exclude congenital syphilis until the infant is 3 to 6 months old, since some infants with congenital infection do not produce IgM antibody until later than normal. In long latency and tertiary syphilis, lipoidal antibodies may fade but FTA-Abs positivity usually persists weakly for 30 or 40 years. Three percent of elderly adults have biologic false-positive serologic findings with these tests, including FTA-Abs.

Direct immunofluorescence or complement fixation tests are of equal sensitivity and specificity and have replaced the Sabin-Feldman dye test for *Toxoplasma.* The latter test used live and potentially infectious organisms, and is no longer generally available.

Complement fixation titers above 256 are consistent with recent infection by cytomegalovirus. Complement fixation tests are greater than 90% reliable for fungal titers (coccidioidomycosis and histoplasmosis), since they are very sensitive. Specificity is somewhat less, however, since *Histoplasma* yeast antigen may cross react with coccidioidomycosis or other fungal infections. High titers may indicate disseminated disease. Latex agglutination tests are less sensitive and may give false-positive and negative results.

28.2   Anti–HIV (HTLV III) Serology

Purpose. AIDS is associated with HIV (human immunodeficiency virus) infection. Patients from high-risk groups who have anti–HIV antibodies should be counseled and monitored about the eventual clinical outcome. Documentation of infection with anti–HIV can support the etiologic diagnosis of lymphopenia or lymphadenopathy. AIDS patients also often have associated fulminant viral infections including CMV, hepatitis B, herpes and EBV. Demonstration of rising antibody titers to any of these viruses is supportive of the diagnosis and may have prognostic implications, since disseminated infection with these viruses may be the terminal event in the immunocompromised patient.

Principle.   Single serum specimens may be tested to document infection with HIV. Anti–HIV testing became available in 1985. Blood donor centers and increasing numbers of reference laboratories or laboratories in large hospitals make the test available. Alternate test sites make the test available to the lay public.

Specimen.   Serum, which can be stored frozen for retrospective studies.

Procedure.   HIV antibody is determined by enzyme-linked immunosorbent assay (ELISA). The patient's serum sample is placed in microtiter plates coated with HIV-sonicated antigen and incubated for 1 hour. The tube is washed free of excess serum and peroxidase-linked goat anti–human IgG is added to the tube. The azo dye and peroxide are added for 10 minutes, and the reaction is then halted with hydrogen fluoride. Color development is determined with a spectrophotometer, and is proportional to the amount of antibody. Concurrently, negative control serum samples are tested and their color development is determined. A positive to negative control ratio determines a cutoff point. All values greater than this point, usually 2.0, are reported as reactive. Repeatedly reactive ELISA test results are confirmed with Western blot or immunofluorescent methods. If the confirmatory test is positive, the patient is regarded as positive for HIV antibody. Confirmatory testing is essential in low-risk groups such as blood donors, but may not be necessary in high-risk groups (male homosexuals, intravenous drug abusers, and hemophiliacs) in whom the ratio is often in a much higher zone.

Confirmatory test methodologies for anti–HIV include indirect fluorescence, radioimmunoprecipitation (RIPA) and Western blot. This procedure is performed by disrupting a cell culture of HIV, separating the viral proteins by polyacrylamide gel electrophoresis, and transblotting the antigens onto a nitrocellulose sheet, which is then cut into strips. Diluted patient serum is incubated with a strip, then stained using peroxidase-conjugated anti-IgG and an azo dye. Viral specific bands arise for antibodies to the envelope, core, reverse transcriptase proteins.

The Western blot test is more specific, but less sensitive, and is technically more difficult to perform than ELISA techniques. Many centralized laboratories have the test available, and a kit test has recently become available. Test procedures

Table 28–2   Diagnostic Methods for Reactive Lymphadenopathy

	Serologic Test		
Disease	CF	IF	HA
Infections			
CMV	>256		
Toxoplasmosis	128		
Tuberculosis			
Histoplasmosis	8–16 (yeast)		
Coccidioidomycosis	4 recent, >16 disseminating		
Lymphogranuloma venereum			
Syphilis		FTA-Abs reactive	
Plaque			256
Tularemia	40–80		
HIV		reactive	
Collagen disease			
RA			
SLE		>80	
Nonspecific			
Cat-scratch hyperplasia			
Sarcoidosis			

ABBREVIATIONS: CF = complement fixation; ELISA = enzyme-linked immunosorbent assay; IF = immunofluorescence; LA = latex fixation; HA = hemagglutination; FLOC = flocculation; CMV = cytomegalovirus; HIV = human immunodeficiency virus; RA = rheumatoid arthritis; SLE = systemic lupus erythematosus; VDRL = Venereal Disease Research Laboratories; RPR = rapid plasma reagin; FTA = fluorescent treponemal antibody.

LA	FLOC	Skin Tests	Comments
		X	
		X	
		X	
		Frei skin test unavailable	
	VDRL, RPR reactive		
			Other tests: ELISA ratio >2.0, or Western Blot reactive
>80			
		Cat-scratch antigen unavailable	
		Kveim skin test unavailable	Angiotensin-converting enzyme elevated

and interpretation for other viruses have been previously described (chapter 25).

Interpretation.   Anti–HIV as determined by ELISA technique with values above the 2.0 cutoff are reactive. Repeatedly reactive ELISA test results are confirmed by the Western blot test and, if the confirmatory test result is reactive, the patient is considered seropositive to HIV. False-negative ELISA results in high-risk patients clinically ill with AIDS have been as high as 4% to 6%. False-positive ELISA results in low-risk blood donors have been 0.14%. There is some variation in test sensitivity because of the differing sources of the cell line in which the virus used in the test is propagated. Dialysis patients may have false-positive reactions due to cross-reaction with HL-A DR antigens derived from the cell culture used to prepare the test reagents. Prominent antibody bands seen in strongly seropositive specimens include: p17, p24, and p55 (core protein products of the *gag* gene); p31, p51, and p66 (reverse transcriptase/endonuclease from the *pol* gene); and gp41, gp120, and gp160 (glycoprotein envelope products of the *env* gene). The FDA criteria for a positive interpretation is quite conservative, requiring band at p24, p31, and either gp41 or gp160. Many researchers interpret any three viral specific bands as a positive result. Blots with one or two bands are considered indeterminate. Patients classified as indeterminate should be retested in 3 to 6 months. ELISA negative specimens can have up to 15% Western blot indeterminate results, commonly from patients with multiple pregnancies, blood transfusions, or organ transplantation. Seroconversion following HIV exposure may require 6 weeks to 6 months. Ninety-three percent to 98% of patients with clinical AIDS are positive for anti–HIV. At least 50% to 70% of high-risk group members are positive, although 15% are asymptomatic. As yet, the clinical course of high-risk patients with anti–HIV is unknown since the disease has a long prodrome; but it would appear that after 5 years, 30% have progressed to AIDS and 30% have ARC. Anti–HIV is associated with viremia in 60% to 70% of cases.

28.3   Lymph Node Culture

Purpose.   Lymph node cultures document the specific organism in infectious lymphadenopathy. They are most applicable for bacterial causes. Infections with *Pneumocystis* or *Mycobacterium avium* in conjunction with lymphadenopathy and other clinical symptoms are included in the Centers for Disease Control definition of AIDS, so that their isolation from lymph nodes and non-nodal tissue is important.

Principle.   Blood cultures are usually not helpful unless obvious systemic symptoms of high fever and leukocytosis are present. Cultures of specific lymph nodes, or of sputum if pulmonary infection is visible on roentgenogram, should be done. *Pneumocystis* is not easily demonstrated in sputum and bronchoscopy is usually necessary. Bone marrow culture is not usually diagnostic because limited numbers of organisms are expected to be present.

Procedure.   Blood or tissue is inoculated on specific media for bacteria, including *Yersinia-Pasteurella,* Sabouraud's agar for fungus, and Löwenstein-Jensen or Middlebrook 7H10 culture medium, or the equivalent, for tuberculosis.

Interpretation.   If the lymph node contains organisms known to cause lymphadenopathy, the culture is diagnostic. Pyogenic organisms such as *Staphylococcus* and *Streptococcus* are probably contaminants from skin in systemic lymphadenopathy.

28.4   Lymph Node Biopsy

Purpose.   Biopsy of the lymph node may provide specific diagnosis and tissue for culture (see chapter 36).

Principle.   Enlarged lymph nodes are biopsied. In venereal disease inguinal lymph nodes may be the only enlarged group. In metastatic carcinoma, there may be only limited regional lymphadenopathy.

Procedure.   Biopsy and culture are taken. The lymph node should be removed intact and submitted to the pathology laboratory unfixed (see chapter 36).

Interpretation.   The presence of follicular hyperplasia, immunoblastic proliferations, acute inflammatory cells, or follicular necrosis suggests a reactive origin. Granulomas, if present, may be epithelioid (in toxoplasmosis, sarcoid, and other diseases) or caseating (in tuberculosis, fungus). Small stellate microabscesses suggest cat-scratch hyperplasia. Geographic necrosis of previous hyperplastic follicles may be seen in fungi and chancroid. Increased plasma cells as a component of lymph-adenitis suggest a venereal origin, especially syphilis. Silver stains may reveal spirochetes. Tumors metastatic to lymph nodes from previously unsuspected malignancy may suggest the primary tumor by their histologic appearance (ie, adenocarcinoma vs squamous carcinoma vs melanoma). Loss of normal lymph node architecture suggests lymphoproliferative neoplasm. Immunoperoxidase studies may be useful in differentiating reactive hyperplasia from malignant lymphoma, and malignant lymphoma from metastatic carcinoma.

28.5   Angiotensin-Converting Enzyme

Purpose.   The angiotensin-converting enzyme test is often positive with pulmonary sarcoidosis, correlating with severity of disease and steroid response. The test is available in reference laboratories.

Principle.   Angiotensin-converting enzyme (ACE) is a glycoprotein present at the surface of capillary endothelial cells. It cleaves peptide substrates, including the decapeptide angiotensin I, converting it to angiotensin II.

$$\text{Angiotensin I} \xrightarrow{\text{Angiotensin-Converting Enzyme}} \text{Angiotensin II} + \text{L-histidyl-L-leucine}$$

ACE is important in the renin-angiotensin system. The enzyme is elevated in many serum samples and particularly in granulomatous lymph nodes of sarcoidosis. It is also elevated in the serum and spleen in Gaucher's disease and in neonatal idiopathic respiratory distress syndrome. It is believed that the sarcoid granulomas secrete the enzyme, increasing its serum as well as tissue levels.

Procedure.   Assay techniques include biologic, spectrophotometric, and spectrofluorimetric assays in which an artificial substrate is substituted. The ultraviolet spectrophotometric method of Cushman and Cheung uses hippuryl-L-histadyl-L-leucine (HHL) as substrate, measuring free hippuric acid released by the enzyme ACE. Hippuric acid is extracted with ethyl acetate from the reaction mixture and quantitated as a measure of enzyme activity. One unit ACE is defined as nanomoles (nmole) hippuric acid released per minute at 37° C under standard assay conditions. Normal values may vary by age and sex, but in active sarcoidosis these differences are no longer significant.

Ancillary Tests

Skin Tests.   Skin tests show strongly positive results in certain infectious diseases with lymphadenopathy, including tuberculosis, histoplasmosis, and coccidioidomycosis (Table 28–2). Frei test antigen (lymphogranuloma venereum), Kveim antigen (sarcoidosis), and cat-scratch antigen are no longer available.

Prolonged stimulation with fungal or tuberculosis organisms provokes a cellular immune response that is recalled when capsular lipid or killed organisms are injected intradermally. T-lymphocytes aggregate at the site of injection, releasing chemotactic factors for monocytes that then release vasoactive amines, producing redness and induration, and, in some cases, necrosis at the injection site. Skin test results become positive 4 to 12 weeks after infection.

Dilute antigen solutions of tuberculin, coccidioidin, and histoplasmin are injected intracutaneously on the forearm. The sites are observed for 48 hours for redness and induration.

Transient redness is not diagnostic. Induration at 48 hours, with or without redness, is interpreted as positive. Negative test results occur with anergy. Anergy can be excluded if the mumps skin test results (to which most adults are sensitive) is positive.

Chest Roentgenograms.   Chest roentgenograms may detect pulmonary hilar lymph nodes or interstitial infiltrates. The procedure is to take an anteroposterior and lateral chest roentgenogram. With sarcoid, a butterfly hilus is seen. With fungal infections, diffuse fibrosis to a cavitary single lesion is found. Interstitial infiltrates are seen with *Pneumocystis,* a common infection in immune deficiency.

Course and Treatment

The clinical course and treatment depends on the cause of lymph node enlargement. In seropositive AIDS, death from infection occurs within 1 to 2 years. AZT delays the final deterioration but is associated with profound anemia. Pentamidine and dapsone, in combination with trimethoprim, have been used to treat *Pneumocystis carinii* pneumonia. In neoplastic disease, radiation or chemotherapy or both are usually indicated.

References

1. Carlson JR, Bryant ML, Hinricks SH, et al: AIDS serology testing in low-risk and high-risk groups. *JAMA* 1985; 253:3405–3408.

2. Daly WJ: Sarcoidosis, in Stein JH (ed): *Internal Medicine.* Boston, Little, Brown & Co, 1983, pp 364–368.

3. Fishbein DB, Kaplan JE, Spira TL, et al: Unexplained lymphadenopathy in homosexual men. *JAMA* 1985; 254:930–936.

4. Ho DD, Pomerantz RJ, Kaplan JC: Pathogenesis of infection with human immunodeficiency virus. *N Engl J Med* 1987; 317:278–286.

5. Jackson JB, Balfour HH: Practical diagnostic testing for human immunodeficiency virus. *Clin Micro Rev* 1988; 1:124–138.

PART 6

Disorders Involving
the Spleen

29

Hypersplenism

Hypersplenism is defined as a reduction in one or more cellular elements in the peripheral blood associated with splenomegaly and corrected by splenectomy.

Pathophysiology

The spleen is a 150-g vascular organ composed of red pulp and lymphoid tissue, or white pulp. The red pulp is a system of sinusoidal blood spaces lined by a fenestrated basement membrane separated by cords of reticuloendothelial cells and macrophages. The lymphoid tissue is found as perivascular sheets of T-lymphocytes and lymphoid follicles of B-lymphocytes. Blood percolates through the sinusoidal spaces into the splenic cords to return through splenic veins to the peripheral circulation. The major functions of the spleen are phagocytosis of damaged red cells, releasing and recycling hemoglobin-bound iron, and reticuloendothelial macrophage ingestion and lymphocyte recognition of antigen, with subsequent production of antibodies. Antigenic stimulation results in follicular hyperplasia with formation of germinal centers composed of immunologically competent T- and B-lymphocytes. The follicular proliferation can result in splenic hyperplasia, with or without splenomegaly. The normally sluggish flow through the 3-μm sinusoidal fenestrations to the splenic cords requires red and white cells

Table 29–1   Mechanisms of Splenic Enlargement and Hypersplenism

Etiology	Mechanism	Disease

Functional	RE hyperplasia or hyperfunction	Hemolytic anemias
		    Immune
		    Thalassemia major
		    Enzyme defects
		    Hereditary spherocytosis
		PA
		Infection
		    Bacterial endocarditis
		    Malaria
		    IM
		    Infectious hepatitis
		    Military tuberculosis
		Collagen disease
		    Felty's syndrome (RA)

Vascular	Portal hypertension	Cirrhosis, liver Portal vein thrombosis
Hematopoietic	Extramedullary hematopoiesis	Myelofibrosis
Metabolic	Macrophage storage of abnormal metabolite	Gaucher's disease Neimann-Pick disease Hemochromatosis
Neoplastic	Malignant proliferations	Chronic leukemias Lymphomas

ABBREVIATIONS: RE = reticuloendothelial; IM = infectious mononucleosis; PA = pernicious anemia; RA = rheumatoid arthritis.

that are properly deformable if they are to make the transit through the spleen. Thus, abnormal red cells, such as spherocytes or target cells, become trapped in the splenic sinusoids and are ingested by macrophages. Increase in the size of the spleen slows the transit time for hematopoietic elements, effectively decreasing their presence peripherally. Even without splenic enlargement, increased activity of phagocytic cells decreases the survival of blood elements. The mechanism for the increase in splenic size varies with the disease (Table 29–1). Red cells that are senescent, damaged, or contain inclusions of nuclear debris, siderotic granules, or denatured hemoglobin (Heinz bodies), are phagocytized by macrophages. The red blood cell is "pitted" when these inclusions are removed, but without lysing the red cell; the resultant notched red cells return to the peripheral circulation (Figure 29–1). After splenectomy the pitting function of the spleen is lost, so that red cells with Howell-Jolly bodies or nucleated red cells are seen circulating in the peripheral blood.

Hypersplenism can produce anemia, leukopenia, or thrombocytopenia or all of these. The mechanisms of cell loss are: macrophage ingestion of damaged cells; macrophage ingestion of globulin-coated cells; mechanical blockade by fibrosis or by splenic cords thickened by reticuloendothelial cells storing mucopolysaccharides, hemosiderin, or other materials; and increased transit time following any increase in spleen size and volume.

Clinical Findings

In most patients with hypersplenism, splenomegaly of varying degree is present, although hypersplenism can result from an overactive reticuloendothelial system with minimal enlargement of the spleen. Early in the course of liver disease, hepatomegaly may be present, but with advancing cirrhosis, the liver may decrease in size. Lymphadenopathy may be present in lymphocytic neoplasms. Jaundice may be secondary to hereditary spherocytosis, malaria, pernicious anemia, or advanced cirrhosis, but it is not a primary symptom of hypersplenism.

Approach to Diagnosis

The diagnosis of hypersplenism is based on "full marrow, empty blood." The approach to diagnosis includes the following:

1. Hematologic findings should show a decrease in 1 or more cell lines in peripheral blood associated with normal or increased production in bone marrow.

2. Splenomegaly is usually determined by physical examination, but in the obese patient, it may be confirmed by radioactive scans of spleen or liver or both using technetium Tc99m.

3. Radioactive studies with chromium-51 determine sites of red cell sequestration and are used if the diagnosis of hypersplenism is in doubt or splenectomy is being considered.

4. Diagnosis of the underlying cause may require liver function tests or radiologic imaging in cirrhosis, blood cultures to diagnose subacute bacterial endocarditis (SBE), or heterophile tests for infectious mononucleosis.

Hematologic Findings

The most common findings in hypersplenism are normochromic anemia and mild to moderate thrombocytopenia. The underlying disease determines the diagnostic approach so that history of alcohol abuse, present or past infection, hepatitis, or a positive family history, as in the storage diseases, are helpful.

In the syndrome of "full marrow, empty blood," cellular elements are generally sequestered in the following order: red cells, platelets, and white cells.

Blood Cell Measurements. Modest decreases in platelet count (100×10^9/L or 100×10^3/µl) to moderately severe decreases (30×10^9/L or 30×10^3/µl) are seen. Normochromic anemia may be present, with levels of hemoglobin at 90 to 110 g/L (9.0 to 11.0 g/dl). Leukocytes are decreased (4.5×10^9/L or 4.5×10^3/µl) with a normal differential count.

Peripheral Blood Smear Morphology. Blood smear morphology varies with the following underlying causes:

1. Spherocytes seen in hereditary spherocytosis.
2. Target cells in liver disease (congestive splenomegaly).
3. Teardrop and hand mirror red cells seen in myelofibrosis.
4. Leukoerythroblastosis with nucleated red cells and immature granulocytes, seen in extramedullary hematopoiesis of myelofibrosis (myeloid metaplasia).
5. Atypical lymphocytes in chronic infections or infectious mononucleosis.

Bone Marrow Examination. Bone marrow aspiration shows normal-to-moderate hypercellularity (80%) with all cell lines increased and maturing normally.

Other Laboratory Tests

29.1 Chromium-51 Labeling

Purpose. Tests with chromium-51–labeled red cells measure red cell survival and splenic uptake of a radioactive label.

Principle Specimen. Chromium-51, a gamma-emitting nuclide with a half-life of 21 to 26 days, can be used to label red cells or platelets. Increased splenic size leads to increased blood flow and increased sequestration of red cells. As labeled red cells are trapped or break down, ^{51}Cr is released at the site of cell sequestration, as detected by external monitoring. Increased splenic sequestration of labeled red cells in the absence of antibody implies hypersplenism. Frequent sampling and gamma counting of the peripheral blood determines the half-life of red cells, which is decreased in hemolysis and in hypersplenism. Radioactive uptake by the spleen is compared to a baseline (precordium) and to the liver to establish ratios of ^{51}Cr uptake. Splenic size can be estimated by radio scan using 1 to 2 mCi of technetium Tc99m, a nuclear medicine procedure requiring only 1 or 2 minutes.

Specimen. Small, equal-volume (3 mL) aliquots of heparinized blood should be refrigerated and counted simultaneously to minimize specimen variability. Specimens can be counted as whole blood or as red cells, excluding counts leaching into plasma as the result of mechanical hemolysis.

Procedure. Performed in a nuclear medicine facility, tests with ^{51}Cr labeled red cells require 3 weeks for the complete study. If hemolysis is present, the study may be completed sooner. A sample of the patient's own red cells is withdrawn, labeled with 50 μCi ^{51}Cr, and reinjected. Serial 3-mL aliquots of blood are drawn over a period of 21 to 26 days to determine the cell half-life. Precordium, spleen, and liver cells are counted for 1 to 3 minutes every 2 days for 3 weeks to determine sites and rate of uptake. Radioactive counts are plotted against time. Ratios of radioactivity between the liver and spleen are calculated for selected points during the three-week period. Suspensions of donor platelets can be labeled similarly and platelet half-life studied. Leukocyte sequestration studies have not been established and are not commonly available.

Interpretation. Normal red cell half-life is 26 days. Normal spleen/liver ratio is 1.0. In hypersplenism the spleen/liver ratio is 1.5 to 2.0, and in hemolysis the spleen/liver ratio is above 3.0.

Normal splenic uptake shows a steady decrease in precordium and peripheral blood radioactivity, with steady, slow increase in spleen and liver (reticuloendothelial) counts. In splenic enlargement caused by hypersplenism peripheral blood radioactivity declines in proportion to decreasing counts in the heart and liver. Since splenic blood flow is increased, counts increase rapidly proportionate to its size and remain constant thereafter, reflecting circulating intact red cells, rather than accumulations seen with red cell degradation as in hemolysis. If radiolabeled donor red cells rather than autologous red cells are used, they must be compatible, since antibody will lead to splenic sequestration and a false interpretation of hyper-splenism.

Notes and Precautions.   The patient's blood volume must remain constant without blood loss or transfusion during the 21 to 26 days of the test. Use of other gamma-emitting radioisotopes as used in lung, liver, or spleen scans must be avoided during the 3 weeks of the test. If platelet concentrates are labeled, they should be relatively free of erythrocytes, which are preferentially labeled.

Course and Treatment

The course of hypersplenism varies with the underlying disorder. Treatment of infectious diseases with the appropriate antibiotic results in resolution of splenic hyperfunction. In cases associated with hereditary diseases of metabolism or of the hemopoietic system, splenic enlargement is usually relentless. Anemia and leukopenia in such disorders may remain moderate, but thrombocytopenia may become severe, $<20 \times 10^9/L$ $(20 \times 10^3/\mu l)$. The secondary hypersplenism of liver disease is of less clinical importance than the potential for exsanguinating hemorrhage from esophageal varices. If severe hypersplenic thrombocytopenia occurs, splenectomy may be considered. Splenectomy is most successful in splenomegaly causing mechanical destruction or sequestration of white cells, red cells, or platelets, as in hereditary spherocytosis or storage diseases. It is of less predictable benefit in immune hemolytic anemia, but succeeds in 50% of patients that respond to steroid therapy. Splenectomy is a temporizing treatment in chronic leukemias. In lymphomas, splenectomy may be part of the diagnostic evaluation. In cirrhosis splenectomy may be necessitated by the surgical shunt procedure that ends in anastomosis of the splenic artery to the renal or mesenteric artery. Splenectomy in myelofibrosis must be weighed between relieving thrombocytopenia and in losing an extramedullary source of hemopoiesis. Without the filtering effect of the spleen, immature granulocytes, including blast cells, appear in increasing numbers in the peripheral blood.

References

1. Boldt DH: Lymphadenopathy and splenomegaly, in Stein JH (ed): *Internal Medicine.* Boston, Little, Brown & Co, 1983, pp 1518–1523.

2. Mollison PL, Engelfreit CP, Contreras M: *Blood Transfusion in Medicine.* London, Blackwell Scientific Publ., 1987, pp 807–809.

3. Bowdler AJ: Splenomegaly and hypersplenism. *Clin Haematol* 1983; 12:467–486.

4. Jandl JH: Spleen and hypersplenism, in *Blood: Textbook of Hematology.* Boston, Little, Brown & Co, 1987, pp 407–432.

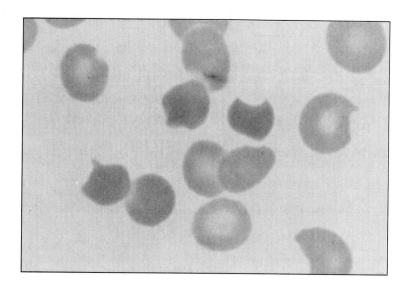

Figure 29-1   Notched red cells or "bite" cells are seen in the Wright stained peripheral smear when Heinz bodies have been removed by the spleen.

30

Liver Disease with Portal Hypertension

Hepatic cirrhosis, regardless of the cause, results in intrahepatic fibrosis with narrowing of the portal vasculature and resultant portal hypertension, one of the most common causes of splenomegaly. Splenomegaly is often associated with hypersplenism, which can result in variable pancytopenia (chapter 29). Table 30–1 lists causes of cirrhosis with the laboratory test or procedure that may be most helpful in making the diagnosis.

Pathophysiology

The functional unit of the liver is the hepatic acinus of Rappaport, differing in histologic landmarks from the lobule. In the acinus, blood flows from the digestive tract by a central axis composed of a portal venule, hepatic arteriole, and a bile ductule, the portal triad. Blood flows peripherally through the acinar sinusoids, between hepatocellular cords, to empty into terminal hepatic veins (central veins). Hepatocellular injury may be presinusoidal or postsinusoidal, resulting in cell death, collapse, and replacement by fibrous tissue (hepatic cirrhosis). The resultant narrowing of portal vasculature increases portal pressure, which is transmitted via the portal and splenic veins to the spleen. The chronic back-pressure leads to chronic congestion and fibrosis and gradual splenic enlargement, and fibrocongestive splenomegaly. Sequestration of red cells, white

Table 30–1   Causes of Hepatic Cirrhosis with Diagnostic Methods

Etiology	Diagnostic Method
Congenital	
Hepatic fibrosis	Biopsy[a]
Metabolic—Nutritional	
Alcoholic cirrhosis	Biopsy
Acute fatty infiltration	Biopsy
Hemochromatosis, idiopathic	Biopsy, iron stain
Hemosiderosis, post-transfusion	Biopsy, iron stain
Hepatolenticular degeneration, Wilson's disease	Serum Ceruloplasmin
Alpha$_1$-antitrypsin deficiency	Serum A$_1$AT
Hematologic	
Extramedullary hematopoiesis	Biopsy
Polycythemia vera	Bone marrow aspiration
Thrombotic thrombocytopenic purpura	Coagulation studies
Infectious	
Syphilis	Syphilis serology
Viral hepatitis	HBsAg, anti-HBc
Chronic active hepatitis	Biopsy, ALT, Alkaline phosphatase
Parasitic	
Schistosomiasis	Biopsy
Clonorchiasis	Biopsy
Vascular	
Post-hepatic congestion (cardiac)	Cardiac history, LD isoenzymes
Hepatic vein obstruction, Budd-Chiari syndrome	Angiography, negative liver biopsy
Toxins	
Alcohol	History
Carbon tetrachloride	
Vinyl chloride	
Methotrexate	
Malignancy	
Hodgkin's disease	Biopsy liver, lymph nodes
Hepatic carcinomatosis	Biopsy

(Continued.)

Table 30–1 *Continued.*

Autoimmune(?)	
Ulcerative colitis	Biopsy liver, colon
Primary biliary cirrhosis	Biopsy, anti-smooth muscle antibody
Lupoid hepatitis	Antinuclear antibody
Miscellaneous Etiology	
Sarcoidosis	Angiotensin converting enzyme, biopsy

ABBREVIATIONS: ALT = alanine transaminase; LD = lactate dehydrogenase.
[a]Unspecified biopsy is of liver

cells, and platelets occurs in the enlarged spleen. Increased pressure in the portal system is transmitted to gastric and esophageal veins, which may bleed chronically or produce a major hemorrhage.

Clinical Findings

Hepatomegaly occurs early in the course of liver disease; a small shrunken liver may result with far advanced cirrhosis. Hepatocellular loss results in abnormal detoxification of metabolites, with an increase in blood ammonia levels and hepatic encephalopathy manifested by tremor, marked confusion, or coma. Portal hypertension also results in ascites.

Approach to Diagnosis

In general, signs or symptoms of altered hepatic function, such as jaundice, malaise, and ascites, lead to the diagnosis of cirrhosis. Many patients with portal hypertension are asymptomatic, and the appearance of hematologic abnormalities due to hypersplenism secondary to cirrhosis leads to evaluation of liver function and morphology.

Hematologic Findings

There is generally normochromic anemia caused by poor nutrition, chronic illness, and hypersplenism. Hypochromic microcytic anemia may result from gastrointestinal bleeding. Deficiency of folate or vitamin B_{12} results in a macrocytic anemia. Rarely there is mild compensated hemolysis with hyperbilirubinemia, reticulocytosis, and an increase in lactic dehydrogenase. Zieve's syndrome, defined by fatty infiltration of the liver, hyperlipidemia, and hemolytic anemia, occurs when liver damage is present, although cirrhosis may not be. Decrease in lecithin cholesterol acyl transferase causes abnormalities in cholesterol transfer from plasma to the red cell membrane resulting in markedly spiculated cells, spur cells. Spur cell anemia, a rare event, is usually seen in alcoholic cirrhosis. Hemolytic anemia has been seen after portocaval shunt and may be severe enough to require transfusion. The cause of such hemolysis may be mechanical turbulence at the anastomotic site or may be intrasplenic.

Polycythemia can be seen in hepatocellular carcinoma that follows cirrhosis.

Coagulopathy is common with liver disease since all factors, except Factor VIII, are manufactured in the liver. The partial thromboplastin and prothrombin times may be markedly prolonged; combined with hypersplenic thrombocytopenia, the potential for hemorrhage is great. Disseminated intravascular coagulation is seen following peritovenous shunt used in the treatment of ascites.

Blood Cell Measurements. The degree of anemia is variable, the hemoglobin level may be 90 to 110 g/L (9 to 11 g/dl) in compensated chronic liver disease, but can be marked following major hemorrhage; in hypochromic microcytic anemia the mean corpuscular volume (MCV) may be <70 fL; in folate or B_{12} deficiency the MCV may be elevated. White cell count is mildly decreased when hypersplenism is present ($\leq 3 \times 10^9$/L or 3×10^3/μl) and the platelet count is moderately decreased (50 to 60 $\times$ 10^9/L or 50 to 60 $\times$ 10^3/μl).

Peripheral Blood Smear Morphology. Morphology is variable. If bleeding, nutritional deficiency, and transfusion therapy have all occurred, the red cell population may be pleomorphic. Morphologic abnormalities of red cells include the following:

1. Target cells in hyperbilirubinemia or cirrhosis.

2. Burr cells in upper gastrointestinal bleeding.

3. Microspherocytes and acanthocytes (spur cells) in abnormal cholesterol exchange between plasma and red cell membranes (Zieve's syndrome).

4. Red cell fragments in hemolysis or severe iron deficiency.

5. Rouleaux secondary to hypoalbuminemia and elevated gamma globulin.

Characteristic peripheral smear red cell morphology in liver disease is "one of everything." Nucleated red cells are uncommon

Table 30–2   Liver Function Tests in Portal Hypertension

Test	Normal Range	Etiology of Change	Comment
Alkaline phospha-tase	44–147 IU/L (37°C)	Intrahepatic fibrosis	Increased in 40% of Laennec's cirrhosis and 100% of biliary cirrhosis; only abnormality in asymptomatic cirrhosis
ALT (SGPT)	6–59 IU/L (37 °C)	Focal recurring cell destruc-tion	Episodic eleva-tion
Bilirubin	0.3–1.9 mg/dL	Intrahepatic fibrosis	Episodic eleva-tion

ABBREVIATIONS: ALT = alanine transaminase; SGPT (-ALT)-serum glutamic pyruvic transaminase.

and, if present, some cause other than portal hypertension with splenomegaly should be considered.

Bone Marrow Examination.   Bone marrow is hypercellular, with normoblastic erythroid hyperplasia of regenerative anemia. Decreased stainable iron reflects chronic blood loss. Megaloblastic changes are present in folate deficiency. Lymphoplasmacytosis of 20% to 25% may be present, and is reflected by the hypergamma-globulinemia seen in cirrhosis.

Hemosiderosis is seen in 25% to 50% of patients with alcoholic cirrhosis, and may indicate generalized hemochromatosis. Hemosiderosis may follow portacaval shunt.

Other Laboratory Tests

30.1   Liver Function Tests

Purpose.   Abnormal liver function supports the diagnosis of cirrhosis as an underlying cause of splenomegaly (see also chapter 29).

Principle.   The most useful tests (Table 30–2) are serum alkaline phosphatase, which is excreted via the intrahepatic biliary tracts; ALT (SGPT), in high concentration in liver cells; and bilirubin conjugated by liver cells and excreted via intrahepatic ducts to the major extrahepatic ducts. Intermittent cell destruction by fatty change releases hepatic cell aminotransferases and causes transient mild hyperbilirubinemia; cirrhosis causes fibrosis of intrahepatic ducts resulting in intrahepatic obstruction and elevation of alkaline phosphatase levels. Bromsulphalein (BSP) dye tests, an allergic dye, is no longer used to evaluate liver function.

Specimen. Serum should be separated from red cells promptly since red cells contain aminotransferases and may cause spurious elevations. Serum samples are stable and can be stored refrigerated or frozen.

Procedure. Most tests of liver enzymes use kinetic methods that measure appearance or disappearance of color in linked enzymatic reactions for which the patient's serum provides the enzyme of interest, as shown in the following prototype reactions:

$$A + B \xrightarrow{\text{Patient Serum Enzyme}} P + Q + (H^+) \qquad (1)$$
$$A, B, Q = \text{Substrates}$$
$$P, R = \text{Products}$$

$$NADH + Q \xrightarrow{(H^+) \text{ Enzyme Z}} NAD + R \qquad (2)$$
$$NAD, NADH, \text{Enzyme Z} = \text{Added Reagents}$$

$$\underset{\text{(Blue)}}{\text{Molybdenum}} \xrightarrow{NAD} \underset{\text{(Colorless)}}{\text{Molybdenum}} \qquad (3)$$

Because the substrates vary with each test and each test modification, results are converted to international units (IU) for uniformity.

Interpretation. Interpretation is summarized in Table 30–2. Abnormal results may be intermittent. Alkaline phosphatase elevation is the most common abnormality and the most persistent.

5′-Nucleotidase is a liver enzyme elevated in a pattern similar to alkaline phosphatase, and is usually available only in reference laboratories. Gamma glutamyl transferase is increased in liver, biliary tract, and pancreatic disease; because of this broad spectrum, it is less helpful than alkaline phosphatase.

30.2 Liver Biopsy

Purpose. Liver biopsy is used to document cirrhosis as an indirect diagnosis of hypersplenism and its associated hematologic abnormalities; it also serves to detect extramedullary hematopoiesis. It is a safer procedure than splenic puncture, but post-biopsy hospital observation for hemorrhage is mandatory.

Specimen. Manipulate the biopsy specimen as little as possible to avoid crushing the tissue. The biopsy specimen should be fixed in formalin and in glutaraldehyde if electron-microscopic examination is to be used. Specimens for culture of acid-fast bacilli and fungus can be taken, but if the specimen is limited, material should be provided for electron-microscopic examination, which can usually identify viruses and other organisms successfully.

Procedure. The biopsy can be obtained percutaneously or by laparoscopy under direct vision. Computed tomographic scanning can be used to direct percutaneous placement of the biopsy needle. Special stains (PAS, silver methenamine) can be applied to histologic sections to identify fungal organisms, and acid-fast stains detect *Mycobacterium tuberculosis*. Masson's stain are used to show increased collagen fibers in cirrhosis.

Interpretation. Biopsy specimens obtained at laparotomy should be obtained early in the procedure to avoid the misleading margination of granulocytes in subcapsular liver, thus suggesting hepatitis. Biopsy specimens taken for the diagnosis of metabolic disease are usually helpful, but biopsy specimens for the diagnosis of infectious or parasitic disease are limited by the focal nature of the underlying illness. For localized lesions, directed biopsy using CAT scans or by laparoscopy are often more productive.

30.3 Radiologic Imaging

Purpose. Imaging techniques include radionuclide scanning with technetium Tc 99m, ultrasonography, computed tomography, and magnetic resonance imaging. Liver/spleen scans with technetium Tc 99m confirm enlargement of these organs; scans may also confirm increased activity of the spleen in the absence of splenomegaly. Ultrasound and CAT scans can detect mass lesions in liver or spleen and, combined with angiography, can detect the site of vascular obstruction. Magnetic resonance imaging will probably replace these techniques.

Other ancillary tests include splenic portography, mesenteric angiography, and hepatic vein wedge pressure, but these are less commonly used.

Course and Treatment

The course of hepatic cirrhosis varies with the underlying disorder. In all cases the cirrhosis is irreversible, although its progression may be stabilized with treatment, as in some metabolic disorders (eg, Wilson's disease, hemosiderosis). Progression of cirrhosis leads to liver failure with portal hypertension and hepatic encephalopathy. Portal hypertension may improve if hepatic function improves. Hepatic encephalopathy may be reversible if diet, gastrointestinal bleeding, and intestinal bacterial flora are controlled.

The hematologic abnormalities of hypersplenism are seldom so severe as to require splenectomy. Splenectomy may correct cytopenias, but often for a very limited time.

Surgical decompression of the portal system by various shunting procedures (portocaval, proximal splenorenal, distal splenorenal) may be necessary to control variceal hemorrhage. The first 2 shunt procedures tend to increase hepatic encephalopathy.

References

1. Combes B, Schenker S: Laboratory tests, in Schiff L, Schiff ER: *Diseases of the Liver,* ed 5. Philadelphia, JB Lippincott Co, 1982, pp 277–278.

2. Conn HO: Cirrhosis, in Schiff L, Schiff ER: *Diseases of the Liver,* ed 5. Philadelphia, JB Lippincott Co, 1982, pp 879–880.

3. Gerber MH, Thung SW: Histology of the liver. *Am J Surg Pathol,* 1987; 11: p 709–722.

4. Schenker S, Hoyumjia AM Jr: Principal complications of liver failure, in Stein JH (ed): *Internal Medicine.* Boston, Little, Brown & Co, 1983, pp 174–183.

5. Zimmerman HJ: Function and integrity of the liver, in Henry JB (ed): *Todd-Sanford-Davidsohn: Clinical Diagnosis and Management by Laboratory Methods,* ed 17. Philadelphia, WB Saunders Co, 1984, pp 217–240.

PART
7

Acute Leukemias

31

Acute Myeloblastic Leukemia

Acute myeloblastic leukemia (AML) is a malignant clonal expansion arising in a single deranged multipotential stem cell and resulting in overgrowth of the granulocytic cell line. The malignant myeloid cells replace the normal bone marrow elements and accumulate in the reticuloendothelial system, including the lymph nodes, liver, and spleen, and eventually may involve any tissue in the body.

Pathophysiology

The cause of acute myeloblastic leukemia remains unknown. It has been clearly established, however, that AML originates from deranged stem cell clones. Cell kinetic studies have shown that the rate of maturation of committed cell lines is markedly reduced, leading to overgrowth of a malignant clonal population that is not programmed to completely differentiate. The variants of AML are thought to represent maturation blocks affecting different stages of the stem cell maturation.

With the arrested maturation of committed cell lines, the malignant clone replaces the normal bone marrow cells, which results in anemia, neutropenia, thrombocytopenia, and an outpouring of immature cells into the peripheral blood. Blasts accumulate in the spleen, liver, and lymph nodes, and frequently invade the meninges, testes, respiratory system, gastrointestinal tract, kidney, skin, and heart. Death does not result from the disease itself but from marrow failure and severe infections born of severe neutropenia.

Clinical Findings

In adults, AML accounts for almost 90% of all acute leukemias. The disease can occur at any age, but the incidence is highest around middle age. The onset of AML may be abrupt, as that of acute lymphoblastic leukemia (ALL) presenting with acute infection or hemorrhage. More commonly, the onset is gradual with fatigue, malaise, weakness, and fever being the most common symptoms. Hemorrhage in the form of petechiae, ecchymosis, or epistaxis is seen in less than 50% of the patients. Bleeding is particularly a problem with one type of AML called acute promyelocytic leukemia (M3), which is frequently associated with disseminated intravascular coagulation.

Physical examination may reveal splenomegaly and lymphadenopathy, but this is usually less remarkable than in ALL. Sternal tenderness is common, and a gingival hyperplasia is especially noticeable in monocytic leukemia (M5). Occasionally, accumulation of blasts may result in the formation of a tumor called "granulocytic sarcoma." Such tumors may be seen in virtually any part of the body and may, occasionally, precede other manifestations of the disease by several months. The presenting clinical features related to pathophysiology are summarized in Table 31–1.

Approach to Diagnosis

After a clinical history and physical examination have been completed, the laboratory diagnosis of acute leukemia proceeds in the following sequence:

1. A complete blood cell count.
2. Examination of the peripheral blood smear for abnormal leukocytes and blasts.
3. Examination of the bone marrow.
4. Cytochemical and immunologic studies.
5. Cytogenetic studies, which may be helpful in the diagnosis and assessment of prognosis.
6. Other studies often performed include coagulation studies, serum biochemistry studies, and febrile evaluation.

Table 31–1   Clinical Features of Acute Leukemia as Related to Pathophysiology

Weakness and pallor
  Anemia

Bleeding or bruising
  Thrombocytopenia (occasionally DIC)

Fever, infections
  Granulocytopenia (immunosuppression)

Bone or joint pain
  Leukemic infiltrates

Neurologic symptoms (headache, vomiting, etc)
  Leukemic cells in CSF

Lymphadenopathy
  Leukemic infiltrates

Hepatosplenomegaly
  Leukemic infiltrates

ABBREVIATIONS: DIC = disseminated intravascular coagulation; CSF = cerebrospinal fluid.

Hematologic Findings

The hematologic findings in AML are variable. In some patients, the diagnosis may be obvious from the examination of the blood count and the peripheral blood smear. In other patients, the leukemic findings may be very subtle and require a careful examination by experienced observers. Since therapy differs significantly, it is essential to be able to differentiate AML from ALL. In addition to a morphologic evaluation of the malignant cells, cytochemical and immunologic studies should be applied in all cases.

Blood Cell Measurements.   Anemia and thrombocytopenia are almost always seen in AML. The leukocyte count is usually elevated, but it is not infrequently normal or decreased.

Peripheral Blood Smear Morphology.   The red cells are usually normochromic and normocytic and occasional nucleated

Table 31–2 Clinical Features, Morphology, and Cytochemistry of Acute Leukemia

Factor	AML	ALL
Age	Common in adults, rare in children	Common in children, rare in adults
Blood	Anemia, neutropenia, thrombocytopenia; myeloblasts and promyelocytes	Anemia, neutropenia, thrombocytopenia; lymphoblasts and prolymphocytes
Morphology	Medium-to-large blasts, more cytoplasm than lymphoblasts, cytoplasmic granules, Auer rods; fine nuclear chromatin and distinct nucleoli	Small or medium blasts, scarce cytoplasm, no granules; fine nuclear chromatin and indistinct nucleoli
Cytochemistry	Positive peroxidase and Sudan Black; negative TdT	Negative peroxidase and Sudan Black; positive TdT
Extramedullary and focal disease	Common in spleen and liver; less common in lymph nodes and CNS; granulocytic sarcoma (chloroma)	Common in lymph nodes, spleen, liver, CNS and gonads

ABBREVIATIONS: AML = acute myeloblastic leukemia; ALL = acute lymphoblastic leukemia; TdT = terminal deoxynucleotidyl transferase; CNS = central nervous system.

red cells are seen, sometimes showing dyserythropoiesis. A variable number of myeloblasts are seen together with promyelocytes and, frequently, decreased numbers of morphologically normal neutrophils. Frequently, neutrophils show dysplastic features in the form of abnormal segmentation of the nucleus and a hypogranular cytoplasm. When only blasts are present, it is often difficult to differentiate AML from ALL without additional studies. Auer rods, pink-staining rods within the cytoplasm, represent the most reliable morphologic feature in distinguishing AML from ALL (Figure 31–1). Auer rods are only found in the granulocytic cell line and represent fused stacks of abnormal primary granules. These stain strongly positive for myeloperoxidase. Table 31–2 summarizes the main differences between AML and ALL.

Bone Marrow Examination. A bone marrow examination should always be performed if a diagnosis of leukemia is being considered. A bone marrow aspirate and biopsy with touch imprints should be performed routinely. Occasionally, the bone marrow aspirate may result in a dry tap. The major reason for difficulty in diagnosis and classification of acute leukemia is improperly prepared bone marrow smears and poor staining quality.

Blasts are increased in number, greater than 30%, even when no blasts are seen in the peripheral blood. A careful search should be made for the presence of Auer rods. Decreased maturation of other myeloid elements and variable degrees of myelodysplasia also occur. Erythroid precursors and megakaryocytes are frequently decreased in number and may show dysplastic features. The bone marrow biopsy specimen is usually hypercellular.

Morphologic Classification of Acute Myeloblastic Leukemia

The most commonly used classification system is the one proposed by the French-American-British (FAB) group using a morphologic and cytochemical classification of AML and ALL (Table 31–3). The morphologic features of the various subtypes of AML are illustrated in Figures 31–2 to 31–9. Recently, modifications of the original classification have been introduced to distinguish AML from myelodysplastic syndrome (Table 31–4). The FAB group specifies that 500 cells should be counted. Furthermore, 2 marrow differential calculations may be required when distinguishing AML from myelodysplastic syndrome. One is based on counting all nucleated cells (excluding lymphocytes, plasma cells, mast cells, and macrophages), and the other on counting all nonerythroid cells, blasts, maturing granulocytes, and monocytes (Table 31–4). In evaluating response to therapy, however, it has been recommended that the blast percentage be based on counting all nucleated cells, because the percentage of erythroblasts and lymphocytes is important for measuring the return of normal marrow. It has also been recommended that the 2 differential counts be used only to separate M6 from myelodysplastic syndrome. It is emphasized that the morphologic classification should be made on the basis of bone marrow examination prior to any treatment. Chemotherapy may rapidly produce considerable changes in cell morphology and complicate the examination.

There is as yet no convincing evidence that subclassification of acute myeloblastic leukemia is of value in selecting treatment or

Table 31–3   FAB Classification of Acute Myeloblastic Leukemia

Type	Characteristic
M1: Myeloblastic leukemia without maturation	Greater than 90% of marrow cells are blasts that are nongranular or contain a few azurophilic granules and/or Auer rods.
M2: Myeloblastic leukemia with maturation	More than 30% to 90% are blasts. More than 10% are granulocytes, with maturation from promyelocytes to PMNs. Fewer than 20% are monocytic cells.
M3: Hypergranular promyelocytic leukemia	Majority of cells are abnormal promyelocytes with numerous bizarre granules and Auer rods. High incidence of DIC. A microgranular variant (M3m) is characterized by clefted nuclei and indistinct granules.
M4: Myelomonocytic leukemia	More than 30% are blasts. Granulocytic and monocytic differentiation. Monocytes and promonocytes exceed 20% but are less than 80%. M4 with eosinophilia is a distinct entity.
M5: Monocytic leukemia	Divided into (a) poorly differentiated (more than 80% monoblasts) and (b) well-differentiated (more than 80% monocytic cells, predominantly promonocytes and monocytes).
M6: Erythroleukemia	Nucleated red blood cells exceed 50% in marrow. Erythroblasts often show bizarre features with multinucleation, giant forms, and megaloblastic features. More than 30% of nonerythroid cells are blasts.

NOTE: Modified French-American-British Cooperative Group Classification. Br J Haematol 1976; 33: 451.

ABBREVIATIONS: PMN = polymorphonuclear leukocyte; DIC = disseminated intravascular coagulation.

Table 31–4   Bone Marrow Analysis to Distinguish Acute
Myeloblastic Leukemia From Myelodysplastic Syndrome

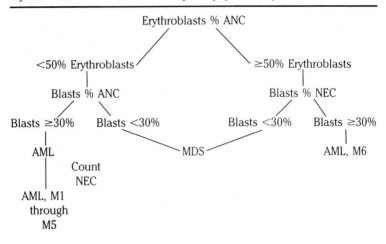

ABBREVIATIONS: AML = acute myeloblastic leukemia; MDS = myelodysplastic
syndrome; ANC = all nucleated cells; NEC = nonerythroid cells.

in predicting prognosis. An exception is promyelocytic leukemia
(M3), which is frequently associated with disseminated intravascular coagulation (DIC) and requires heparin therapy.

Special Types of Acute
Myeloblastic Leukemia

Acute Megakaryoblastic Leukemia (M7).   Acute megakaryocytic leukemia is thought to represent 4% to 8% of acute
leukemias. Its frequency may be more common because it is
often difficult to recognize. The blasts, which often display
lymphoid morphology, are 10 to 20 μm in diameter with round-to-oval nuclei. The latter are centrally or eccentrically located
and show very little chromatin clumping with 1 or more small,
indistinct nucleoli. Some blasts have nuclear lobation or are
multinucleated. The cytoplasm is scant, basophilic, and frequently
shows blebs (buds) or projections sometimes resembling platelet
formation (Figure 31–10). Atypical megakaryocytes are often admixed with the blasts.

The blasts stain negative with myeloperoxidase and Sudan
black. The acid phosphatase stain is usually diffusely positive, and
there is granular PAS positivity. The nonspecific esterase stain often

shows characteristic features depending on the substrate used. The combination of positive staining with acetate esterase and negative staining with butyrate esterase is almost pathognomonic, but the presence of megakaryoblasts cannot be ruled out, even if acetate esterase is not clearly positive. The most reliable method for identifying megakaryoblasts appears to be electron microscopy or the use of monoclonal antibodies. Platelet peroxidase, as demonstrated with the electron microscope, is distinct from granulocytic peroxidase. The former is detected in the nuclear envelope and endoplasmic reticulum. If a platelet peroxidase test is to be performed, the laboratory must be notified in advance to handle the specimen appropriately. Antiplatelet monoclonal antibodies (platelet glycoprotein Ib, IIb, and/or IIIa) parallel the findings using platelet peroxidase in the identification of megakaryoblasts. Antibody to factor VIII has also been used successfully in identifying megakaryoblasts.

Microgranular Promyelocytic Leukemia (M3m).

This variant of acute promyelocytic leukemia (M3) deserves special notice because it is frequently mistaken for other types of leukemia. The mean leukocyte count is significantly higher in the microgranular variant than in the usually promyelocytic leukemia. The blasts characteristically have a deeply notched, "monocytoid" nucleus (Figure 31–5). The cytoplasm is abundant and may contain no granules or a fine dusting of minute granules, and a few cells contain prominent azurophilic granules and Auer rods. The peroxidase reaction is strongly positive and the nonspecific esterase reaction is negative or weakly positive. The disease may be mistaken for myelomonocytic (M4) or monocytic leukemia (M5), lymphosarcoma cell leukemia or occasionally Sézary syndrome. The incidence and severity of DIC are the same as that of typical promyelocytic leukemia, and cytogenetic studies reveal the same chromosomal abnormality, ie, chromosomal translocation [t(15;17)]. Patients with the M3m variant of promyelocytic leukemia may have a shorter survival than those with typical M3.

Myelomonocytic Leukemia (M4) with Eosinophilia.

M4 with eosinophilia, which is associated with an inversion of chromosome 16,inv(16) (p13q22), appears to be a distinct entity. The marrow eosinophils, which are increased (from 6% to 35%), contain a mixture of eosinophilic and basophilic granules and stain positive with PAS and the specific esterase (chloroacetate esterase) stains. Normal granulocytes stain negative with specific esterase. These patients are highly responsive to induction chemotherapy, but also appear to have increased incidence of central nervous system involvement.

Myelodysplastic Syndromes

The term "myelodysplastic syndrome" has replaced what was previously called "pre-leukemia" and refers to a state of abnormal division, maturation, and production of erythrocytes, granulocytes, monocytes, and platelets. In general, it is characterized by qualitative and quantitative abnormalities of the hematopoietic cells. The myelodysplastic syndromes are mainly observed in patients exceeding 50 years of age, but recently it has also been observed in children. Though myelodysplastic syndromes are usually associated with the possible development of AML, they have also been associated with ALL. It is important to be able to identify this entity since several cancer study groups have introduced treatment protocols for myelodysplastic syndrome, utilizing drugs that promote in vitro differentiation, such as low-dose cytosine arabinoside.

Anemia is the major manifestation and is usually normochromic with reticulocytopenia though reticulocytosis may also be present. A variable degree of anisocytosis and poikilocytosis is present. Neutropenia is common, and the granulocytes are often poorly granulated with decreased peroxidase and leukocyte alkaline phosphatase (LAP) activity. Pseudo–Pelger-Huët anomaly and other abnormalities in nuclear segmentation are frequently present (Figure 31–11). These abnormalities in the granulocytes are referred to as dysgranulopoiesis. Thrombocytopenia is common, as is abnormal platelet morphology. Dysmegakaryocytopoiesis, in the form of micromegakaryocytes, large or small mononuclear forms or cells with multiple small nuclei, are not uncommon (Figure 31–12). The bone marrow is usually hypercellular, and morphologic abnormalities such as megaloblastoid features, cytoplasmic vacuolization, abnormal granulation, and ring sideroblasts, are often observed (Figure 31–13). The characteristic hematologic features are summarized in Table 31–5. A variety of cytogenetic abnormalities have been described; the most common recurring abnormalities are -5, 5q-, -7, +8.

The FAB group has published a scheme for the classification of the myelodysplastic syndromes. Several studies have shown good correlation between this classification system and the prognosis. This scheme stresses the importance of recognizing two types of blasts that differ primarily in their cytoplasmic characteristics. Type I blasts are the "typical" myeloblasts that have a fine nuclear chromatin pattern, prominent nucleoli, and absence of cytoplasmic granules. Type II blasts, in contrast, have few primary granules and slightly more cytoplasm, but the nucleus is still centrally located. The so-called nonblasts are the usual promyelocytes or myelocytes that have an eccentric nucleus, a developed Golgi apparatus, a

Table 31-5 Hematologic Findings for Myelodysplastic Syndromes

Dyserythropoiesis

Peripheral Blood	Bone Marrow
Normochromic, normocytic, or macrocytic anemia	Erythroid hypo-, normo-, or hyperplasia
Decreased absolute reticulocyte count	Erythroblasts may demonstrate: megaloblastic or megablastoid changes
Nucleated red cells	
Dual red cell population	nuclear budding
Anisocytosis	karyorrhexis
Poikilocytosis	multinucleation
Oval macrocytes	internuclear bridging
Polychromasia	Vacuolated erythroblasts
Basophilic stippling	Ring sideroblasts
Siderocytes	PAS-positive erythroblasts
	Abnormal mitotic figures

Dysgranulopoiesis

Peripheral Blood	Bone Marrow
Neutropenia	Myeloid hyperplasia with partial maturation arrest
Monocytosis	
Pseudo-Pelger-Huët	Diminished or absent secondary granules
Hypogranular PMNs	
Immature granulocytes	Myeloperoxidase deficient neutrophils
Decreased myeloperoxidase activity	Abnormal granulation
	Irregular cytoplasmic basophilia
	Increased blasts
	Abnormal localization of immature precursors
	Abnormal mitotic figures

Dysmegakaryocytopoiesis

Peripheral Blood	Bone Marrow
Thrombocytopenia	Macro- or micro-megakaryocytes
Micromegakaryocytes	Mononuclear megakaryocytes
Large, atypical platelets	Abnormal granulation
Abnormal granulation	
Vacuolization of platelets	

ABBREVIATIONS: PAS = periodic acid-Schiff; PMN = polymorphonuclear leukocyte.

dense or clumped chromatin pattern, numerous primary or secondary granules, and abundant cytoplasm. Hypogranular cells should not be called blasts if the rest of the features of nonblasts are apparent.

Table 31–6 FAB Classification of Myelodysplastic Syndromes

Refractory anemia (RA)

  <1% blasts in peripheral blood, <5% blasts in bone marrow

  Hypercellular bone marrow with erythroid hyperplasia and/or
    dyserythropoiesis

  Normal granulocytes and megakaryocytes

Refractory anemia with ring sideroblasts (RARS)

  Same as above with >15% ring sideroblasts

Refractory anemia with excess of blasts (RAEB)

  Cytopenia affecting two or more cell lines

  <5% blasts in peripheral blood and <20% blasts in bone marrow

  Hypercellular bone marrow with erythroid or granulocytic hyperplasia

  Dysgranulopoiesis, dyserythropoiesis, and/or dysmegakaryocytopoiesis

RAEB in transformation (RAEB-T)

  >5% blasts in peripheral blood and/or 20% to 30% blasts in bone
    marrow

  Auer rods may be present

Chronic myelomonocytic leukemia (CMML)

  Monocytes $>1 \times 10^9/L$

  Often associated increase in mature granulocytes

  <5% blasts in peripheral blood, and 5% to 20% blasts in bone
    marrow

The following conditions are included in the myelodysplastic
syndrome by the FAB group (see also Table 31–6):

1. Refractory Anemia (RA)—RA is characterized by persistent anemia, reticulocytopenia, variable degrees of dyserythropoiesis,
   and infrequent dysgranulopoiesis. The blasts should not exceed
   1% in the peripheral blood and 5% in the bone marrow. The
   bone marrow is normal to moderately hypercellular with erythroid hyperplasia or dyserythropoiesis or both. The granulocytic
   and the megakaryocytic cell lines are usually normal in appearance.

2. Refractory Anemia With Ring Sideroblasts (RARS)—This entity
   is synonymous with acquired idiopathic sideroblastic anemia. It
   differs from RA in that 15% or more of the nucleated red blood
   cells in the bone marrow are ring sideroblasts.

3. Refractory Anemia With Excess Blasts (RAEB)—This is the most common myelodysplastic syndrome. Anemia is the prominent feature but, in addition, neutropenia or thrombocytopenia or both are common. Dysgranulopoiesis in the peripheral blood is common. The percentage of Type I and Type II blasts is between 5% and 20% in the bone marrow and less than 5% in the peripheral blood. The bone marrow is hypercellular with granulocytic or erythroid hyperplasia or both. There is almost always evidence of granulocytic maturation.

4. Chronic Myelomonocytic Leukemia (CMML)—This entity is similar to refractory anemia with excess blasts, except that there is a prominent monocytic component of greater than 1×10^9 L in the peripheral blood (Figure 31–14).

5. Refractory Anemia With Excess Blasts in Transformation (RAEB-T)—These patients have more than 5% blasts in the peripheral blood and between 20% and 30% blasts in the bone marrow.

It should be noted that patients treated with radiotherapy or chemotherapy or both may have findings indistinguishable from the myelodysplastic syndromes described above; thus, in such cases the disorder is referred to as secondary myelodysplastic syndrome. Such patients often differ, however, in having variable degrees of myelofibrosis with a hypocellular marrow and a variable number of ring sideroblasts. These patients also have an increased incidence of AML. Myelodysplastic features may also be seen in bone marrow from patients with AIDS.

The prognosis in the myelodysplastic syndrome is extremely variable, but poor risk factors include: severe cytopenia, increased blast count, dysgranulopoiesis and dysmegakaryocytopoiesis, impairment of erythroid and granulocyte-macrophage colony formation, marked, ineffective erythropoiesis, chromosomal abnormalities (especially acquisition of new karyotype anomalies during the course of the disease), and abnormal localization of immature granulocyte precursors (myeloblasts and promyelocytes) in the bone marrow. The latter refers to clustering of myeloblasts and promyelocytes centrally in the bone marrow biopsy, instead of along endosteal surfaces where they usually reside.

Transformation to AML occurs in about 30% of patients, varying from approximately 12% in RARS to about 75% in RAEB-T. The median survival has been reported to range from 2 to 3 months in RAEB-T, 12 to 18 months in RAEB and CMML, and 36 to 54 months in patients with RA and RARS. Thus, in terms of survival, there appears to be 3 distinct groups. Patients who do not die from leukemia die from complications of bone marrow failure, ie, infection and bleeding.

The FAB group has revised the criteria to distinguish M6 from myelodysplastic syndrome. In patients where 50% or more of the nucleated bone marrow cells are erythroid, the separation is made by counting the percentage of blasts within the nonerythroid series. When 30% or more of the nonerythroid cells are blasts, the diagnosis is M6, and when less than 30% of the nonerythroid cells are blasts, the diagnosis is myelodysplastic syndrome (Table 31–4).

It may be difficult to distinguish myelodysplastic syndrome from acute leukemia when the blast count approaches the 20% to 30% range. Repeated bone marrow examinations will, however, resolve this, since acute leukemia is usually a rapidly progressive disease.

Other Laboratory Tests

31.1 Cytochemistry

Purpose. Cytochemistry is helpful in differentiating AML from ALL, and in identifying various subtypes of AML. It may also be useful in predicting the prognosis. It is particularly useful when no identifiable features, such as granules or Auer rods, are seen in the leukemic cells.

Principle. Enzymatic activity in the cytoplasm is demonstrated by means of specific substrates and appropriate "couplers" to provide localized color in the area of enzyme activity. The color is produced by union of one of the products of the enzyme action with the coupler.

Specimen. Smears of good quality are made from blood and bone marrow. Capillary blood from a fingerstick or anticoagulated blood may be used. Special fixatives are recommended with many stains. Satisfactory preparations can, however, be made from smears that have only been air dried. Ideally, all cytochemical stains should be made on fresh specimens. Since this is often not practical, unstained smears can be stored, covered, and kept away from light in a refrigerator. For the peroxidase stain, however, a fresh smear is preferred.

Procedure. A variety of cytochemical stains are available and a specific cytochemical profile exists for each hematopoietic cell line (Table 31–7). Myeloperoxidase, present in primary granules, Sudan black B (SBB), and specific esterase stains (naphthol AS-D chloroacetate esterase) show positive results in the granulocytic cell series, but negative results in the lymphocytic cell line. These stains are, therefore, useful in differentiating

Table 31–7 Cytochemical Studies to Differentiate Acute Myeloblastic Leukemia from Acute Lymphoblastic Leukemia

	Peroxidase/Sudan Black	NSE	TdT
AML: Myeloblasts	+	−	−
Monoblasts	+ / −	+	−
ALL: Lymphoblasts	−	−	+

NOTE: + indicates positive reaction, − indicates negative reaction

ABBREVIATIONS: NSE = nonspecific esterase; TdT = terminal deoxynucleotidyl transferase; AML = acute myeloblastic leukemia; ALL = acute lymphoblastic leukemia.

AML from ALL. Sudan black B stains a variety of lipids in granulocytes. It is especially useful when fresh smears are not available, since freshly made smears are preferred for the peroxidase stain. The specific esterase stain is less sensitive than SBB and peroxidase reactions, but is very useful for paraffin-embedded tissue sections in separating granulocytic from lymphocytic cell proliferations.

Nonspecific esterase (using alpha-naphthyl acetate or alpha-naphthyl butyrate as substrates) stains monocytes and histiocytes diffusely and is used to identify monocytic leukemias (M4 and M5) (Table 31–8). Nonspecific esterase does not stain granulocytes.

The periodic acid–Schiff (PAS) reaction is not very useful in differentiating acute leukemias. The typical block staining of lymphoblasts in ALL may occasionally be seen in AML and is frequently observed in acute monocytic leukemia.

Terminal deoxynucleotidyl transferase (TdT) is a DNA-polymerase enzyme present in immature lymphocytes but absent in normal myeloid cells. It may be helpful in separating ALL from AML.

Interpretation. The interpretation and usefulness of the special stains described above are indicated in Tables 31–7 and 31–8. The nonspecific esterase stain, using butyrate as substrate, produces a dot of dense, localized positivity in the cytoplasm of most mature T-lymphocytes, but not in ALL, and may be diffusely positive in epithelial cell malignancies. Positive staining by nonspecific esterase occurs also in erythroblasts in megaloblastic anemia. In megakaryoblastic anemia (M7) the nonspecific esterase stain is often positive using alpha-naphthyl acetate, but negative with butyrate as substrate. PAS diffuse staining in erythroblasts is seen in approximately 60% of pa-

Table 31–8   Cytochemical Reactions in Acute
Myeloblastic Leukemia

FAB Classification	M1	M2
Peroxidase or Sudan Black	>3%	>50%
Nonspecific esterase	<20%	<20%

tients with erythroleukemia (M6). TdT is found in 95% of patients with ALL and in 5% to 10% of patients with AML. TdT positivity in ALL is, however, usually uniformly strong in 80% to 100% of the blasts, while in AML the activity is weaker and present in a smaller percentage of cells.

Notes and Precautions.   Many of the stains require considerable technical expertise to be performed well; experience with interpretation of cytochemical stains in acute leukemia is necessary. Leukemic cells may not stain the same way as their normal counterparts. Thus, one may observe neutrophils from patients with AML (and myelodysplastic syndrome) that stain negative with peroxidase and SBB. Occasionally, the immature cells in AML are negative with peroxidase stains, but SBB is positive. Rare cases of SBB-positive granules in ALL have also been observed.

For therapeutic purposes, it is essential to be able to distinguish AML from ALL. One should not rely on the morphologic features observed in a Romanovsky-type stain only to distinguish ALL from AML. A peroxidase or Sudan Black stain and the nonspecific esterase stain should be done in all cases. If cytochemcial studies are negative, immunologic markers should be performed. If these are not available in the local laboratory, appropriate specimens should be sent to a specialty laboratory.

Ancillary Tests

Immunologic Cell Marker Studies.   Though immunologic markers in AML are not as important as in ALL, in cases where the cytochemical markers are negative or equivocal, monoclonal antibodies reactive with myeloblasts and monoblasts can be very helpful. Multiple commercially available monoclonal antibodies reactive with AML cells have become available (eg, My4, My7, My8, My9, Mo1, Mo2). The common ALL antigen (CALLA), which is present in the majority of cases of ALL, is usually absent in AML. There is

M3	M4	M5	M6
near 100%	20% to 80%	variable	>3%
variable	20% to 80%	>80%	variable

evidence that immunologically defined subgroups of patients with AML, which are of a potential clinical significance, can be identified with monoclonal antibodies.

Conflicting cytochemical and immunologic marker study results may be seen in cases of mixed or hybrid leukemia where there is an apparent mixture of myeloid and lymphoid cells. The cases that are TdT positive may benefit from treatment with vincristine sulfate and prednisone.

Cytogenetics. The majority of patients with AML can be shown to have chromosome abnormalities when sensitive techniques are utilized. The most common structural aberrations are translocations. The morphologic subtypes of AML have been associated with several distinct chromosomal abnormalities (Table 31–9). In AML the incidence of Philadelphia chromosome is 2% to 3%.

Recent studies suggest that AML, ALL, and myelodysplastic syndrome can be divided into low-, intermediate-, and high-grade disease subgroups according to the type of chromosome abnormality detected. Thus in AML inversion 16 and a single miscellaneous defect are considered low-grade; trisomy 8 and translocations t(6;9), t(8;21), t(9;22), t(15;17) are intermediate-grade; and monosomy 7 or deletion 7q or four or more chromosomal defects are associated with a high-grade or poor prognostic group. In myelodysplastic syndrome, normal chromosome or deletion 5q is low-grade; trisomy 8 is intermediate-grade; and monosomy 7, deletion 7q, or four or more chromosome defects are high-grade or associated with a poor prognosis.

The technique for detecting abnormal chromosomes in the marrow in AML or myelodysplastic syndrome is different from that in ALL. In the former, overnight culture stimulates myeloblasts to divide, and cell synchronization with methotrexate shows finely banded chromosomes. In ALL, a direct marrow technique is preferable since, in this disease, the blasts do not grow well in standard cultures.

It would appear then that the best method for typing acute leukemia is to use a combination of morphology, cytochemistry,

Table 31–9   Common Chromosomal Abnormalities in Acute Leukemia and Myelodysplasia

AML–M2	t(8;21)(q22;q11), −y
AML–M3	t(15;17)(q22;q21)
AML–M4	del(11)(q23)
AML–M4 with eosinophilia	inv(16)(p13;q22),del(16)(q22)
AML–M5	t(9;11)(q22;q23; or q24)
ALL–L1 & L2	t(9;22)(q34;q11), t(4;11)(q21;q23)
ALL–L3	t(8;14)(q24;q32) t(2;8)(p12,q24) t(8;22)(q24;q11)
Myelodysplasia (de novo and therapy related)	−5/5q −,20q −,−7/7q − del(5)(q13;q33) del(7)(q22;q34)

ABBREVIATIONS: AML = acute myeloblastic leukemia; ALL = acute lymphoblastic leukemia.

immunophenotyping, and cytogenetics. It is possible in the future that leukemias may be classified in terms of the genes that are abnormally regulated or that encode an abnormal product.

Coagulation Studies.   Bleeding in AML is usually caused by thrombocytopenia. In patients with severe bleeding, however, DIC should be considered. DIC is associated particularly with acute promyelocytic leukemia (M3) probably caused by thromboplastic material released from leukemic promyelocytes.

Serum Biochemistry.   Serum uric acid levels are frequently elevated, especially in patients with high white cell counts and during chemotherapy. Uric acid is the end-product of nucleic acid degeneration. Elevated serum levels of calcium and magnesium may also be seen. Similarly, serum lactate dehydrogenase (LD) levels are usually elevated.

Febrile Evaluation.   The incidence of infection in AML increases with the degree of neutropenia. Any patient with fever should be assumed to have an infection until proven otherwise (see chapter 32).

Biopsy of Other Tissue.   Even though the initial diagnosis of AML is usually made by examining blood and bone marrow, occasionally leukemia may present initially as a tumor. Such tumors are made up of myeloblasts and occur in skin, testicles, ovaries, bone, lymph nodes, orbit, gastrointestinal tract, and breast. In AML such tumors are called granulocytic sarcoma or chloroma, and the tumors may precede the development of AML by weeks or by more than a year. A specific esterase stain of the histologic sections will usually identify the cells as being of myeloid origin. The initial site of relapse in AML may also be in an extramedullary location, and a biopsy specimen of the lesion will usually demonstrate the leukemic infiltrate.

Course and Treatment

The therapeutic approach to AML is similar to that used for ALL, but the results are usually not as good. The most commonly used treatment for AML is a combination of cytosine arabinoside, daunorubicin, and 6-thioguanine. All AML subtypes are treated similarly, except those in patients with promyelocytic leukemia (M3) who also receive anticoagulants and blood products as needed for treatment of DIC. The remission rate in AML is usually 60% to 80%. Bone marrow failure is usually severe, and prolonged intensive care is necessary. Approximately half the patients continue in the first remission for 3 to 10 years. Bone marrow transplantation results are encouraging with close to 50% long-term survival in younger patients. Supportive care in patients with AML consists of treatment and prophylaxis of hemorrhage with various blood products, plus treatment and prophylaxis of infection.

References

1. Bennet JM, Catovsky D, Daniel HT, et al: Proposals for the classification of the myelodysplastic syndromes. *Br J Haematol* 1982; 51:189–199.

2. Bennet JM, Catovsky D, Daniel MT, et al: Proposed criteria for the classification of acute myeloid leukemia. *Ann Intern Med* 1985; 103:626–629.

3. Bitter MA, LeBeau MM, Rowley JD, et al: Associations between morphology, karyotype, and clinical features in myeloid leukemias. *Hum Pathol* 1987; 18:211–225.

4. Dewald GW, Pierre RV: Cytogenetic studies in neoplastic hematologic disorders. *Current Hematol Oncol* 1988; 6:231–266.

5. Foucar K, Langdon RM, Armitage JO, et al: Myelodysplastic syndromes: A clinical and pathologic analysis of 109 cases. *Cancer* 1985; 56:553–561.

6. Gale RP: Acute myelogenous leukemia: Recent advances in therapy, in Fairbanks VF (ed): *Current Hematology and Oncology,* vol. 5, Chicago, Year Book Medical Publishers, Inc, 1987.

7. Griffin JD, et al: Use of surface marker analysis to predict outcome of adult acute myeloblastic leukemia. *Blood* 1986; 68:1232–1241.

8. Huang M, Li C, Nichols WL, et al: Acute leukemia with megakaryocytic differentiation: A study of 12 cases identified immunocytochemically. *Blood* 1984; 64:427–439.

9. International Committee for Standardization in Haematology (ICSH): Recommended methods for cytological procedures in hematology. *Clin Lab Haematol* 1985; 7:55–74.

10. McKenna RW, Parkin J, Bloomfield CD, et al: Acute promyelocytic leukemia: A study of 39 cases with identification of a hyperbasophilic microgranular variant. *Br J Haematol* 1982; 50:201–214.

11. Pui CH, Dahl GV, Melvin S, et al: Acute leukemia with mixed lymphoid and myeloid phenotype. *Br J Haematol* 1984; 56:121—130.

12. Yunis JJ: Should refined chromosomal analysis be used routinely in acute leukemias and myelodysplastic syndrome? *N Engl J Med* 1986; 315:322–323.

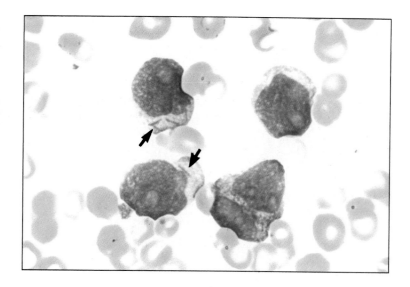

Figure 31–1   Myeloblasts with Auer rods (arrows).

Figure 31–2   AML, M1. Multiple myeloblasts without granules and no evidence of maturation.

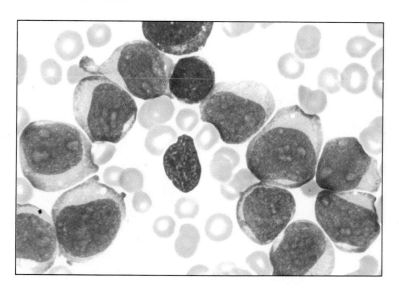

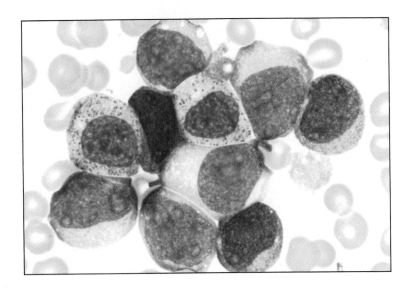

Figure 31–3   AML, M2. Myeloblasts, promyelocytes, and myelocytes.

Figure 31–4   AML, M3. Two hypergranular promyelocytes filled with Auer rods (arrows).

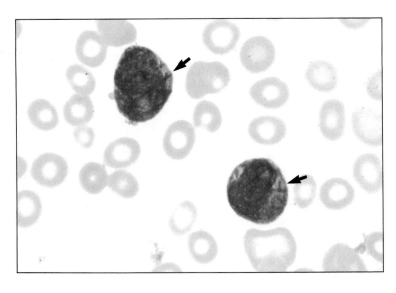

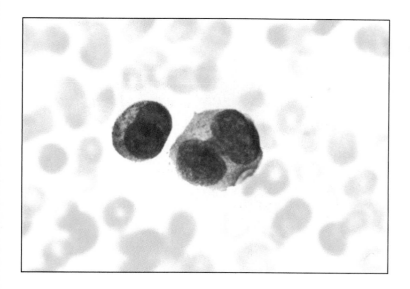

Figure 31–5 AML, M3m. Characteristic clefted promyelocytes containing indistinct granules.

Figure 31–6 AML, M4. Multiple myeloblasts and monocytoid cells.

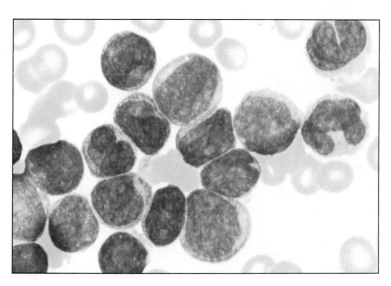

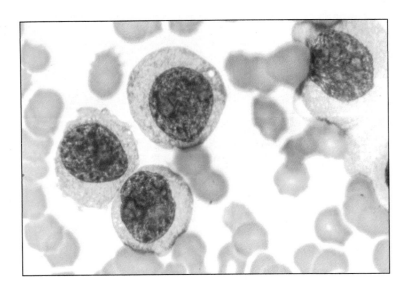

Figure 31–7   AML, M5a. Several monoblasts.

Figure 31–8   AML, M5b. Several promonocytes and monocytes.

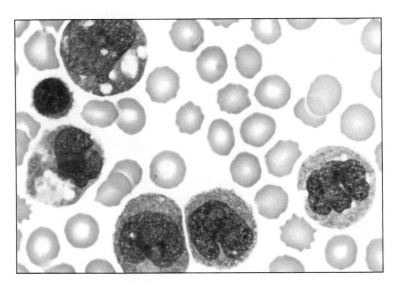

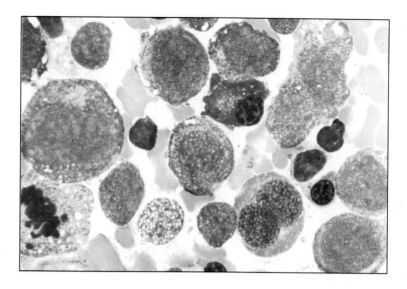

Figure 31–9   AML, M6. Binucleated erythroblasts, increased blasts, and an atypical mitotic figure.

Figure 31–10   AML, M7. Micromegakaryoblasts with scant-to-moderate cytoplasm containing irregular cytoplasmic "blebs," and large platelet forms.

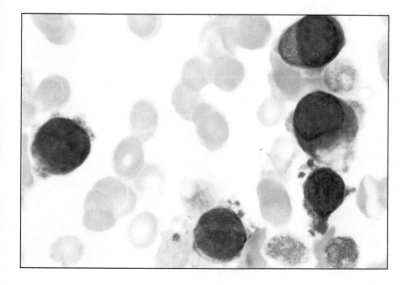

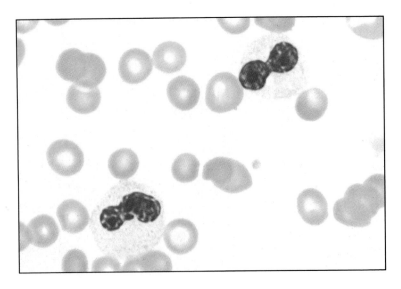

Figure 31–11   Myelodysplastic syndrome. Two hypogranular pseudo–Pelger-Huët cells.

Figure 31–12   Myelodysplastic syndrome. A mononuclear megakaryocyte.

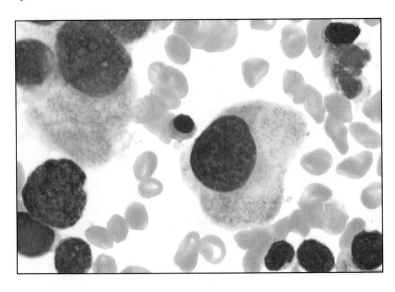

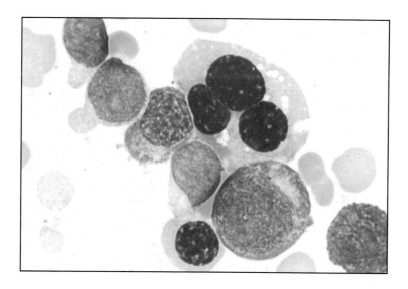

Figure 31–13   Myelodysplastic syndrome. A multinucleated megaloblastoid erythroid precursor and increased blasts.

Figure 31–14   Myelodysplastic syndrome. CMML. Two atypical monocytes and a hypogranular, hypersegmented neutrophil.

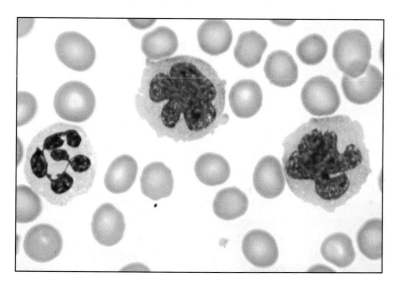

32

Acute Lymphoblastic Leukemia

Acute lymphoblastic leukemia (ALL) is a malignant clonal expansion arising from lymphocytic precursors in the bone marrow, thymus, and lymph nodes. It is the most frequent malignancy of childhood and the second leading cause of death in children less than 15 years of age.

Pathophysiology

The etiology of acute lymphoblastic leukemia remains unknown. In contrast to acute myeloblastic leukemia (AML), the clonal abnormality in ALL is thought not to arise in multipotential stem cells, but to originate in committed lymphoid stem cells. The majority, approximately 80% of cases, represent expansion of a heterogeneous group of B-cells varying in maturity; approximately 20% are T-cell leukemias.

The malignant lymphoid cells replace the normal bone marrow cells, resulting in anemia, neutropenia, thrombocytopenia, and an outpouring of immature cells into the peripheral blood. In addition, lymphoblasts accumulate in the reticuloendothelial system, including the lymph nodes, liver, and spleen, and frequently invade meninges and testis, eventually involving potentially any tissue in the body. Death in ALL is usually related to bone marrow failure and marked neutropenia resulting in severe infections.

The presenting clinical features of acute leukemia as related to pathophysiology are summarized in Table 31–1.

Clinical Findings

ALL is most common between the ages of 2 and 10 years, with an incidence of 27 cases per 1 million children. There is a low frequency after 10 years of age, with a secondary rise after the age of 40. In adults, however, AML is much more common than ALL. The onset of ALL is usually acute, and the presenting symptoms usually include fatigue, malaise, and listlessness. Fever, hemorrhage, and bone pain are common findings. Physical examination frequently reveals moderate lymphadenopathy, splenomegaly and hepatomegaly, and petechiae, or ecchymosis or both. Approximately 5% of patients with ALL have central nervous system (CNS) disease at diagnosis, and 1% of patients have testicular involvement. CNS and the testicles are major sites of potential relapse in ALL.

Approach to Diagnosis

After a clinical history and physical examination have been completed, the laboratory diagnosis of ALL proceeds in the following sequence:

1. A complete blood count.
2. Examination of the peripheral blood smear for abnormal leukocytes and blasts.
3. Examination of the bone marrow.
4. Cytochemical and immunological studies as needed for a correct diagnosis.
5. Cytogenetic studies, which may be helpful in diagnosis and assessment of prognosis.
6. Other studies often performed include serum biochemistry analyses, cerebrospinal fluid (CSF) analysis, and febrile evaluation.

Hematologic Findings

In some patients, the diagnosis of ALL may be readily apparent from the examination of the blood cell count and peripheral blood smear. In many patients, however, there is a variable degree of pancytopenia, and blasts may be difficult to detect in the peripheral blood smear. The examination of the bone marrow, at the time of diag-

Table 32–1 Morphologic Features to Differentiate Acute Myeloblastic Leukemia from Acute Lymphoblastic Leukemia

	ALL[a] Lymphoblast	AML[a] Myeloblast
Blast size	Small	Large
Cytoplasm	Scant	Moderate
Chromatin	Dense	Fine, lacy
Nucleoli	Indistinct	Prominent
Auer rods	Never present	Present in 50%

ABBREVIATIONS: AML = acute myeloblastic leukemia; ALL = acute lymphoblastic leukemia.

[a]These are general features. The morphology may vary considerably

nosis, will usually show a predominance of lymphoblasts. With proper therapy more than 50% of children with ALL can now be cured. It is therefore essential that ALL be distinguished from AML, and that a correct subclassification of ALL be made. This requires a careful morphologic evaluation of the leukemic cells, together with cytochemical and immunological studies.

Blood Cell Measurements. A normochromic, normocytic anemia with reticulocytopenia is usually present and may be severe. The leukocyte count may be decreased, normal, or increased. The leukocyte count in ALL represents an important prognostic indicator. White blood cell counts less than $10 \times 10^9/L$ ($10 \times 10^3/\mu l$) at diagnosis are associated with a good prognosis, white blood cell counts between $10 \times 10^9/L$ and $50 \times 10^9/L$ ($10 \times 10^3/\mu l$ and $50 \times 10^3/\mu l$) are associated with intermediate prognosis, and patients with white blood cell counts above $50 \times 10^9/L$ ($50 \times 10^3/\mu l$) have the poorest prognosis. The platelet count may be normal, but is commonly decreased.

Peripheral Blood Smear Morphology. The red cells are usually normochromic and normocytic and, occasionally, a leukoerythroblastic response may be seen with nucleated red blood cells and immature granulocytes. Neutropenia and a variable number of lymphoblasts are common. Occasionally, eosinophilia may be present, which, in some cases, has given rise to hypereosinophilic syndrome. Lymphoblasts characteristically have scant agranular cytoplasm with a round-to-ovoid nucleus having a fine chromatin pattern and indistinct nucleoli. As described below, however,

Table 32–2   FAB Classification of Acute
Lymphoblastic Leukemia

Cell Characteristics	L1	L2	L3
Cell size	Predominantly small blasts, homogeneous	Large, heterogeneous	Large, homogeneous
Nuclear chromatin	Homogeneous	Heterogeneous	Stippled, homogeneous
Nuclear shape	Regular, round, occasional clefting	Irregular, clefting	Regular, round-to-ovoid
Nucleoli	Inconspicuous	One or more, may be large	One or more, prominent
Cytoplasm	Scanty	Variable, moderately abundant	Moderately abundant
Cytoplasmic vacuolation	Usually absent	Variable	Prominent

NOTE: French-American-British Cooperative Group. *Br J Haematol* 1976; 33: 451.

the morphologic features of the lymphoblasts may vary. Occasionally in ALL, lymphoblasts contain azurophilic cytoplasmic granules (mainly in L2 subtype). Such cases may be mistaken for acute myeloblastic leukemia. The granules in ALL, however, are negative for peroxidase (Table 32–1).

It is essential to have a technically well-prepared smear, one preferably made from nonanticoagulated blood.

Bone Marrow Examination.   The site from which a bone marrow specimen is obtained is not usually important, since leukemia is a diffuse disease. It may be easier to obtain marrow particles from the sternum, but for safety reasons and the advantage of being able to make a biopsy specimen, the posterior iliac crest is preferred. Multiple smears should be made. One is stained with a Romanovsky stain and the rest should be left unstained for cytochemical and immunologic procedures. If uncertain about the type of fixation to use for cytochemical stains, it is best to leave the slides air-dried and unfixed. Heparinized bone marrow aspirate should be obtained routinely for immunologic cell marker studies. Occasionally, the bone marrow aspirate results in a dry tap, and

Table 32–3   Incidence of Morphologic Subtypes of Acute Lymphobastic Leukemia

	Children	Adults
L1	85%	35%
L2	13%	63%
L3	2%	2%

the diagnosis has to be made based on the bone marrow biopsy specimen. Imprints of the bone marrow biopsy specimen should routinely be made by touching the biopsy specimen gently on several glass slides. The latter should then be stained with a Romanovsky stain and other stains as needed. Immunologic cell marker studies can also be performed on such imprints using the immunoalkaline phosphatase technique. The bone marrow biopsy specimen and histologic sections of the aspirate are particularly useful for evaluation of cellularity. Multiple bone marrow studies should be done during treatment to follow efficacy of chemotherapy.

In the majority of patients, the bone marrow is extremely hypercellular, consisting almost entirely of lymphoblasts. In children in particular, many of the lymphoid cells have the appearance of small lymphocytes. Occasionally, necrosis may be present and, rarely, the marrow is hypocellular.

Morphologic Classification of Acute Lymphoblastic Leukemia

The French-American-British (FAB) classification has proven to be very useful in ALL (Table 32–2). The most helpful features in distinguishing L1 from L2 are the nuclear to cytoplasmic ratio and the presence or absence of nucleoli. In children, the majority of ALLs are classified as L1; in adults, a classification of L2 morphology is more common (Table 32–3). This classification scheme correlates well with relapse-free survival. "Pure" L1 (90% or more L1 cells) patients have the best prognosis and "pure" L2 (50% or more L2 cells) patients have a worse prognosis. Patients who have mixed-cell types (L1 and L2) have intermediate relapse-free survival. L3 ALL is associated with the worst prognosis. L3 ALL cells have surface immunoglobulin indicating a B-cell line, but otherwise the L1 and L2 types do not correlate well with cell surface markers. The morphologic features of ALL are illustrated in Figures 32–1 to 32–3.

Meticulous attention should be paid to preparing a "perfect" bone marrow aspirate smear and biopsy specimen. Because it is so important for therapy that an accurate diagnosis be made, cytochemical and immunologic studies should be performed routinely. Cytogenetic studies may also be very useful.

Other Laboratory Tests

32.1 Cytochemistry

Purpose. The addition of cytochemistry is helpful in differentiating ALL from AML (Table 31–7).

Principle, Specimen, and Procedure. See Test 31.1.

Interpretation. Myeloperoxidase and Sudan Black B stains are negative in ALL. The PAS stain may show block staining in lymphoblasts, but it should not be relied on to distinguish ALL from AML, since similar staining patterns may be seen in both types of leukemia.

Terminal deoxynucleotidyl transferase (TdT) is a DNA-polymerase enzyme normally present only in immature, cortical thymic, and bone marrow lymphocytes. TdT can be identified in blasts on blood smears, bone marrow smears, and imprints. The ideal specimen is a cytocentrifuge preparation of bone marrow aspirate. The specimen should be no longer than 1 week old. Both immunofluorescent and immunoenzymatic techniques are used with commercially available antibodies.

TdT is found in 95% of patients with ALL and is present in T-cell and common ALL types (Figure 32–4). TdT has also been identified in a small number of patients with AML. The latter cases may, however, represent mixed leukemias (AML and ALL). It is possible that the latter patients also may benefit from treatment similar to that used in ALL.

Caution should be exercised in interpreting a small number of positive TdT cells as evidence of relapse in post-treatment bone marrow from patients with ALL. Small numbers of positive cells have been observed in normal bone marrow donors. The identification of TdT in blasts may be helpful in detecting minimal central nervous system (CNS) leukemia and differentiating a reactive from a leukemic process. Identification of TdT may also be useful in identifying ALL infiltrates in testicular biopsy specimens.

Table 32–4 Markers of Differentiation in Recognized Subgroups of Acute Lymphoblastic Leukemia

Phenotype	SIg	CIg	B4	T Antigen	CALLA	TdT
Null cell	−	−	+ / −	−	−	+
[a]Common (non–B, non–T-cell)	−	−	+	−	+	+
T-cell	−	−	−	+	− (+)	+
Pre–B-cell	−	+	+	−	+	+
B-cell	+	+	+	−	+	−

NOTE: + indicates positive reaction, − indicates negative reaction.

ABBREVIATIONS: SIg = surface immunoglobulins; CIg = intracytoplasmic immunoglobulins; CALLA = common ALL antigen; TdT = terminal deoxynucleotidyl transferase; B4 = B-cell antigen; ALL = acute lymphoblastic leukemia.

[a]With B-cell monoclonal antibodies or gene rearrangement studies, more than 90% of these subtypes are shown to be of B-cell lineage (B-cell precursor ALL)

32.2 Immunologic Cell Marker Studies

Purpose. In addition to study of cell morphology and cytochemical markers, an immunologic classification is important for the correct diagnosis and prognosis in acute lymphoblastic leukemia.

Principle. Immunologic characterization of lymphoid malignancies is based on identification of cell surface or cytoplasmic antigens or both (Table 32–4). The B-lymphocyte is a lymphoid cell that produces immunoglobulin bound to the plasma membrane surface (SIg) or within the cytoplasm (CIg). The T-lymphocyte is a lymphoid cell that possesses receptors for sheep erythrocytes (E-rosettes) or specific surface T-cell antigens or both. Lymphocytes that cannot be classified as B- or T-cells using the classic methods of surface immunoglobulin and E-rosettes are called non-B, non-T cells. The non-B, non-T cell ALLs have been divided into common ALL (CALL) and null cell ALL. CALL is characterized by the presence of a surface marker referred to as the common ALL antigen (CALLA), which is a transient marker of early lymphoid cell differentiation. CALL accounts for approximately 70% of all cases of childhood ALL. It is less frequent in adult ALL (Table 32–5). Null cell ALL lacks the common ALL antigen. With monoclonal B-cell antibodies

Table 32–5 Incidence of Immunologic Subgroups of Acute Lymphoblastic Leukemia

Phenotype	Children	Adults
Null	5%	33%
Common (non–B, non–T-cell)	68%	45%
T-cell	10%	20%
Pre–B-cell	15%	NA
B-cell	2%	2%

ABBREVIATIONS: NA = not available.

and gene rearrangement studies, it has been shown that most non-B, non-T cell ALLs are neoplastic counterparts of early B-cell differentiation.

T-cell ALL is found in 10% to 20% of patients with ALL. Monoclonal T-cell antibodies have demonstrated that the majority of T-cell ALL belongs to the prothymocyte or, rarely, thymocyte stage of differentiation.

B-cell ALL (L3) accounts for approximately 2% of the cases of ALL and has blasts with identical morphology to Burkitt's lymphoma. The cells are characterized by the presence of surface immunoglobulin (SIg).

Specimen. Immunologic cell marker studies can be performed on cell suspensions made from peripheral blood, bone marrow aspirates, and body fluids using immunofluorescent manual techniques or flow cytometry. Immunoenzymatic methods (immunoalkaline phosphatase), frozen sections, peripheral blood smears, bone marrow smears, touch imprints or, ideally, cytocentrifuge preparations can be used.

It is essential that the laboratory performing the marker studies be notified prior to obtaining the specimen to determine their preference of specimen and how it should be best handled.

Procedure. The markers of differentiation in the recognition of major subgroups of ALL are shown in Table 32–4. The sheep red blood cell rosette method has now been replaced with T-cell specific antisera. Monoclonal antibodies are commercially available for identifying a spectrum of T-cell subsets. The immunologic marker studies can be performed by the fluorescent method using a UV light microscope or by automated

methods using flow cytometry. The immunoalkaline phosphatase method has the advantage that live cell suspensions are
not required and the cells can readily be visualized using a
light microscope.

Interpretation.   With the use of good morphologic preparations,
together with cytochemical and immunologic methods, the
number of cases classified as undifferentiated acute leukemia
should be very small. The clinically important immunologic
groups are the early pre–B-cell (most of the common ALLs),
pre–B-cell, B-cell, and T-cell. The common ALL group that accounts for approximately 70% of all cases of ALL is associated
with the best prognosis. These patients are usually children, a
mediastinal mass is not usually present, and the leukocyte count
is not markedly elevated.

The T-cell ALL, which accounts for 10% to 20% of cases of
ALL, is more commonly seen in older children and adults and
is frequently associated with a mediastinal mass, hepatosplenomegaly, early CNS involvement, and a high peripheral white
blood cell count. These patients often have a poor prognosis,
but in the absence of mediastinal mass, CNS involvement, and
high peripheral leukocyte count, they may respond well to therapy similar to those patients who have common ALL.

B-cell ALL, which is morphologically very similar to Burkitt's
lymphoma, is very rare and is usually associated with a poor
prognosis. The cells are usually TdT-negative and often associated with the t(8;14) chromosome abnormality. Null cell ALL
appears to represent a heterogeneous group. Some of these
cases may be myeloid or monocytoid, and some may have
blasts at the stage of bifurcation of lymphoid and myeloid differentiation.

It is essential that the results of the immunologic studies
always be correlated with morphologic characteristics and cytochemical stains to ensure the accuracy of cell identification.

Table 32–6 is a list of monoclonal antibodies used in immunologic marker studies.

Ancillary Tests

Cytogenetics.   High-resolution banding techniques have revealed clonal chromosomal abnormalities in over 90% of patients
with ALL (Table 32–7). The three most common types of reciprocal
translocations (t(9;22), t(4;11), and t(8;14)) have been reported in
approximately a third of adults and a tenth of children. Such chromosomal defects have been associated with a median survival of

Table 32–6 Monoclonal Antibodies for Lymphoid and Granulocytic Malignancies

CD	Common Names	Spectrum of Activity
CD1	Leu6, T6, OKT6	Immature thymocytes, Langerhans' cells, hairy cells
CD2	Leu5, T11, OKT11	Pan–T-cells (E-Rosette receptor)
CD3	Leu4, T3, OKT3	Pan–T-cells
CD4	Leu3, T4, OKT4	T-helper cells
CD5	Leu1, T1, OKT1	Pan–T-cells, rare B-cells, B-cell CLL
CD6	T12, TU33, T411	Pan–T-cell, rare B-cells
CD7	Leu9, 3A1, 4A	T-cell and NK cells
CD8	Leu2, T8, OKT8	T-suppressor cells
CD9	J2, BA2	T-cells, B-cells early myeloid, monocytes, platelets
CD10	CALLA, J5, BA3	Pre–B-cells, pre–T-cells, common ALL
CD11	Leu15, Mo1, OKM1, Mo5	T-suppressor cells, monocytes, granulocytes
CDw14	My4, Mo2	Monocytes, immature granulocytes
CD15	Leu M1, My1, X-hapten	Granulocytes, monocytes, RS cells
CD16	Leu11, VEP 13	Fc IgG receptor on NK cells and neutrophils
CDw17	T5A7	Granulocytes, monocytes
CD19	Leu12, B4	Pan–B-cells, not plasma cells
CD20	Leu16, B1	Pan–B-cells, not plasma cells
CD21	B2, CR2	Mature B-cells in blood, germinal centers and mantle zone
CD22	Leu14, SHCL-1, T015	Pan–B-cells
CD23	Tu1, PL13, Blast 2	B-cells in mantle zone, not in blood
CD24	BA1	Pan–B-cells, granulocytes, plasma cells
CD25	Interleukin-2, Tac	Activated B- & T-cells, interleukin-2 receptor
CD30	Ki-1, BerH2	RS cells, activated B- & T-cells
—	TdT	B- & T-cell precursors, cortical thymocyte

(Continued.)

Table 32–6 *Continued.*

CD	Common Names	Spectrum of Activity
—	HLA-DR (Ia-like)	B-cells, activated T-cells, not plasma cells, monocytes
CD33	My9, L4F3	Immature granulocytes
CDw41	J15, gpIIb/IIIa	Megakaryocytes
CD45	LCA, T200, T29/33	Leukocytes, usually not plasma cells, sometimes not lymphoblasts

ABBREVIATIONS: CD = cluster designation; CLL = chronic lymphocytic leukemia; NK = natural killer; CALLA = common ALL antigen; ALL = acute lymphoblastic leukemia; RS = Reed-Sternberg.

less than 12 months, whereas there is an association of over 4 years remission and possible cure in a third to half of patients without such translocations. The highest response rates to treatment and the best survival rates are seen in patients with either diploid or markedly hyperdiploid karyotypes.

The Philadelphia chromosome (Ph^1) has been reported to be present in 17% of adult ALL patients and 6% of child ALL patients. In adults especially, the Ph^1 chromosome has been associated with a poor prognosis.

Cerebrospinal Fluid Analysis. Infiltration of meninges is the most important extramedullary manifestation of acute lymphoblastic leukemia. It has particularly been associated with T-cell ALL. Without treatment directed against the CNS the incidence of meningeal involvement in ALL may be as high as 80%. The CNS is also one of the most common sites of relapse in children. The cytocentrifuge method has proven to be very effective in providing satisfactory smears of CSF in patients with leukemia. At least 2 mL of CSF should be obtained. When the CSF is involved, the cell count may vary from few blasts to numerous blast cells. When only an occasional blast is found, it may be extremely difficult to be certain whether it is a leukemic cell or an atypical mononuclear cell. Identification of TdT or use of immunologic marker studies (if an adequate number of cells are present) may be helpful in identifying leukemic cells in CSF.

Febrile Evaluation. Fever in a patient with ALL should be assumed to be caused by infection until proven otherwise. In addition to neutropenia, the cellular and humoral immunity are frequently abnormal. The patient should be examined for localizing

Table 32–7 Correlation of Morphology, Immunology, and Cytogenetics in Acute Lymphoblastic Leukemia

Type	Morphology	Immunophenotype	Cytogenetics
Common	L1 or L2	CALLA +, Ia +, B4 +, TdT +	Normal, t(4;11), t(9;22)
Pre–B-cell	L1 or L2	CALLA +, Ia +, B4 +, CIg +, TdT +	Normal, t(1;19), t(9;22)
T-cell	L1 or L2	CALLA –, T antigen +, Ia –, B4 –, TdT +	Normal, t(11;14)
B-cell	L3	CALLA +, Ia +, B4 +, SIg +, TdT –	t(8;14)

ABBREVIATIONS: CALLA = common acute lymphoblastic leukemia antigen.

symptoms and signs of infection; urine and sputum should be examined, and blood cultures should be obtained. Infections caused by *Pseudomonas, Staphylococcus aureus,* and gram-negative enteric organisms are particularly common. In addition, infections with opportunistic organisms such as *Candida* and *Aspergillus* occur. *Pneumocystis carinii* infection of the lung is seen with increasing frequency; the diagnosis is made by identifying the organism in a lung biopsy specimen.

Serum Biochemistry.   Serum uric acid levels are elevated in about half of the patients, especially in patients with a high white blood cell count undergoing chemotherapy. Prophylactic hydration plus allopurinol are important precautions. Serum lactic dehydrogenase (LD) is frequently elevated.

Course and Treatment

The prognosis in ALL ranges from approximately 70% complete remission at 5 years for the "good" prognosis group to approximately 35% complete remission at 5 years for the "poor" prognosis group. The best prognosis is associated with the 2- to 9-year-old group with leukocyte counts of less than 10×10^9/L (10×10^3/μl) and with less than 10% L2 marrow blast cells. A poor prognosis has been associated with those under 1 year of age and over the age of 10 years, with white cell counts greater than 10×10^9/L (10×10^3/μl) (especially when greater than 50×10^9/L or 50×10^3/μl) and more than 10% L2 lymphoblasts. T-cell ALL patients with a high white cell count and a mediastinal mass have a poor prognosis.

Patients with the B-cell ALL have the poorest prognosis. In addition to age, leukocyte counts, FAB lymphoblast morphology and immunologic phenotypes, and chromosome studies have been shown to be of prognostic importance. As mentioned above, children whose blasts contain more than 50 chromosomes have a good prognosis, while those with specific translocations such as t(9;22), t(4;11), and t(8;14) have a poorer prognosis.

Therapy in ALL may be divided into three parts; remission induction, central nervous system prophylaxis, and maintenance in remission. Remission induction with a combination of vincristine sulfate and prednisone usually results in an 85% to 90% remission rate. The patient in a poorer prognostic group may, in addition to vincristine and prednisone, be given L-asparaginase or anthracycline or both. Maintenance therapy usually consists of mercaptopurine administered orally on a daily basis and methotrexate administered orally on a weekly basis with prednisone and vincristine reinforcements. This treatment is maintained during 2 to 3 years of continuous remission. CNS prophylaxis consists of cranial irradiation plus intrathecal methotrexate. Bone marrow transplantation may be useful in children who have relapses of ALL while receiving therapy.

Treatment of ALL is steadily improving as we develop better definition of high-risk groups and apply early intensification of chemotherapy for such cases. More than 50% of children with ALL may now be cured of their disease. In those who cannot be cured, the major cause of death is infection or, less commonly, hemorrhage.

References

1. Bennet JM, Catovsky D, Flandrin G, et al: The morphological classification of acute lymphoblastic leukemia: Concordance among observers and clinical correlations. *Br J Haematol* 1981; 47:553–561.

2. Foon K, Todd RF: Immunologic classification of leukemia and lymphoma. *Blood* 1986; 68:1–31.

3. Lilleyman JS, Hann IM, Stevens RF: French-American-British (FAB) morphological classification of childhood lymphoblastic leukemia and its clinical importance. *J Clin Pathol* 1986; 39:998–1002.

4. Look AT: The emerging genetics of acute lymphoblastic leukemia: Clinical and biologic implications. *Semin Oncol* 1985; 12:92–104.

5. Pinkel D: Curing children of leukemia. *Cancer* 1987; 59:1683–1691.

6. Pui CH, Williams DL, Raimondi SC, et al: Unfavorable presenting clinical and laboratory features are associated with CALLA negative non-T, non-B lymphoblastic leukemia in children. *Leukemia Res* 1986; 10:1287–1292.

7. Smithson WA: Childhood acute lymphocytic leukemia, in Fairbanks VF (ed): *Current Hematology and Oncology.* Chicago, Yearbook Medical Publisher Inc, 1987, vol 5.

8. Sobol RE, Boyston I, LeBien TW, et al: Adult acute lymphoblastic leukemia defined by monoclonal antibodies. *Blood* 1985; 65:730–735.

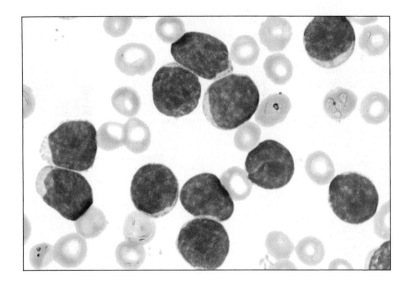

Figure 32-1 ALL, L1. The blasts are small with scant cytoplasm and indistinct nucleoli.

Figure 32-2 ALL, L2. The blasts are larger than L1 blasts, have moderately abundant cytoplasm, and distinct nucleoli.

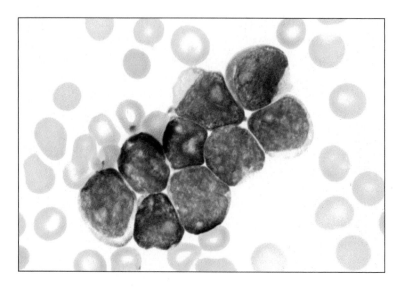

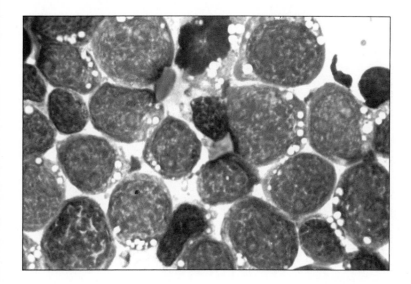

Figure 32–3   ALL, L3. The blasts have blue cytoplasm with characteristic vacuoles, moderately coarse or clumped chromatin pattern, and distinct nucleoli.

Figure 32–4   (TdT). Immunofluorescent study shows nuclear staining in lymphoblasts in patient with ALL.

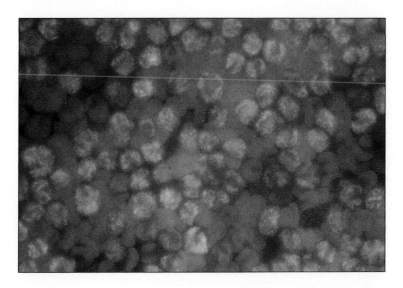

PART
8

Chronic Leukemias

33

Chronic Myelogenous Leukemia

Chronic myelogenous leukemia (CML) or chronic granulocytic leukemia (CGL) is a myeloproliferative disorder characterized by a clonal proliferation of granulocytic cells, which results in a large increase in total body granulocyte mass. In the majority of patients, there is a terminal blastic metamorphosis. CML comprises approximately 20% of all leukemias and is seen most frequently in the middle aged, but rarely in children.

Pathophysiology

CML is a clonal disorder having its origin from multipotential stem cells. More than 95% of patients with CML have a translocation of one of the long arms of chromosome 22, usually to one of the 9 chromosomes. The presence of this abnormal chromosome, the Philadelphia chromosome (Ph[1]), in a patient with leukocytosis and granulocytic hyperplasia in the bone marrow, is diagnostic of CML. In CML, chromosomal rearrangements are associated with translocation and activation of cellular oncogenes. The protooncogene c-abl is located on chromosome 9. This oncogene is translocated to chromosome 22. The breakpoint on chromosome 22 occurs within the bcr gene. The final result is a chimeric gene bcr-c-abl. The clonal nature of CML has been confirmed by studies of the distribution of isoenzymes of G6PD.

The granulocytic hyperplasia, at all stages of maturation within the bone marrow, can be explained by a combination of stem cell expansion and a delay in cell cycle, maturation-division, and compartmental transit time. The average half-life of granulocytes in the blood in patients with CML is 5 to 10 times longer than normal. At the same time, the granulocyte turnover rate may be increased tenfold. Thus, CML is characterized by major regulatory defects that are probably due to abnormalities in the multipotential stem cells.

Clinical Findings

CML is most frequently seen in patients between 50 and 60 years of age, and is usually associated with an insidious development. The initial symptoms may include malaise, fatigue, weight loss, and, as the disease progresses, upper abdominal discomfort. Physical examination usually reveals splenomegaly. Hepatomegaly is less common and lymphadenopathy is very unusual; when present, it is often associated with an accelerated phase (acute transformation) of the disease. As the disease progresses, the spleen may become markedly enlarged and in general, the magnitude of splenomegaly correlates with the leukocyte count.

Approach to Diagnosis

Following clinical history and physical examination, the laboratory diagnosis of CML proceeds in the following sequence:

1. A complete blood count.
2. Examination of the peripheral blood smear.
3. Examination of the bone marrow.
4. Cytochemical studies (leukocyte alkaline phosphatase, TdT) as needed.
5. Cytogenetic studies for the Philadelphia chromosome.

A comparison of the major findings in chronic and acute leukemia is seen in Table 33–1.

Hematologic Findings

The hematologic findings in CML are quite characteristic, but not diagnostic. Severe leukemoid reactions, eg, due to infections, can mimic CML, and myeloproliferative disorders such as myelofibrosis may have similar blood and bone marrow findings.

Table 33-1   Comparison of Acute and Chronic Leukemia

	Acute	Chronic
Age	All ages	Adults
Clinical onset	Sudden	Insidious
Lymphadenopathy	Mild	Moderate
Splenomegaly	Mild	Moderate to prominent
Anemia and thrombocytopenia	Prominent	Mild
Leukemic cells	Immature	Mature
Course (untreated)	6 months or less	2–6 years

Blood Cell Measurements.   The majority of patients have mild normochromic, normocytic anemia at the time of diagnosis. The anemia becomes more severe as the leukocyte count increases. The rise in leukocyte count is gradual, the majority of patients having counts ranging between $20 \times 10^9/L$ and $500 \times 10^9/L$ ($20 \times 10^3/\mu l$ and $500 \times 10^3/\mu l$) at the time of diagnosis. In contrast to AML, the platelet count is normal or often elevated.

Peripheral Blood Smear Morphology.   The diagnosis of CML can usually be suspected from an examination of the peripheral blood. The striking feature is granulocytosis with the entire spectrum of granulocytic precursors being present (Figure 33–1). Mature granulocytes and metamyelocytes predominate. Promyelocytes and myeloblasts do not usually exceed 10% in the chronic phase. An increased number of eosinophils and basophils is characteristic in CML, and is a useful marker in distinguishing CML from a leukemoid reaction. Occasional nucleated red blood cells are not uncommon.

Bone Marrow Examination.   The bone marrow is markedly hypercellular with a large increase in the myeloid:erythroid (M:E) ratio. As in the peripheral blood, all stages of maturation of the granulocytic series are present, and there is usually an increased number of basophils and eosinophils. The number of erythroid precursors is often decreased. The megakaryocytes are usually increased in number and frequently show dysplastic features. The latter is a common feature of the myeloproliferative disorders (see chapter 35). The bone marrow biopsy specimen often reveals mild myelofibrosis, which may become more severe as the disease progresses. Bone marrow fibrosis is associated with a poor prognosis because major fibrotic changes are often associated with the ac-

Table 33–2   Conditions Associated with Abnormal Leukocyte Alkaline Phosphatase

Decreased	Increased
Chronic myelogenous leukemia	Myelofibrosis (rarely low)
Paroxysmal nocturnal hemo-globinuria	Polycythemia vera
	Leukemoid reaction
Hypophosphatemia	Pregnancy and oral contraceptive intake
ITP	
Sarcoidosis	Hodgkin's disease
Infectious mononucleosis	Multiple myeloma
Pernicious anemia	
Myelodysplastic syndrome	

ABBREVIATIONS: ITP = idiopathic thrombocytopenic purpura.

celerated or blastic phase of the disease. The number of megakaryocytes often correlates with the degree of myelofibrosis.

It should be noted that bone marrow examination per se is often of little help in making the diagnosis of CML. It is indicated, however, to obtain material for cytogenetic studies (Philadelphia chromosome) and to evaluate the degree of bone marrow fibrosis because of its prognostic importance.

Other Laboratory Tests

33.1   Leukocyte Alkaline Phosphatase (LAP)

Purpose.   Together with cytogenetics, LAP is the most useful confirmatory test in CML.

Principle, Specimen, and Procedure.   See Test 18.1.

Interpretation.   In CML, the LAP score is zero or markedly decreased. The diagnostic value of a low score in patients with CML is increased by the fact that the LAP scores are usually elevated in the conditions with which CML is most commonly mistaken, such as granulocytic leukemoid reactions, polycythemia vera, and myelofibrosis with myeloid metaplasia (Table 33–2). It should be noted, however, that the LAP score in CML may be normal or increased in the presence of infection and pregnancy, and after a splenectomy. Also, during the accelerated or blastic phase, the LAP may be normal or elevated.

33.2 Cytogenetics

Purpose. The Philadelphia chromosome (Ph[1]) is present in more than 95% of patients with CML. It is diagnostic of CML in the presence of granulocytosis in the peripheral blood and bone marrow.

Principle. The Ph[1] chromosome abnormality results from translocation of the greater part of the long arm of chromosome 22 to another chromosome, usually chromosome 9. This is an acquired somatic mutation of a common stem cell of granulocytes, erythroid cells, megakaryocytes, and monocyte cell lines. The Ph[1] chromosome persists throughout the course of the disease.

Specimen. Bone marrow is the tissue of choice. A buffy coat preparation of peripheral blood may be used if no bone marrow can be obtained and if the peripheral blood contains an adequate number of cells of the myelocytic stage or younger. Bone marrow is aspirated directly into a syringe that has been rinsed with heparin. An aliquot of 0.5 to 1.0 mL of bone marrow is transferred immediately into (1) a sterile screw-top vial containing 2 mL of sterile tissue culture medium, or (2) a sterile small (2- to 3-mL) plain (red top) vacuum tube. This specimen should not be refrigerated. The sample can be transported to a reference laboratory with satisfactory results if the specimen arrives within 24 hours. Lymph node biopsy specimen and splenic tissue may also be subjected to chromosome analysis under special circumstances.

Procedure. Chromosome charts are prepared by examining metaphase spreads of leukocytes from blood or bone marrow or both. Chromosome analysis is performed following 24 to 48 hours of incubation at 37° C without phytohemagglutinin stimulation. Many techniques are available by which chromosomes can be studied. The simplest type is termed a "direct study." A cell suspension is made of leukocytes from blood or bone marrow and incubated with colchicine to arrest cell division at the metaphase stage. The cells are swollen by hypotonic saline treatment and fixed. The fixed cells are placed on a slide, flattened, and dried. The metaphase spreads are then stained, examined under the microscope, and photographed.

Cell culture techniques are employed when the cells have a low mitotic index. Malignant leukocytes grow in vitro without stimulation, and peak cell division occurs at 24 to 48 hours after onset of cell culture. G and Q banding is utilized for detailed karyotypic analysis.

Interpretation. The Ph¹ chromosome is present in more than 95% of patients with CML, both in relapse and in apparent remission of the disease. During accelerated phase or blast crisis, additional chromosome abnormalities are frequently found. A small number of patients lack the Ph¹ chromosomes. These patients may have a disease different than classic CML (see below).

Although the Ph¹ chromosome translocation is the cytogenetic hallmark of CML, molecular detection of rearrangement of the genes involved in the translocation breakpoint (the bcr locus on chromosome 9 and the abl proto-oncogene on chromosome 22) is a more sensitive and specific marker for CML. Bcr/abl rearrangements may be present in suspected cases of CML that are cytogenetically normal.

Ancillary Tests

Terminal Deoxynucleotidyl Transferase (TdT). TdT is a marker for early lymphoid cells (see chapter 32). In approximately 30% of patients with CML in blast crisis, TdT is present. The reason for performing a TdT in CML is that patients with a positive TdT test result respond more frequently to vincristine and prednisone, drugs normally used for treatment of ALL. Identification of TdT can be done on blasts in peripheral blood (if an adequate number of blasts are present), on bone marrow aspirate material, or on imprints from a biopsy specimen. With the use of an immunoperoxidase technique, TdT can also be demonstrated in histologic sections.

Course and Treatment

CML has a constant, predictive course during the chronic phase, with a median survival of 3 to 4 years. Approximately 20% of the patients survive 7 years or more. The majority of patients die from complications associated with blast crisis, usually infection or hemorrhage or both.

The principle of therapy in CML is to reduce the total granulocyte

Table 33–3   Characteristics of Chronic Myelogenous Leukemia

Age	30–50 years, rarely in children
Physical examination	Splenomegaly
Leukocyte count	50–200 × 10⁹/L
Blood findings	Granulocytosis with entire spectrum of precursors from myeloblasts (<2%) to mature neutrophils; eosinophilia and basophilia; platelet count normal or increased
Bone marrow findings	Granulocytic hyperplasia, eosinophilia and basophilia; megakaryocytic hyperplasia and variable degree of myelofibrosis
Leukocyte alkaline phosphatase	Markedly decreased
Chromosome analysis	Philadelphia chromosome
Course	After 2–3 years, disease usually terminates in an accelerated phase with an increase in blasts (blast crisis), and/or myelofibrosis

mass and relieve symptoms of hyperleukocytosis, thrombocytosis, and splenomegaly. The alkylating agent, Busulphan, is the most commonly used chemotherapeutic agent. Though Busulphan is an effective therapy during the chronic phase of the disease, no effective therapy is available yet for blast crisis. The only definitive prospect for curing CML at this time appears to be marrow transplantation.

Table 33–3 is a summary of the characteristic features in CML.

Special Diagnostic Considerations

Accelerated Phase and Blast Crisis in CML.   There are 3 phases in the biologic natural history of CML: the chronic phase, the accelerate phase, and the terminal blastic phase or crisis. The metamorphosis from the chronic phase to blast crisis can occur very rapidly or gradually over several months. The less fulminant transition is referred to as the accelerated phase or acute transformation. The development of blast crisis occurs in the majority of patients with CML between 2 and 6 years from the time of diagnosis. The accelerated phase and blast crisis are associated with a maturation block similar to that seen in AML. Features associated with the accelerated phase include increased number of basophils, additional chromosome abnormalities, and myelofibrosis.

Blast crisis is usually associated with a predominance of granulocytic blasts (60% of cases), but blast crisis associated with lymphoblasts (30% of cases), monoblasts, erythroblasts, and megakaryoblasts have also been described (Figure 33–2). In some instances, myeloid-lymphoid hybrid blasts or granulocytic blast mixtures may be present. This mixture of blast crisis is not surprising as CML represents a lesion in the multipotential stem cells. Stem cells and blast crisis are associated with a clonal expansion of any or several potential progeny. The type of blasts present usually does not influence therapy except if lymphoid blast crisis is identified (TdT-positive cells), in which case therapy normally used for ALL is indicated. Lymphoid blast crisis may be seen in approximately 30% of patients with CML. These blasts usually have lymphoblastic morphology, are positive with TdT, and have the CALLA antigen.

Clinically the accelerated phase and blastic crisis are associated with marked malaise, fatigue, anorexia, and weight loss. Lymphadenopathy may develop, and biopsy of such lymph nodes reveals a predominance of blasts (granulocytic sarcoma) such that it may be mistaken for large-cell lymphoma. Increasing anemia and thrombocytopenia are other common features.

Atypical CML.   In 5% to 10% of the patients who show a CML-like picture, the Philadelphia chromosome is absent. This so-called "Ph[1]–negative CML" appears to be a distinct hematologic entity representing 10% to 15% of the total CML population. Compared to classic CML, the patients are usually older, have a higher incidence of anemia, thrombocytopenia, monocytosis, marrow blasts, decreased marrow megakaryocytes, and a lower incidence of basophilia and thrombocytosis. Atypical CML is associated with a poor prognosis (median survival, 14 months). Some investigators believe that this entity is related to the myelodysplastic syndrome, chronic myelomonocytic leukemia. Thus, Ph[1]–negative CML may be a nonentity.

References

1. Bernstein R: Cytogenetics of chronic myelogenous leukemia. Seminars in Hematol 25:20–34, 1988.
2. Bloomfield CD (ed): *Chronic and Acute Leukemias in Adults.* Boston, Martinus Nijhoff Publishers, 1985.

3. Champlin RE, Golde DW: Chronic myelogenous leukemia: Recent advances. *Blood* 1985; 65:1039–1047.

4. Dekmezian R, Kantarjian HP, Keating MJ, et al: The relevance of reticulin stain-measured fibrosis at diagnosis in chronic myelogenous leukemia. *Cancer* 1987; 59:1739–1743.

5. Dreazen O, Cannani E, Gale RP: Molecular biology of chronic myelogenous leukemia. Seminars in Hematol 25:35–49, 1988.

6. Jacknow G, Frizzera G, Gajl-Peczalska K, et al: Extramedullary presentation of the blast crisis of chronic myelogenous leukemia. *Br J Haematol* 1985; 61:225–236.

7. Jandl JH: Chronic myeloproliferative syndromes, in *Blood: Textbook of Hematology*. Boston, Little, Brown & Co, 1987, pp 671–726.

8. Kantarjian HM, Keating MJ, Walters RS, et al: Clinical and prognostic features of Philadelphia chromosome–negative chronic myelogenous leukemia. *Cancer* 1986; 58:2023–2030.

9. Kantarjian HM, Keating MJ, Talpaz M, et al: Chronic myelogenous leukemia in blast crisis. *Am J Med* 1987; 83:445–454.

10. Muehleck SD, McKenna RW, Arthur DC: Transformation of chronic myelogenous leukemia: Clinical, morphologic, and cytogenetic features. *Am J Clin Pathol* 1984; 82:1–14.

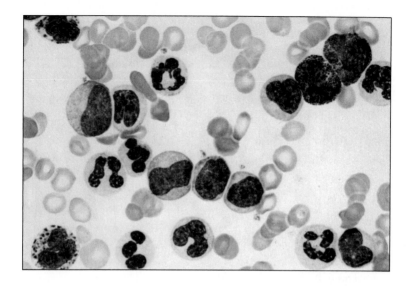

Figure 33–1 CML. A spectrum of granulocytes, from immature to mature, together with basophils and an eosinophil, are seen in a peripheral blood smear.

Figure 33–2 CML in blast crisis. Many blasts and a few mature cells are seen in a peripheral blood smear.

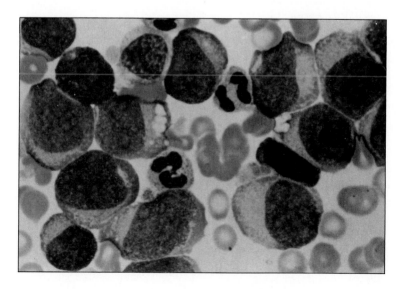

34

Chronic Lymphocytic Leukemia and Other Lymphoid Leukemias

Chronic lymphocytic leukemia (CLL) is an acquired clonal lympho-proliferative disorder characterized by an accumulation of small lymphocytes in the peripheral blood, bone marrow, lymph nodes, and spleen. In the United States and Europe, CLL accounts for approximately 30% of all leukemia, while in the Orient CLL is rarely seen.

Pathophysiology

CLL is an acquired clonal lymphoproliferative disorder of small, immunologically incompetent lymphocytes. Immunologic studies reveal surface immunoglobulin, intracytoplasmic immunoglobulin, or both of the leukemic cells in over 95% of patients, indicating that the majority of CLL originates from a clone of cells arrested at an early stage of B-cell differentiation. The cells from these patients show clonal immunoglobulin gene rearrangement. In approximately 5% of the cases, however, the cells have a T-cell phenotype demonstrating clonal rearrangements of the T-beta and T-gamma chains of the T-cell antigen receptor. Evidence indicates that B-cell CLL derives from a committed B-cell precursor stem cell compartment and not from the multipotent compartment as in acute lympho-blastic leukemia. Similarly, T-cell CLL originates in a committed stem cell compartment. This clonal restriction to a single committed cell line possibly explains the rarity of blast transformation in CLL in contrast to CML.

Genetic factors may play an important role in CLL. The trisomy 12 is the most common numerical chromosome abnormality, and its presence is considered to be evidence of aggressive disease. The most common structural chromosome abnormality is 14q + , and patients with this abnormality have a high incidence of prolymphocytic leukemia or Richter transformation.

B-cell CLL is usually associated with excessive T-suppressor activity, which may contribute to the immunologic impairment commonly seen in CLL. Hypogammaglobulinemia, which is seen in approximately 50% of patients, is due to an intrinsic B-cell defect caused by an imbalance in immunoglobulin chain synthesis.

Clinical Findings

The majority of patients with CLL are over 60 years of age, but the disease may also occur in individuals younger than 30 years of age. The disease may be discovered by chance, by blood examination, or by the finding of an enlarged lymph node or spleen during examination for an unrelated complaint. Other patients may seek advice because of enlarged lymph nodes or complaints related to anemia. Physical examination usually shows generalized lymphadenopathy, and hepatosplenomegaly is common. Lymphadenopathy may wax and wane over several months. During the course of the disease, extranodal involvement, including the gastrointestinal tract and lungs, is not unusual.

The physical examination, together with results of a blood cell count, is the basis of Rai's staging system, which has been shown to be useful in predicting the course of the disease (Table 34–1).

Approach to Diagnosis

Following a clinical history and physical examination, the approach to the laboratory diagnosis of CLL proceeds in the following sequence:

1. A complete blood count.
2. Examination of the peripheral blood smear.
3. Examination of the bone marrow.
4. Immunologic cell marker studies when needed for diagnosis.
5. Cytogenetic studies, which may be useful for prognosis and perhaps therapy.
6. Ancillary studies such as serum immunoglobulins and Coombs' antiglobulin test.

Table 34–1   Rai's Staging System for Chronic Lymphocytic Leukemia

Stage 0	Absolute lymphocytosis of >15 × 10^9/L and 40% or more lymphocytes in bone marrow
Stage I	Absolute lymphocytosis plus enlarged lymph nodes
Stage II	Absolute lymphocytosis plus enlarged liver and/or spleen; lymphadenopathy may or may not be present
Stage III	Absolute lymphocytosis plus anemia (Hgb <110 g/L or hematocrit <0.33%); lymph nodes, spleen, or liver may or may not be enlarged
Stage IV	Absolute lymphocytosis and thrombocytopenia (platelet count, <100 × 10^9/L); anemia and organomegaly may or may not be present

Hematologic Findings

The diagnosis of CLL can usually be suspected from the peripheral blood findings. Bone marrow examination is indicated to confirm the diagnosis and as an indicator of prognosis. Other disorders that may be associated with small-cell lymphocytosis include infectious disorders such as pertussis, infectious mononucleosis, and tuberculosis. These entities are usually easily distinguishable from CLL, and should not represent a diagnostic problem. Several other malignant lymphoproliferative disorders, however, such as lymphosarcoma cell leukemia, prolymphocytic leukemia, T-cell lymphocytosis, and hairy cell leukemia may closely resemble CLL, and are discussed later in this chapter.

Blood Cell Measurements.   Anemia is found at presentation in approximately 50% of patients. The anemia may be due to autoimmune hemolytic anemia, which occurs in approximately 20% of patients, or associated with bone marrow failure due to CLL involvement or hypersplenism. The Coombs'-positive autoimmune hemolytic anemia in CLL can be quite severe, necessitating blood transfusions.

The absolute lymphocyte count is above 15 × 10^9/L (15 × 10^3/μl) and, in most patients, it is between 30 and 300 × 10^9/L (30 and 300 × 10^3/μl). In some patients, the lymphocyte count may undergo cyclic fluctuations. Mild thrombocytopenia may be seen in approximately 40% of patients at time of diagnosis.

Peripheral Blood Smear Morphology. The red blood cells are usually normochromic and normocytic, although polychromasia and spherocytes may be seen in patients who have hemolytic anemia. In most patients, the leukemic cells appear as small- and medium-sized normal lymphocytes (Figure 34–1). A variable number of large lymphocytes may be present. Ruptured lymphocytes or so-called basket or smudge cells are common. When more than 15% to 20% of the lymphocytes have the appearance of prolymphocytes, which are characterized by large cells with moderately abundant cytoplasm and prominent nucleoli, the patient is said to have developed prolymphocytic transformation. The latter is usually associated with an accelerated phase of the disease. In addition, patients with more aggressive disease, instead of having a homogeneous lymphocyte population, may have pleomorphic lymphocytes, which often contain cleaved nuclei that resemble so-called lymphosarcoma cells in malignant lymphoma of the follicular small cleaved-cell variety.

Bone Marrow Examination. Initially the marrow may show only slight lymphocytosis. Histologic sections of the aspirate or preferably a biopsy specimen, are usually more helpful in identifying the lymphocytosis than are aspirate smears at the early stage of the disease. There is significant correlation between the infiltration patterns and clinical stage and survival. Thus, a diffuse infiltrative pattern is usually associated with a more rapidly progressive course than a nondiffuse pattern (Figure 34–2).

Other Laboratory Tests

34.1   Cell Surface Markers

Purpose.   Cell surface marker studies may be useful in early diagnosis of CLL and may be of prognostic importance.

Principle, Specimen, and Procedure.   See Test 32.2.

Interpretation.   B-lymphocytes in B-CLL express a single immunoglobulin light chain (either kappa or lambda, but not both) on their surface membrane. In addition, the lymphocytes usually have IgM and IgD heavy chains on their surface. IgG or IgA are much less common. Characteristically the surface membrane–bound immunoglobulin is present in very small amounts. In addition, B-CLL lymphocytes cross-react with the monoclonal antibody T101 or Leu-1, a Pan–T-cell antibody. The latter is not present on normal B-cells and is predominantly expressed on small lymphocytic malignancies such as CLL, small lymphocytic lymphoma, and intermediate lymphocytic lymphoma of B-cell phenotype.

In the majority of patients, cell surface marker studies are not needed to make a diagnosis of CLL. In patients who present with persistent mild idiopathic lymphocytosis, however, the documentation of monoclonicity, ie, the presence of only one light chain, is helpful in the diagnosis of CLL. This may be especially helpful in younger individuals with persistent lymphocytosis.

Cell surface markers are necessary to make a diagnosis of persistent T-cell lymphocytosis or T-cell CLL, as will be discussed later.

34.2 Cytogenetics

Purpose. Chromosome studies may be useful in the prognosis and perhaps therapy in patients with CLL.

Specimen and Procedure. See Test 33.2.

Interpretation. Chromosome studies of PHA-stimulated lymphocytes in CLL usually reveal normal karyotypes. If lymphocyte cultures are stimulated by B-cell mitogens, however, clonal chromosomal abnormalities are revealed in about half the patients. The most common numerical chromosome abnormality is trisomy 12, a karyotypic change thought to be a marker of aggressive disease. The most common structural chromosome abnormality is the marker 14q + . Patients with the 14q + marker chromosome usually show high leukocyte counts, advanced clinical staging, and are refractory to therapy.

Ancillary Tests

Coombs' Antiglobulin Test. Autoimmune hemolytic anemia develops in approximately 20% of the patients with CLL at some stage, and approximately one third develop serious hemolysis. Occasionally, the hemolytic anemia may antedate CLL by months or years. The Coombs' direct antiglobulin test is usually positive, and the antibody is of the IgG type.

Serum Immunoglobulin. Hypogammaglobulinemia is seen in at least 50% of patients with CLL and may increase in severity as the disease progresses. Usually all immunoglobulin classes are depressed. In approximately 5% of the patients with CLL, a monoclonal hypergammaglobulinemia is present. Because this is usually IgM, the disease may be difficult to distinguish from Waldenström's macroglobulinemia.

Lymph Node Biopsy. Lymphadenopathy is common in CLL. A lymph node biopsy is not indicated for the diagnosis of CLL, but may be useful in the diagnosis of Richter's syndrome, which is a transformation to a large cell lymphoma occurring in about 5% to 10% of CLL patients. In other uncomplicated CLL patients, the lymph node biopsy specimen shows complete replacement of the normal architecture with small lymphocytes. Scattered throughout the lymph node, however, are variably sized clusters of transformed lymphocytes referred to as "immature foci" or "pseudofollicular proliferation centers," which are also characteristic of small lymphocytic lymphoma.

Course and Treatment

The clinical course of CLL is variable. Many patients have relatively good health, living more than 10 years, while some patients die within 1 year. The staging system in Table 34–1 is useful for predicting the course of the disease. Good prognosis is associated with stage 0, intermediate prognosis with stages I and II, and poor prognosis with stages III and IV. Additional prognostic indicators include the pattern of lymphocytic infiltration in the bone marrow biopsy and the degree of absolute lymphocytosis and chromosomal abnormalities. The vulnerability to bacterial, viral, and fungal infections is most often the cause of morbidity and mortality of advanced-stage patients.

Richter's syndrome is defined as the development of large-cell lymphoma in the course of CLL. The transformation to large-cell lymphoma usually begins in the lymph nodes, but the disease eventually involves extranodal tissue, including the bone marrow. The development of large-cell lymphoma in CLL is usually associated with a poor prognosis.

Some patients with CLL develop what has been termed prolymphocytic transformation. This refers to a condition where more than 20% of the total lymphocytes have the appearance of prolymphocytes. The latter are large lymphocytes with abundant cytoplasm and round-to-oval nuclei with prominent nucleoli. This transformation is frequently, but not always, associated with aggressive disease.

Most therapy in CLL is palliative and not curative. In general, the treatment is started in the presence of any of the following: autoimmune hemolytic anemia, progressive marrow failure, massive splenomegaly, "bulky" disease, progressive hyperlymphocytosis, or increased susceptibility to bacterial infections. Corticosteroids and alkylators such as chlorambucil are the most widely used treatment. Intensive combination chemotherapy and total body radiation may be useful in advanced disease.

Other Chronic Lymphoid Leukemias

T-Cell CLL.   T-cell CLL represents 2% to 5% of all CLL cases, and may be divided into T-CLL with helper phenotype (marked by an aggressive course), and T-CLL with suppressor phenotype (marked by an indolent course).

T-CLL with helper phenotype has been reported most commonly in young adults (<40 years of age) who present with marked lymphocytosis (30 to 700 × 10^9/L or 30 to 700 × 10^3/μl), lymphadenopathy, skin involvement, diffuse marrow infiltration, and relatively frequent central nervous system involvement. The leukemic cells are small, the cytoplasm is agranular, and the nuclei are often irregular and without nucleoli. The disease is usually aggressive, with median patient survival of 15 months.

Chronic T-Cell Lymphocytosis (Suppressor T-Cell CLL). This disorder has been variably called chronic T-cell lymphocytosis, granulated T-cell lymphocytosis, T-gamma lymphocytosis with neutropenia, leukemia of large granular lymphocytes, and chronic suppressor T-cell CLL. It is a clinically and morphologically distinct syndrome with a particular constellation of biologic features. The disease is characterized by a moderate lymphocytosis (rarely >15 × 10^9/L or 15 × 10^3/μl), severe neutropenia, and mild anemia. The peripheral white blood cells are replaced to a variable degree with a population of large- to medium-sized granular lymphocytes with round-to-irregular nuclear contours, condensed chromatin, and prominent, variably sized, reddish granules in abundant cytoplasm (Figure 34–3). Lymphocytes in the bone marrow range from 20% to 40%. Immunologic phenotyping of the lymphocytes reveals mature, suppressor phenotype.

Physical examination reveals splenomegaly with little or no lymphadenopathy. Some patients have rheumatoid arthritis or other autoimmune disease.

There is controversy whether chronic T-cell lymphocytosis is a reactive or malignant process. The clinical behavior of this disorder is usually indolent with periods of infection, but in some patients it is more aggressive and suggestive of a malignant process, eg, T-cell CLL.

Prolymphocytic Leukemia.   Prolymphocytic leukemia is characterized by marked splenomegaly, minimal lymphadenopathy, marked leukocytosis (often $>100 \times 10^9/L$ or $100 \times 10^3/\mu l$) consisting predominantly of prolymphocytes, and variable degrees of thrombocytopenia. The prolymphocytes are larger and have more cytoplasm than small lymphocytes in B-cell CLL. Their nuclear chromatin pattern is moderately coarse and there is a prominent nucleolus (Figure 34–4). The patients do not respond to treatment that is usually effective in CLL, and the prognosis is considerably worse than CLL.

In addition to this apparent denovo prolymphocytic leukemia, there is also, in a small number of patients, B-cell CLL that transforms into prolymphocytic leukemia (prolymphocytic transformation). These patients have an increasing number of prolymphocytes ($>20\%$) that have the same immunologic phenotype as the small CLL lymphocytes. This transformation is usually associated with increasing splenomegaly and lymphadenopathy. In most patients prolymphocytic transformation is associated with a poor prognosis.

While the majority of the prolymphocytic leukemias are of B-cell origin, a small number of T-cell types have also been described. The clinical manifestations in T-cell prolymphocytic leukemia are similar to the B-cell types, except that skin involvement appears to be more common in the former. Morphologically and ultrastructurally, T- and B-prolymphocytes are indistinguishable. The T-prolymphocytes stain positive with acid phosphatase and nonspecific esterase in a focal pattern. Immunologic studies have shown both mature helper and mature suppressor phenotypes. T-cell prolymphocytic leukemia is an aggressive disease with a median patient survival of less than 1 year.

Hairy Cell Leukemia.   Hairy cell leukemia is a rare form of leukemia characterized by splenomegaly, minimal lymphadenopathy, cytopenia, and the presence of atypical mononuclear cells in the blood and bone marrow.

The mononuclear cells ("hairy" cells), as seen in the blood smear, have features of both lymphocytes and monocytes (Figure 34–5). The nuclear chromatin pattern has a ground-glass or spongy appearance. The light, gray-blue cytoplasm is moderately abundant and usually has characteristic "hairy" projections. The morphology may, however, vary considerably, and the number of malignant cells in the peripheral blood may be very small. Thus, the diagnosis may be missed even by a relatively experienced observer. The size of the cell varies from 10 to 20 μm in diameter and the nucleocyto-plasmic ratio is also variable. In some cases the cells have multiple, thin, irregular cytoplasmic projections, in other cases the cytoplasm is abundant with blunt and broad cytoplasmic projections, and occasionally the cytoplasmic projections may be indistinct. The nuclei may be ovoid, clefted, or sometimes convoluted (Figure 34–5).

In most patients the malignant cells are positive with the tartrate-resistant acid phosphatase (TRAP) stain, though the degree of positivity varies. It should be noted that TRAP positive cells may also be seen occasionally in CLL, in prolymphocytic leukemia, lympho-sarcoma cell leukemia, and in "reactive" lymphocytes. The non-specific esterase is often moderately positive in a crescent-like fashion, and S100 has been demonstrated within the cytoplasm.

The cell of origin of hairy cell leukemia has been the source of much controversy. There is good evidence that the hairy cells belong to the B-cell lineage. Surface marker studies usually reveal a monoclonal B-cell population.

A bone marrow aspirate often results in a dry tap, but the bone marrow biopsy specimen reveals a focal or diffuse infiltrate of mono-nuclear cells, which characteristically are less densely packed than the malignant cells in other leukemias or lymphomas (Figure 34–6). The bland, uniform mononuclear cells have well-defined nuclei and a clear cytoplasm that gives them a halo-like appearance. Since the leukemic cells in the peripheral blood may be few and difficult to recognize, and because a bone marrow aspirate frequently reveals a dry tap, the bone marrow biopsy is the most useful examination for the diagnosis of hairy-cell leukemia.

Hairy cell leukemia has in the past been, and probably still is, frequently misdiagnosed as chronic lymphocytic leukemia, malignant lymphoma, aplastic anemia or, rarely, chronic monocytic leukemia. It is important to recognize this disease, because the patients usually do not respond to conventional chemotherapy used in CLL, and most do not tolerate aggressive chemotherapy. Splenectomy, however, appears to be of benefit in patients with large spleens and severe cytopenia. Interferon and deoxycoformycin are showing considerable promise as therapeutic agents.

Lymphosarcoma Cell Leukemia. The term lymphosar-coma cell leukemia (LCL) is used to describe involvement of the peripheral blood by lymphoma cells. The white blood cell count is usually not greater than $25 \times 10^9/L$ ($25 \times 10^3/\mu l$). Hodgkin's disease hardly ever involves the blood. However, involvement of the blood with non-Hodgkin's lymphoma is not unusual.

Using sensitive flow cytometric methods, it can be shown that circulating malignant cells are present in most patients with non-Hodgkin's lymphoma. In such studies there may be no correlation with morphologic evidence of bone marrow involvement by lymphoma, but there is usually a strong correlation with clinical staging. The morphologic features of LCL depend on the type of lymphoma the patient has. In patients with small cleaved cell (poorly differentiated lymphocytic) lymphoma, the malignant cells appear as medium-sized lymphocytes, with scant cytoplasm, and a nucleus that has a moderately clumped chromatin pattern and characteristic nuclear cleavage ("buttock cells") (Figure 34–7). In small lymphocytic (well-differentiated) lymphoma the malignant cells have an appearance identical to those seen in CLL. In lymphoblastic lymphoma the malignant cells are similar to ALL, except that nuclear convolutions are usually more prominent. In large cell ("histiocytic") lymphoma the malignant cells appear as large lymphocytes, with moderately abundant blue cytoplasm, a round-to-ovoid nucleus with a variable, clumped chromatin pattern, and nucleoli that may or may not be prominent depending on the subtype of large cell lymphoma.

Sézary's Syndrome. In Sézary's syndrome, which is a form of mycosis fungoides (cutaneous T-cell lymphoma), the malignant T-cells (usually mature helper T-cells) are present in the skin as well as in the blood. The so-called Sézary cells have the appearance of medium-sized lymphocytes, moderate-to-scant cytoplasm, and a nucleus that has characteristic brainlike convolutions (cerebriform nucleus) (Figure 34–8). A small number of Sézary-like cells may be seen in normal blood, but if they constitute greater than 15% of the lymphocytes, they are considered to represent circulating malignant cells. The acid phosphatase and the nonspecific esterase stains both usually stain positive in a dotlike fashion in Sézary cells.

Circulating Sézary cells in mycosis fungoides is usually associated with aggressive disease that may require systemic chemotherapy.

Adult T-Cell Leukemia/Lymphoma (ATLL). ATLL was initially described in Japan, and, more recently, in the Caribbean and United States, and is characterized by malignant T-lymphocytes in peripheral lymph nodes, skin, spleen, and peripheral blood. The disease is transmitted by human T-cell lymphotropic virus (HTLV-1). The malignant cells have scant cytoplasm and a lobated or "knobby" nucleus with clumped chromatin (Figure 34–9). In the majority of patients, these cells are mature postthymic (TdT-negative and T6-negative), activated helper or sometimes suppressor T-cells. The patients frequently have hypercalcemia and respond poorly to current therapy.

Table 34–2 presents a summary of the characteristic clinical and laboratory features of the chronic lymphoid leukemias.

Table 34–2   Clinical and Laboratory Features of Chronic Lymphoproliferative Disease[a]

Type	Leukocyte Count × 10⁹/L	Cell Morphology
B-cell (CLL)	50–150	Similar-to-normal, small lymphocytes
T-cell lymphocytosis	15–30	Medium-to-large lymphocytes with azurophilic cytoplasmic granules Nuclear folding or convolutions unusual
B-cell PLL	75–100	Moderate-to-large lymphocytes with clumped chromatin and prominent nucleoli
T-cell PLL	75–100	Same as B-cell PLL
Lymphosarcoma cell leukemia	10–30	Medium-to-large lymphocytes often with clefted nucleus
Hairy cell leukemia	4–30	Small-to-medium lymphocytes with moderate to abundant cytoplasm with hairlike projections
CTCL	12–20	Medium lymphocytes with cerebriform nuclei
ATLL	5–30	Medium lymphocytes with lobated or "knobby" nuclei

ABBREVIATIONS: PPL = prolymphocytic leukemia; CTCL = cutaneous T-cell lymphoma; ATLL = adult T-cell leukemia/lymphoma; HTLV = human T-cell leukemia virus; CLL = chronic lymphocytic leukemia; TdT = terminal deoxynucleotidyl transferase.

[a]It should be noted that several of the disorders (T- and B-cell PLL and ATLL) listed as chronic lymphoproliferative disorders have, in fact, an aggressive course similar to acute leukemia

Lymphadenopathy	Splenomegaly	Special Features
1 + –2 +	1 + –3 +	Hypogammaglobulinemia and Coombs' positive hemolytic anemia common
0–1 +	1–3 +	Frequent neutropenia; usually suppressor T-cells; occasionally dermal invasion
0 + –1 +	2 + –3 +	Aggressive disease
0 + –1 +	2 + –3 +	Aggressive disease; helper or suppressor phenotype; dermal invasion not uncommon; TdT negative
2 + –3 +	1 + –2 +	Non-Hodgkin's lymphoma; diagnosis by lymph node biopsy
0–1 +	2 + –3 +	Cells contain tartrate resistant acid phosphatase; bone marrow biopsy diagnostic
0–1 +	0	Skin involvement; bone marrow usually negative; usually mature, helper phenotype, sometimes suppressor cells
2 + –3 +	0–1 +	Dermal invasion, hypercalcemia, often associated with HTLV; mature helper or suppressor phenotype, TdT negative

References

1. Golomb HM: Diagnosis and treatment of hairy cell leukemia, in Gale RP, Golde DW (eds): *Leukemia: Recent Advances in Biology and Treatment.* New York, Alan R Liss Inc, 1985, 121–133.

2. Han T: Prognostic importance of cytogenetic abnormalities in patient with chronic lymphocytic leukemia. *N Engl J Med* 1984; 310:288–292.

3. Han T, Barcos M, Emrich H, et al: Bone marrow infiltration patterns and their prognostic significance in chronic lymphocytic leukemia: Correlations with clinical, immunologic, phenotypic, and cytogenetic data. *J Clin Oncol* 1984; 2:562–570.

4. Harousseau JL: Malignant lymphoma supervening in chronic lymphocytic leukemia and related disorders: Richter's syndrome: A study of 25 cases. *Cancer* 1981; 48:1302–1308.

5. Jaffe E, Blattner WA, Blayney DW: The pathologic spectrum of adult T-cell leukemia/lymphoma in the United States. *Am J Surg Pathol* 1984; 8:263–275.

6. Jandl JH: Chronic lymphatic leukemia: Prolymphocytic leukemia and hairy cell leukemia, in *Blood: Textbook of Hematology.* Boston, Little Brown & Co, 1987, 751–800.

7. Melo JV, Catovsky D, Galton DAG: The relationship between chronic lymphocytic leukemia and prolymphocytic leukemia. *Br J Haematol* 1986; 63:377–387.

8. Newland AC, Catovsky D, Linch D, et al: Chronic T-cell lymphocytosis: A review of 21 cases. *Br J Haematol* 1984; 58:433–446.

9. Rai KR, Sawitsky A, Jagathambal K: Chronic lymphocytic leukemia. *Med Clin North Am* 1984; 68:697–711.

10. Sandberg AA, Abe S: Cytogenetic techniques in haematology. *Clin Haematol* 1980; 9:19–38.

11. Semenzato G, Pandolfi F, Chisesi T, et al: The lymphoproliferative disease of granular lymphocytes: A heterogeneous disorder ranging from indolent to aggressive conditions. *Cancer* 1987; 60:2971–2978.

12. Spier C, Kjeldsberg CR, Head D: Chronic lymphocytic leukemia in young adults. *Am J Clin Pathol* 1985; 84:675–678.

13. Volk JR, Kjeldsberg CR, Eyre H: T-cell prolymphocytic leukemia: Clinical and immunologic characterization. *Cancer* 1983; 52:2049–2054.

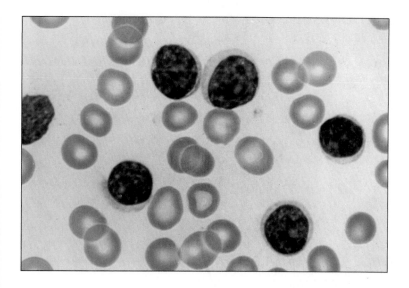

Figure 34–1　CLL. Several small, normal-appearing lymphocytes in the peripheral blood smear.

Figure 34–2　CLL. A nodular pattern of involvement is seen in this bone marrow biopsy.

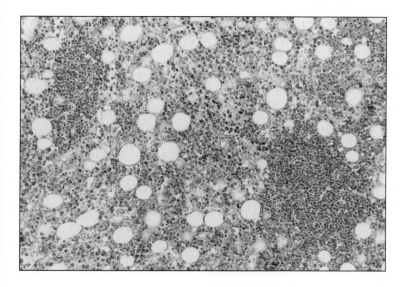

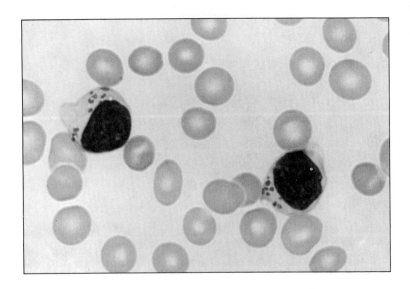

Figure 34–3   Chronic T-cell lymphocytosis. Two lymphocytes containing variably sized cytoplasmic granules.

Figure 34–4   Prolymphocytic leukemia. Four prolymphocytes characterized by abundant cytoplasm and a round nucleus with a prominent nucleolus.

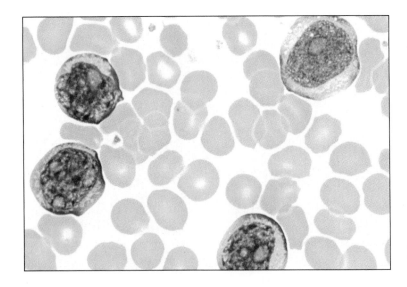

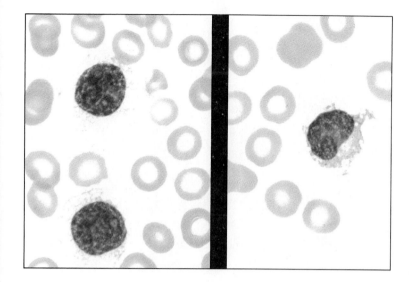

Figure 34–5 Hairy cell leukemia. Peripheral blood smear from two patients showing the variable morphology of hairy cells.

Figure 34–6 Hairy cell leukemia. Sheets of characteristically loosely packed cells in a bone marrow biopsy specimen.

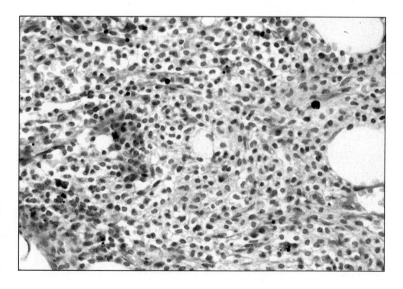

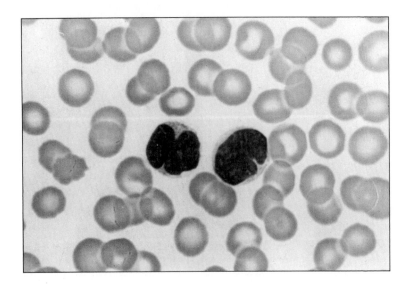

Figure 34–7   Lymphosarcoma cell leukemia. Two lymphocytes in the peripheral blood show characteristic nuclear cleavage. From a patient with malignant lymphoma, small cleaved-cell type.

Figure 34–8   Sézary syndrome. The Sézary cell has moderate-to-scant cytoplasm and a cerebriform nucleus.

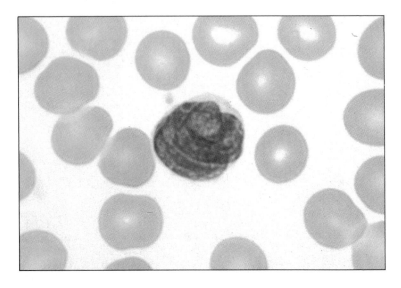

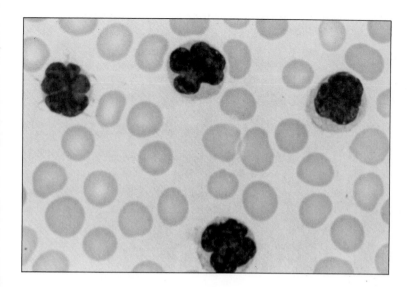

Figure 34–9   Adult T-cell leukemia/lymphoma. The leukemic lymphocytes have scant cytoplasm and a lobated or "knobby" nucleus with
clumped chromatin.

PART 9

Myeloproliferative
Disorders

35

Myeloproliferative Disorders: Myelofibrosis and Thrombocythemia

The term "myeloproliferative disorder" was introduced to describe a group of closely related syndromes such as chronic myelogenous leukemia, polycythemia vera, myelofibrosis with myeloid metaplasia, and essential thrombocythemia (Table 35–1). These disorders have similar clinical and hematologic manifestations at some stage in the disease process (Table 35–2). Chronic myelogenous leukemia (CML) and polycythemia vera are described in chapters 33 and 17, respectively, and this chapter will be confined to a discussion of myelofibrosis with myeloid metaplasia and essential thrombocythemia.

Pathophysiology

A large number of synonyms have been used for myelofibrosis with myeloid metaplasia, including idiopathic myelofibrosis, chronic myelosclerosis, agnogenic myeloid metaplasia, aleukemic megakaryocytic myelosis, and leukoerythroblastic anemia. These names usually indicate the feature of the disease that appears most striking to the observer. The disorder is clonal in nature, arising from an abnormal, multipotent hematopoietic stem cell. No specific cytogenetic abnormality has been described, but 13q− is common. There are variable degrees of fibrosis in the bone marrow and a variable proliferation of the granulocytic, erythrocytic, and mega-

Table 35–1   Classification of Myloproliferative Disorders

Polycythemia vera
Chronic myelogenous leukemia
Myelofibrosis with myeloid metaplasia
Essential thrombocythemia

Table 35–2   Common Features of Myeloproliferative Disorders

Similar clinical manifestations

   Asymptomatic, or fatigue, bleeding, splenomegaly

Peripheral blood

   Anemia with variable red cell changes

   Variable degrees of leukocytosis with immature cells

   Variable degrees of eosinophilia and basophilia

   Qualitative and quantitative platelet abnormalities

Bone marrow

   Panmyelosis with variable degrees of myelofibrosis

Spleen

   Extramedullary hematopoiesis

Apparent "transitional" forms between various types

Accelerated phase or "blastic" crisis common in terminal stages

---

karyocytic series in the bone marrow, spleen, liver, and lymph nodes. It is thought that abnormal megakaryocyte precursors release growth factors (platelet factor IV and PDGF) that stimulate fibroblasts, causing the fibrosis seen in the bone marrow. It must be known that myelofibrosis is not secondary to some known cause, such as metastatic carcinoma. Patients suffering from this disease characteristically have an enlarged spleen, caused by extramedullary hematopoiesis. Splenic enlargement may be considerable and is caused by a combination of vascular expansion, tremendous red cell pooling, hematopoietic hyperplasia, and fibrosis.

Recent studies have not demonstrated the correlation between the extent of marrow fibrosis and duration of disease, splenic weight, or degree of splenic myeloid metaplasia. Likewise, studies have been unable to document a progression of marrow fibrosis as a cause for the increase in splenomegaly.

Table 35-3   Characteristics of Idiopathic Myelofibrosis

Insidious onset with weakness, weight loss, pallor

Splenomegaly

Normochromic anemia

Red cell morphology
  Prominent poikilocytosis (tear drop forms) and anisocytosis

Nucleated red cells common in peripheral blood

White cell count
  Elevated ($<30 \times 10^9$/L), normal or rarely decreased, immature granulocytes, occasional myeloblasts, mild eosinophilia and basophilia

Platelet count
  Increased, normal or decreased, giant platelets, micromegakaryocytes, and megakaryocytic fragments

Bone marrow
  Panmyelosis with increasing myelofibrosis

The myelostimulatory theory is the most widely held theory that explains extramedullary hematopoiesis in myelofibrosis with myeloid metaplasia. This theory suggests a myelostimulatory factor that results in a proliferation of the hematopoietic and stromal cell lines in the bone marrow as well as in organs that were previously hematopoietic in the fetus. More recent studies suggest that distended, altered sinusoids containing intravascular hematopoietic cells provide these cells access to the circulation, resulting in the leukoerythroblastosis characteristic of this disorder. These hematopoietic cells are filtered from the peripheral blood by the spleen and accumulate in that organ. Autonomous hematopoiesis may occur late in the course of the disease. The characteristic features of this disorder are listed in Table 35-3.

Essential (primary, idiopathic) thrombocythemia, the least common of the myeloproliferative disorders, is marked by megakaryocyte proliferation, and overproduction of the platelets is the predominant feature. The recurrent hemorrhage and thrombosis sometimes observed in patients suffering from this disorder are caused by the marked elevation in the platelet count associated with abnormal platelet function. Hence, this entity has also been called "hemorrhagic thrombocythemia." Iron deficiency anemia

Table 35–4 Characteristic Features of Essential Thrombocythemia

Insidious onset

Bleeding and thromboembolic phenomena

Splenomegaly

Platelet count
Sustained thrombocytosis in excess of $1,000 \times 10^9/L$

White cell count
Neutrophilic leukocytosis ($<30 \times 10^9/L$), mild shift to left

Anemia
Normochromic, normocytic or microcytic, hypochromic

Bone marrow
Marked megakaryocytic proliferation

may develop as a result of chronic gastrointestinal hemorrhage. Between hemorrhages, there may be a tendency toward polycythemia. As with other myeloproliferative disorders, essential thrombocythemia has been shown to be a clonal abnormality of the multipotential stem cell. The main features of this disorder are listed in Table 35–4.

Clinical Findings

The myeloproliferative disorders usually have an insidious onset; the patient may present with a long history of weakness or may be relatively asymptomatic. In myelofibrosis with myeloid metaplasia, the patients develop a variety of symptoms, including malaise, weight loss, bleeding, diarrhea, and fever. Splenomegaly is the main physical finding and may be associated with abdominal discomfort, pain, indigestion, or dyspnea. Other features that may be present include: hepatomegaly, petechiae, and bleeding (usually secondary to thrombocytopenia caused by splenic trapping, or abnormal platelet function, or both), ascites, jaundice, portal hypertension, cirrhosis, and, rarely, lymphadenopathy.

In essential thrombocythemia, the patients may be asymptomatic or may complain of weakness, headache, parasthesias, and dizziness. Bleeding may be seen in the gastrointestinal tract and, less commonly, in the urinary tract or the skin. Other features may include thrombosis and peptic ulceration in the esophageal varices. Splenomegaly is seen in approximately 60% of patients but is usually not as prominent as in myelofibrosis with myeloid metaplasia. The liver may be slightly enlarged, but only rarely is there lymph node enlargement.

Approach to Diagnosis

Following a clinical history and physical examination, the laboratory diagnosis of myeloproliferative disease proceeds in the following sequence:

1. A complete blood count.
2. Examination of the peripheral blood smear.
3. Examination of the bone marrow.
4. Testing for leukocyte alkaline phosphatase.
5. Cytogenetic studies.

Hematologic Findings

The hematologic findings in myelofibrosis and essential thrombocythemia are variable and depend on the stage of the disease. As expected, there is considerable overlap between the different types of myeloproliferative disorders. Myelodysplastic syndrome may be extremely difficult to differentiate from myelofibrosis with myeloid metaplasia. The former usually does not have significant splenomegaly or the teardrop-form red cell morphology typically seen in myelofibrosis. In the differential diagnosis of myelofibrosis with myeloid metaplasia, other conditions associated with bone marrow fibrosis and leukoerythroblastosis must be considered (Table 35–5). In the differential diagnosis of essential thrombocythemia, other disorders associated with elevated platelet count should be considered (Table 35–6).

Blood Cell Measurements. In myelofibrosis with myeloid metaplasia, initially mild normochromic, normocytic anemia is present that becomes progressively more severe. The leukocyte count is often slightly increased, usually $<30 \times 10^9$/L (30×10^3/ μl), or is occasionally decreased. The platelet count is initially normal or high. As the disease progresses, thrombocytopenia and leukopenia are common.

In essential thrombocythemia, a mild normochromic, normo-

Table 35–5 Conditions Possibly Associated with Myelofibrosis and Leukoerythroblastosis

Non-Malignant	Malignant
Gaucher's disease	Myeloproliferative disorders
Paget's disease	Leukemias, acute and chronic
Granulomatous disorders	Hodgkin's disease
Renal osteodystrophy	Non-Hodgkin's lymphoma
	Multiple myeloma
	Metastatic carcinoma

Table 35–6 Causes of Elevated Platelet Count

Endogenous	Reactive
Essential thrombocythemia	Hemorrhage
Occasionally in polycythemia vera, myelo-fibrosis, and chronic myelocytic leukemia	Chronic iron deficiency Malignancy Postsplenectomy Chronic infections

cytic anemia is usually present. The anemia may become microcytic hypochromic if the patient has chronic bleeding. Almost one third of patients, however, may show a normal or elevated hematocrit value, in which case the patient may be misdiagnosed as having polycythemia vera. The leukocyte count may be normal but is usually moderately increased. The striking feature in essential thrombocythemia is the markedly elevated platelet count, usually exceeding 1 million/μL.

Peripheral Blood Smear Morphology. In myelofibrosis, the whole spectrum of granulocytic precursors may be seen, and the blood smear resembles a granulocytic leukemoid reaction. The percentage of blasts may vary from 0% to 10%, and the presence of blasts in the peripheral blood does not necessarily indicate an accelerated phase or blast crisis. Eosinophilia and basophilia may be present but are usually less severe than in CML. In addition to immature granulocytes, there is usually a small number of nucleated red blood cells, which, together with the immature granulocytes, constitute the so-called leukoerythroblastic picture (Figure 35–1). The red cell morphology usually includes a significant degree of anisocytosis, poikilocytosis, and polychromasia. Teardrop forms (dacryocytes) and ovalocytes are common in myelofibrosis. Hypochromic microcytic cells may be seen in patients who have developed iron deficiency caused by bleeding. Platelets will often exhibit abnormal morphology and may be extremely large in size. Fragments of megakaryocytes or micromegakaryocytes may also be seen.

In essential thrombocythemia, large clumps of platelets are usually seen. In addition, the platelets show a marked variation in size and shape, including giant platelets, microplatelets, and platelets showing abnormal granularity. The leukocytes that are usually increased in number show a shift to the left, but promyelocytes and myeloblasts are unusual. As with myelofibrosis, mild eosinophilia and basophilia are not uncommon. The red cells are usually normochromic and normocytic, but microcytic hypochromic red cells may be found in patients who have chronic blood loss.

Bone Marrow Examination. In myelofibrosis, aspiration of the bone marrow often results in a dry tap. A bone marrow biopsy must always be performed in patients in whom a myeloproliferative disorder is being considered. Early in the course of myelofibrosis, the bone marrow may not show striking abnormalities, except for hypercellularity with an increased number of all cell lines. All stages of maturation are represented. This is the so-called cellular phase of myelofibrosis (Figure 35–2). Usually an increased proportion of neutrophil precursors and megakaryocytes are seen. The megakaryocytes occur in clusters, are frequently abnormal in size and shape, and may sometimes be difficult to recognize as megakaryocytes. The marrow sinusoids characteristically become distended.

A reticulin stain is necessary to detect early myelofibrosis. The degree of myelofibrosis increases as the disease progresses. The marrow gradually becomes less cellular, and the megakaryocytes remain until myelofibrosis becomes the predominant feature (Figure 35–3). Formation of collagen in the marrow is associated with the appearance of extramedullary hematopoiesis of spleen, liver, and sometimes lymph nodes. The degree of marrow fibrosis does not, however, necessarily correlate with the duration of the disease and splenic myeloid metaplasia. In addition to myelofibrosis, increasing osteosclerosis may be seen.

In essential thrombocythemia, the bone marrow also shows panmyelosis. There is a preponderance of megakaryocytes, that frequently occur in clusters showing extensive platelet production. The megakaryocytes vary considerably in size and shape (Figure 35–4). In general, the bone marrow findings in essential thrombocythemia are difficult to separate from those of myelofibrosis, and as the disease progresses, a transition from essential thrombocythemia to myelofibrosis frequently occurs.

Other Laboratory Tests

35.1 Leukocyte Alkaline Phosphatase (LAP)

Purpose. The LAP score may be useful in differentiating CML from other myeloproliferative disorders.

Principle, Specimen, and Procedure. See Test 18.1.

Interpretation. In CML, the LAP score is characteristically zero or markedly decreased. It is usually elevated in the other myeloproliferative disorders, though in myelofibrosis with myeloid metaplasia, the LAP score may be high, normal, or low. Low scores are particularly seen in patients with low white counts. Therefore, a low LAP score does not rule out myelofibrosis with myeloid metaplasia. In essential thrombocythemia, the LAP score is usually normal or elevated.

35.2 Cytogenetic Studies

Purpose. Cytogenetic studies may be useful in distinguishing CML from the other myeloproliferative disorders.

Principle, Specimen, and Procedure. See Test 33.2.

Interpretation. The Philadelphia (Ph[1]) chromosome, which is present in all cases of CML, is absent in both myelofibrosis and essential thrombocythemia. Several chromosome changes have been observed in the myeloproliferative disorders, but none is specific, except for the Ph[1] chromosome.

Ancillary Tests

Bleeding Test. Bleeding problems may occur in myeloproliferative disorders, particularly in essential thrombocythemia and less frequently in myelofibrosis with myeloid metaplasia. The bleeding may be caused by thrombocytopenia or a defect in platelet function. When the latter is present, prolonged bleeding time and impairment of in vitro platelet aggregation often occurs. The cause of bleeding in essential thrombocythemia, however, is poorly understood, and the bleeding time may be normal.

Blood Biochemistry. Serum uric acid level is frequently elevated and may lead to gouty arthritis, urate stones, and nephropathy, particularly in patients with a high leukocyte count. In addition, the serum alkaline phosphatase level may be elevated, which may be a reflection of extramedullary hematopoiesis in the liver. Increased lactic dehydrogenase (LD) level also is seen.

Radiology. Osteosclerosis has been demonstrated in approximately 50% of patients with myelofibrosis and myeloid metaplasia; it is not seen in patients with CML. The bones most frequently affected are (in order of frequency): femur, pelvis, vertebrae, radius, tibia, and sternum. Foci of rarification may also be seen.

Biopsy of Tissue Other Than Bone Marrow. Extramedullary hematopoiesis may be associated with lymph node enlargement. Biopsy of a lymph node usually reveals normal architecture and a mixed proliferation of hematopoietic cells in the sinuses. Atypical megakaryocytes may predominate. In myelofibrosis with myeloid metaplasia, extramedullary tumors rarely develop. These tumors may occur in the pleura, spinal cord, spleen, liver, mesentery, or retroperitoneal cavity, and are composed of immature hematopoietic cells. The extramedullary hematopoiesis seen in lymph nodes or as tumors may sometimes exhibit such bizarre morphology that it may be mistaken for a malignant lymphoma or metastatic carcinoma. A specific esterase stain is helpful in confirming the presence of granulocytic cell precursors.

Course and Treatment

Patients exhibiting myelofibrosis with myeloid metaplasia usually show a gradual progressive deterioration that is associated with increasing splenomegaly and fibrosis of the bone marrow. The median survival is 4 to 5 years, but many patients live 10 years or longer. In approximately 10% of patients, there is an expansion of the malignant clone in form of an accelerated phase or blastic crisis. The picture in the peripheral blood and bone marrow may then be indistinguishable from acute myeloblastic leukemia. Anemia becomes progressively more severe, requiring multiple blood transfusions.

In essential thrombocythemia, a number of patients go for years without requiring therapy. Other patients may experience repeated hemorrhagic and thromboembolic episodes. In rare patients, blastic crisis or pure red cell aplasia develops.

Therapy for myelofibrosis with myeloid metaplasia is mainly for the treatment of symptoms. Androgen therapy has been used to stimulate erythropoiesis in patients who are markedly anemic. In patients who have marked leukocytosis, thrombocytosis, and splenomegaly, chemotherapy with alkylating agents may be helpful. Splenectomy is beneficial in approximately one half of patients with marked thrombocytopenia, anemia, or splenic pain. Local radiation may be useful for those patients who are not candidates for splenectomy. Allopurinol therapy may be indicated in patients who have a high serum uric acid level.

In essential thrombocythemia, therapy may not be needed. When a patient develops a thrombotic or bleeding episode, however, treatment is indicated and usually consists of an alkylating agent or P-32 to reduce the platelet count. Occasionally, thrombocytophoresis may be useful. In addition, drugs that interfere with normal platelet function, such as aspirin, may be useful with or without anticoagulants. Splenectomy is usually contraindicated.

Special Diagnostic Considerations

Acute Myelofibrosis (Myelosclerosis). Acute or malignant myelofibrosis is a rare disease characterized by pancytopenia, minimal poikilocytosis and anisocytosis (in contrast to myelofibrosis with myeloid metaplasia), bone marrow fibrosis, and panmyelosis. Most of the cells present are immature, and megakaryocytes or megakaryoblasts are prominent. Also, in contrast to myelofibrosis with myeloid metaplasia, splenomegaly is minimal or absent. The disease is fulminant and usually fatal. It may be impossible to distinguish acute megakaryocytic leukemia (M7—see chapter 32 for classification schema) from acute myelofibrosis, and they may be variants of the same disease process.

Undifferentiated or Atypical Myeloproliferative Syndrome. Approximately one third of the patients may have to be categorized as having so-called undifferentiated or atypical myeloproliferative syndrome because their laboratory findings do not fit into a specific disease entity. Thus, some patients exhibit myeloid metaplasia in the spleen and liver, with a classical leukoerythroblastic blood smear, but the bone marrow shows only panmyelosis with minimal fibrosis. This may closely resemble CML, but in contrast to CML, these patients have normal or elevated LAP scores and lack the Ph[1] chromosome. To exclude polycythemia vera, the red cell mass must be normal. Still other patients may have severe myelofibrosis but only minimal myeloid metaplasia. A summary of the differential

Table 35–7 Differential Characteristics of Chronic Myeloproliferative Syndromes

	Myelofibrosis Myeloid Metaplasia
Hemoglobin	Decreased
Leukocyte count	Usually <30 × 10⁹/L
Differential count	Moderate number of immature granulocytes
Eosinophilia and/or basophilia	Usually present
Red cell morphology	Anisocytosis and teardrop poikilocytosis
Nucleated red cells in blood	Common
Platelet count	Normal, increased, or decreased
Bone marrow	Hypercellular with increasing fibrosis
LAP	Variable, usually increased
Ph¹	Absent
Splenomegaly	Marked

ABBREVIATIONS: CML = chronic myelogenous leukemia; LAP = leukocyte alkaline phosphatase; Ph¹ = Philadelphia chromosome.

characteristics of the various myeloproliferative syndromes is shown in Table 35–7.

References

1. Frisch B, Bartz R: Histology of myelofibrosis and osteomyelosclerosis, in Lewis SM (ed): *Myelofibrosis: Pathophysiology and Clinical Management.* New York, Marcel Dekker Inc, 1985, pp 51–86.
2. Iland HJ: Essential thrombocytosis: Clinical and laboratory characteristics at presentation. *Trans Assoc Physiol* 1983; 96:165–174.
3. Jandl HJ: Blood, in *Textbook of Hematology.* Boston, Little Brown & Co, 1987.

Essential Thrombocythemia	CML	Polycythemia Vera
Normal or decreased	Decreased	Normal or increased
Usually $<20 \times 10^9$/L	Usually $>50 \times 10^9$/L	Usually $<20 \times 10^9$/L
Usually normal	Many immature granulocytes	Usually normal
May be present	Present	May be present
Normal or hypochromic, microcytic	Usually normal	Normal or hypochromic, microcytic
Rare	Rare	Rare
Increased	Normal, increased, or decreased	Normal or increased
Hypercellular with megakaryocytosis	Marked myeloid hyperplasia	Hypercellular with decreased iron stores
Usually normal	Decreased	Usually increased
Absent	Present	Absent
Absent or mild	Moderate	Absent or mild

4. Lewis SM: Myelofibrosis: Pathophysiology and clinical management. Marcel Dekker Inc, New York, 1985, vol 4.

5. Reed RE: Polycythemia vera and agnogenic myeloid metaplasia. *Med Clin North Am* 1980; 64:667–681.

6. Silverstein MN: Myeloproliferative disease, in Fairbanks V (ed): *Current Hematology and Oncology,* vol 6. Chicago, Year Book Medical Publishers, 1988, pp 163–184.

7. Wolf BC, Neiman RS: Hypothesis-splenic infiltration and the pathogenesis of extramedullary hematopoiesis in agnogenic myeloid metaplasia. *Hematol Pathol* 1987; 1:77–80.

8. Wolf BC, Neiman RS: Myelofibrosis with myeloid metaplasia: Pathophysiologic implications of the correlation between bone marrow changes and progression of splenomegaly. *Blood* 1985; 65:803–809.

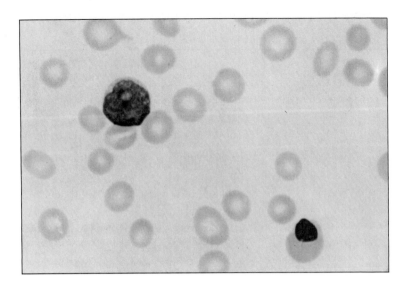

Figure 35–1 Peripheral blood smear from patient with myelofibrosis showing a myeloblast, a nucleated red blood cell, and a rare teardrop form red cell.

Figure 35–2 Bone marrow biopsy from patient with early myelofibrosis showing panhyperplasia.

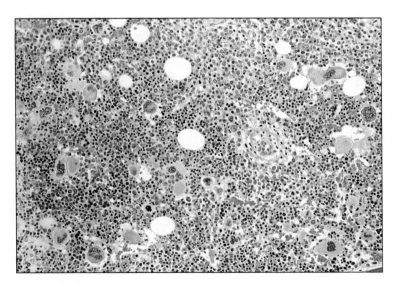

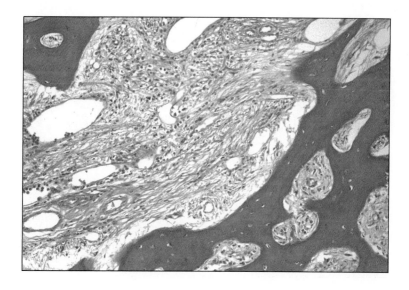

Figure 35–3   Prominent fibrosis, osteosclerosis, and dilated sinuses are seen in the bone marrow biopsy from patient with advanced myelofibrosis.

Figure 35–4   Bone marrow biopsy from patient with thrombocythemia showing increased megakaryocytes that vary in size and shape.

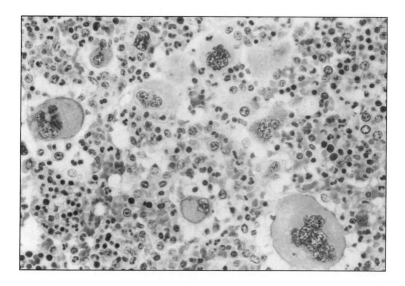

PART 10

Lymphomas

36

Non-Hodgkin's Lymphoma

"Malignant lymphoma" is the generic term for malignant neoplasms of lymphoid tissue. This chapter concerns malignant lymphomas other than Hodgkin's disease, or non-Hodgkin's lymphomas (NHL). Hodgkin's disease differs considerably from the other lymphomas and will be described in chapter 37. This chapter also features a brief discussion of disorders that may be misdiagnosed as malignant lymphoma.

Pathophysiology

Immunologic studies have revealed that malignant lymphomas are neoplasms of the immune system. They arise from their normal cell counterparts within the lymphoreticular system and are caused by derepression of lymphocyte transformation as a consequence of molecular genetic changes. The cells involved are B- and T-lymphocytes and histiocytes. The neoplastic cell proliferation occurs in lymph nodes and lymphoid components of other tissues. The disease usually starts in the lymph nodes, but when the patient is first seen, evidence of lymphoma in other sites, such as the spleen, liver, and bone marrow, frequently exists. Less common is extranodal lymphoma, in which the disease is initially confined to areas such as the alimentary tract, thyroid, breast, gonads, bone, or skin.

Malignant lymphoma differs from leukemia mainly in the distribution of the cell proliferation. Leukemia implies involvement of the bone marrow and the peripheral blood, while lymphoma denotes a malignant neoplasm initially confined to lymphoid tissue. As the lymphoma spreads, however, the bone marrow is often involved, and lymphoma cells may also be seen in the peripheral blood. When the latter occurs, the term "lymphosarcoma cell leukemia" is commonly used.

The malignant lymphomas are a heterogeneous group of disorders and consist of many subtypes. Over the years, numerous classifications of malignant lymphoma have been introduced. In contrast to Hodgkin's disease, unfortunately, no international agreement exists about histopathologic classification. As a direct consequence of advances in immunology, our understanding of the function and morphology of the lymphoid system is changing. Most of the lymphoid neoplasms can be divided into B- and T-cell proliferations, and we have learned to appreciate the wide range of morphologic expressions that lymphocytes and histiocytes may have. Thus, the "histiocyte" in Rappaport's classification is now recognized as being a transformed lymphocyte rather than a true histiocyte. The controversy regarding the correct or best classification system will, undoubtedly, continue as more information becomes available regarding the function and morphology of lymphocytes and histiocytes. Ultimately the disease may be defined by changes that have occurred in the molecular genetics of the cell.

Clinical Findings

The clinical manifestations of malignant lymphoma are varied, but the most common presenting complaint is the discovery of enlarged, usually painless, lymph nodes or an abdominal mass. Extranodal disease brings about one third of patients to the physician and is especially common in children. The most frequent extranodal site of presentation is the gastrointestinal tract. Fever, weight loss, and anorexia are less common manifestations. Lymphomas may have atypical clinical presentations, such as symptoms secondary to compression of vital organs, eg, spinal cord compression, ureteral compression, thoracic outlet syndrome, intestinal obstruction, or airway obstruction.

A careful investigation of the extent of the patient's disease before treatment is important for proper management. Extensive clinical staging should also be done. The extent of the staging procedure should be decided by consultation involving the primary physician, an oncologist, a radiotherapist, a surgeon, a pathologist,

Table 36–1   Staging Procedures in Non-Hodgkin's Lymphoma

1. Clinical history and physical examination, with description of all superficial lymph nodes

2. Lymph node biopsy; fine needle aspirate and/or true-cut needle biopsy

3. Radiologic studies: chest x-ray; computed tomography scan, lymphangiography, intravenous pyelogram, skeletal survey, etc, as indicated)

4. Bone marrow biopsy (bilateral needle or open)

5. Complete blood counts with evaluation of blood smear

6. Liver and renal function tests

7. Serum protein electrophoresis

8. Cytologic examination of any effusion

9. Lumbar puncture with cytologic CSF examination as indicated

10. Radioisotopic evaluation as clinically indicated

11. Laparotomy and splenectomy, if information is likely to affect therapy

ABBREVIATIONS: CSF = cerebrospinal fluid.

and a radiologist. Clinical staging includes: physical examination; bone marrow aspiration and biopsy; radiologic studies to detect disease in the mediastinum, retroperitoneum, and bones; certain laboratory tests; and, in selected cases, exploratory laparotomy. A detailed physical examination must be done, during which all enlarged lymph nodes should be reported and measured and the size of the spleen noted. The clinical staging procedures are summarized in Table 36–1.

The staging sequence is also important. Thus, following bone marrow biopsy in follicular, small cleaved cell lymphoma, 50% to 70% of patients will be shown to have marrow involvement and would therefore be classified as having stage IV disease. Therefore, except for in the large cell lymphomas, laparotomy is rarely necessary. Table 36–2 shows the clinical classification of the extent or stage of disease.

Classification of Non-Hodgkin's Lymphoma

The histologic features of a lymphoma are characterized by a proliferation of malignant lymphocytes or histiocytes that partially or completely obliterate the normal lymph node architecture. The non-

Table 36–2   Lymphoma Stages

Stage I	Disease limited to 1 anatomic region or 2 contiguous anatomic regions on the same side of the diaphragm
Stage II	Disease in more than 2 anatomic regions or in noncontiguous regions on the same side of the diaphragm
Stage III	Disease on both sides of the diaphragm but limited to involvement of the lymph nodes and spleen
Stage IV	Disease of any lymph node region with involvement of liver, lung, or bone marrow

Hodgkin's lymphomas are separated into those with a follicular (nodular) architectural pattern and those with a diffuse pattern. It is important to be able to differentiate a follicular from a diffuse pattern, because the former indicates a better prognosis. Further classification depends on the predominant cell type present.

In recent years, many new classifications have been added to this complicated and controversial field of pathology. In this chapter, the terminology used is that of the Working Formulation of Non-Hodgkin's Lymphomas. The advances made in immunology, cytochemistry, and electron microscopy have produced several changes in our understanding of the function and morphology of the lymphoreticular system. As discussed in the Pathophysiology section, two principal classes of lymphocytes have been identified, namely, B- and T-lymphocytes, with multiple subtypes. The B- and T-cell lymphocyte systems encompass a spectrum of morphologic entities. Furthermore, it has become apparent that morphologic heterogeneity in malignant lymphoid cells may not relate to degrees of differentiation. Thus, terms such as "well-differentiated" or "poorly differentiated" lymphocytic lymphomas are scientifically inaccurate. It has been shown that the follicular lymphomas arise from B-lymphocytes in the germinal centers, and that the histiocytic lymphomas are rarely true histiocytes but are instead transformed B-lymphocytes or less common T-lymphocytes that morphologically resemble histiocytes.

Three major classifications are now in use: the Rappaport, the Lukes and Collins, and the Kiel (Lennert) classification systems (Tables 36–3, 36–4, 36–5), all of which have been shown to be equally clinically useful. The Working Formulation for Clinical Usage was proposed as a common language to be used by clinical investigators to translate from one classification scheme to another (Table 36–5). The malignant lymphomas may also be separated on the basis of immunologic phenotype (Table 36–6).

Table 36–3   Rappaport Classification of Non-Hodgkin's
Lymphoma (Modified)

Nodular

   Lymphocytic, poorly differentiated

   Mixed, lymphocytic and histiocytic

   Histiocytic

Diffuse

   Lymphocytic, well-differentiated

   Lymphocytic, well-differentiated with plasmacytoid features

   Lymphocytic, poorly differentiated

   Lymphoblastic

   Mixed, lymphocytic and histiocytic

   Histiocytic

   Undifferentiated Burkitt's

   Undifferentiated non-Burkitt's

Malignant lymphoma, unclassified

It is important to have the correct histopathologic diagnosis established before treatment, because the pathologic findings will predict several clinicopathologic factors. Thus, a patient diagnosed as having small cleaved cell lymphoma, or mixed small and large cell lymphoma, has an 80% probability of having a follicular lymphoma and only a 20% chance of having a diffuse lymphoma. In contrast, <10% of large cell lymphomas are follicular. About 90% of patients with small cleaved cell or mixed small and large cell lymphomas have stage III or IV disease.

If a lymphoma is first diagnosed in an extranodal site (eg, bone marrow or liver) and an assessment of the histologic pattern is to be made (ie, follicular or diffuse), a careful search should yield a lymph node for biopsy. This is important because the pattern of involvement (follicular or diffuse) has an important influence on the prognosis, and this pattern is difficult to assess outside the lymph node.

Over time, sequential biopsies may show a change in histologic type, usually toward a more malignant form, eg, a change from follicular to diffuse lymphoma or small cleaved cell to large cell lymphoma.

Table 36–4 Lukes and Collins Classification of Non-Hodgkin's Lymphoma

---

Undefined cell type

T-cell type
  Small lymphocytic
  Sézary syndrome/mycosis fungoides
  Convoluted lymphocytic
  Immunoblastic sarcoma

B-cell type
  Small lymphocytic
  Plasmacytoid lymphocytic
  Follicular center cell, small cleaved
  Follicular center cell, large cleaved
  Follicular center cell, small noncleaved
  Follicular center cell, large noncleaved
  Immunoblastic sarcoma

Subtypes of follicular center cell lymphomas
  Follicular
  Follicular and diffuse
  Diffuse
  Sclerotic with follicles
  Sclerotic without follicles

Histiocytic

Malignant lymphoma, unclassified

Histopathologic and Clinicopathologic Features

Follicular Lymphomas. The follicular lymphomas account for approximately 50% of all non-Hodgkin's lymphomas in the United States. They occur predominantly in the older age group, are rarely seen in individuals younger than 35 years of age, and occur with equal frequency in both sexes. Patients with follicular lymphoma usually have a better prognosis than those with diffuse

Table 36–5 Working Formulation of Non-Hodgkin's Lymphomas for Clinical Usage and the Kiel Classification

Working Formulation	Kiel Equivalent or Related Term
Low grade	
Malignant lymphoma Small lymphocytic Consistent with CLL Plasmacytoid	ML lymphocytic, CLL ML lymphoplasmacytic/ lymphoplasmacytoid (immunocytoma)
Malignant lymphoma, follicular Predominantly small cleaved cell Diffuse areas Sclerosis	ML centroblastic-centrocytic (small), follicular, follicular and diffuse, or diffuse
Malignant lymphoma, follicular Mixed, small cleaved and large cell Diffuse areas Sclerosis	
Intermediate grade	
Malignant lymphoma, follicular Predominantly large cell Diffuse areas	ML centroblastic-centrocytic (large), follicular, follicular and diffuse, or diffuse
Sclerosis	
Malignant lymphoma, diffuse Small cleaved cell Sclerosis	ML centrocytic (small)
Malignant lymphoma, diffuse Mixed, small and large cell	ML centroblastic-centrocytic (small), diffuse
Sclerosis	ML lymphoplasmacytic/ -cytoid polymorphic
Epithelioid cell component	

(Continued.)

Table 36–5   *Continued.*

Working Formulation	Kiel Equivalent or Related Term
Malignant lymphoma, diffuse	
Large cell	ML centroblastic-centrocytic (large), diffuse
Cleaved cell	ML centrocytic (large)
Noncleaved cell	ML centroblastic
Sclerosis	

High grade

Malignant lymphoma	
Large cell, immunoblastic	ML immunoblastic
Plasmacytoid	
Clear cell	
Polymorphous	T-zone lymphoma
Epithelioid cell component	Lymphoepithelioid cell lymphoma
Malignant lymphoma	
Lymphoblastic	
Convoluted cell	ML lymphoblastic, convoluted cell type
Non–convoluted cell	ML lymphoblastic, unclassified
Malignant lymphoma	
Small non–cleaved cell	
Burkitt's	
Follicular areas	ML lymphoblastic, Burkitt type, and other B-lymphoblastic

Miscellaneous

Composite	
Mycosis fungoides	Mycosis fungoides
Histiocytic	None
Extramedullary plasmacytoma	ML plasmacytic
Unclassifiable	None
Other	None

ABBREVIATIONS: ML = malignant lymphoma; CLL = chronic lymphocytic leukemia.

Table 36–6 Malignant Lymphoproliferative Disorders and
Related Immunologic Phenotype

B-Cell Neoplasms

    Follicular lymphoma

    Small lymphocytic lymphoma/CLL (95%)

    Immunocytoma

    Small non–cleaved cell lymphoma

    Large cell lymphoma (70%)

    Plasmacytoma, myeloma

    Hairy cell leukemia

    Intermediate lymphocytic lymphoma, mantle zone lymphoma

T-Cell Neoplasms

    Lymphoblastic lymphoma (90%)

    Large cell lymphoma (15%)

    Small lymphocytic/CLL (2%)

    Adult T-cell leukemia/lymphoma

    Mycosis fungoides and Sézary syndrome

Histiocytic Neoplasms

    Malignant histiocytosis

    True histiocytic lymphoma

    Dendritic reticulum cell

    Interdigitating reticulum cell

    Fibroblastic reticulum cell

ABBREVIATIONS: CLL = chronic lymphocytic leukemia.

lymphoma, even though in the latter the disease is more frequently
disseminated at the time of diagnosis. Gastrointestinal involvement
is less common in follicular than in diffuse lymphoma.

    The follicular lymphomas are characterized by a follicular (nod-
ular) growth pattern and must be distinguished from reactive follicular hyperplasia (Figure 36–1), which may be difficult, particularly in technically poor preparations. They are neoplasms of
B-lymphocytes originating in the germinal centers and are divided
into three major subtypes: small cleaved cell type, large cell type,
and mixed small and large cell type. A case is classified as small
cleaved cell type when the estimated percentage of large cells is

<25%, and large cell type when the large cells approximate <50% or more. If the estimate of large cells is between 25% and 50%, the case is classified as mixed cell type. The small cleaved cell type is most common, and the large cell type is the least common of the follicular lymphomas.

The follicular large cell lymphomas have a poorer prognosis than the other two types and are more prone to progress into a diffuse lymphoma. Not infrequently, one observes both follicular and diffuse patterns in the same lymph node, which usually indicate a poorer prognosis than a pure follicular type.

Patients with follicular, small cleaved cell lymphoma or mixed small and large cell lymphoma usually have involvement of the bone marrow and liver, and lymphoma cells may be seen in the blood (lymphosarcoma cell leukemia). In contrast, the follicular large cell lymphoma, which usually is a more aggressive tumor, is rarely seen in the blood and less commonly involves the bone marrow.

Diffuse Lymphomas. The diffuse lymphomas are a heterogeneous group of tumors occurring in both young and old patients and are twice as common in men as in women. In contrast to the follicular lymphomas, constitutional symptoms are common. The diffuse lymphomas may present with intra-abdominal disease or mediastinal involvement, particularly with large cell lymphoma, Burkitt's lymphoma, and lymphoblastic lymphoma. Except for small lymphocytic lymphoma, the prognosis in cases of diffuse lymphoma is usually less favorable than in follicular lymphoma.

Small lymphocytic lymphoma characteristically reveals diffuse infiltration of the lymph node by small, normal-appearing lymphocytes (Figure 36–2). The histologic features are indistinguishable from those observed in chronic lymphocytic leukemia. This type of lymphoma may be misdiagnosed as Hodgkin's disease (lymphocyte predominance type). The latter disease should be suspected in a patient younger than 40 years of age who has a lymph node showing diffuse involvement by small, normal-appearing lymphocytes; a careful search for Reed-Sternberg cells must be made in such cases. Immunologic markers may be helpful in the differential diagnosis, as a small lymphocytic lymphoma in >90% of cases is made up of monoclonal B-cells. In Hodgkin's disease, there is a mixture of polyclonal B- and T-cells.

In a small percentage of patients with small lymphocytic lymphoma, the cell proliferations consist of a mixture of lymphocytes, plasma cells, and plasmacytoid lymphocytes. If, in addition, the cells secrete monoclonal IgM into the serum and the patient has hyperviscosity syndrome, the disease is referred to as Waldenström's macroglobulinemia; lymphoplasmacytic proliferations are referred to as immunocytomas in the Kiel classification.

Intermediate lymphocytic lymphoma is not represented in most classification schemes. Morphologically, this disease lies between small lymphocytic and small cleaved cell lymphoma, featuring a diffuse proliferation of small lymphoid cells (usually monoclonal B-cells) having slightly irregular or indented nuclei. The median age of patients is 65 years, and the majority have stage III or IV disease. It appears to be a low-grade lymphoma. Immunophenotyping and cytogenetic findings suggest a close relationship to small lymphocytic lymphomas.

Mantle-zone lymphoma is believed to be a follicular variant of intermediate lymphocytic lymphoma. This lymphoma appears to have a predilection for the gastrointestinal tract. The lymphoma is characterized by the proliferation of small atypical lymphoid cells that appear as wide mantles surrounding small benign-appearing germinal centers. Because of its benign appearance, it may be misdiagnosed as benign lymphoma hyperplasia.

Diffuse, small cleaved cell lymphoma (Figure 36–3) is almost never seen in children and is also uncommon in adults. The disease more frequently originates in B-cells but may also be of T-cell origin.

Diffuse, mixed small and large cell lymphoma is composed of a mixture of small cleaved lymphocytes and large lymphocytes (Figure 36–4). No uniform agreement exists, however, on the histopathologic definition of mixed cell lymphoma. In general, this is primarily a disease of adults and is rare in children. Immunologic studies have shown that they constitute a heterogeneous group of B- and T-cell neoplasms.

Diffuse, large cell lymphomas are characterized by a proliferation of large mononuclear cells. The nuclei of large cell lymphomas are equal in size to or larger than a macrophage nucleus, or 3 times the size of a small lymphocyte. Large cell lymphomas represent approximately 30% of the diffuse, aggressive non-Hodgkin's lymphomas in adults. They consist of a heterogeneous group of lymphomas, the majority of which are composed of lymphocytes at various stages of transformation and are associated with subtle morphologic variations (Figures 36–5, 36–6, 36–7). Only a small percentage are composed of "true" histiocytes (Figures 36–8, 36–9). Distinguishing between the subtypes of large cell lymphomas is often difficult and depends on the quality of the material available. Little evidence exists that the morphologic subclassification of large cell lymphomas can be correlated with survival.

In contrast to follicular lymphomas, the diffuse large cell lymphomas are frequently limited to one side of the diaphragm. About 30% of the patients are found to have localized disease (ie, stage I or II). Large cell lymphomas are more frequently present in extranodal sites than the other lymphomas and include the naso-pharynx, gastrointestinal tract, skin, soft tissues, bone, lungs, and mediastinum; involvement of the peripheral blood is rare. In addition, the pattern of involvement in the spleen and liver is different in the large cell lymphomas. Small cleaved cell lymphomas are usually distributed in small, uniform nodules throughout; large cell lymphomas produce large, irregular, often destructive tumors in the spleen and liver.

Large cell lymphomas may both grossly and microscopically bear close resemblance to metastatic carcinoma. Cytochemistry, immunologic cell markers, and electron microscopy may be helpful in distinguishing between lymphoma and epithelial or other non-lymphoid neoplasms. It is therefore important that appropriate specimens be routinely set aside for immunologic study or electron microscopic study or both.

About 65% to 70% of large cell lymphomas are composed of B-lymphocytes, approximately 10% to 15% have T-cell markers, and around 5% are "true" histiocytic tumors. To date, immunologic phenotyping of large cell lymphomas has not been successful in predicting survival differences.

Small, noncleaved cell ("undifferentiated") lymphomas have been divided into Burkitt's and non-Burkitt's type. The histopathologic distinction between the two is often subtle and subjective. In Burkitt's lymphoma, the cells are uniform in size and shape, while in the non-Burkitt's type, the cells vary more in the size and shape of the nuclei. As yet, no clear-cut cytochemical or immunologic method exists for separating the two types. Furthermore, there is question as to the clinical usefulness of distinguishing these two lymphomas.

The small, noncleaved cell lymphomas feature cell nuclei that are larger than those in the small lymphocytes of small lymphocytic lymphoma or chronic lymphocytic leukemia (CLL), but smaller than the nuclei of large cell lymphoma (Figure 36–10). The nuclei of the "starry-sky" macrophages are useful as a guide to size, because the nuclei of small noncleaved cells should be slightly smaller than the nuclei of macrophages (Table 36–7). The moderately abundant cytoplasm of the cells often contains lipid-laden vacuoles, which are most readily seen in Romanovsky-stained imprints of the tumor (Figure 36–11). The small noncleaved cell lymphomas are of B-lymphocytic origin. The cells are characteristically negative with PAS stain and strongly positive with methyl green pyronine stain. In contrast to lymphoblastic lymphoma, the cells do not usually contain terminal deoxynucleotidyl transferase (TdT).

In Central Africa, where Burkitt's lymphoma is endemic, the disease frequently presents as a maxillomandibular lesion. In non-African patients, the disease is frequently localized to the abdomen,

Table 36–7 Comparison of Morphologic, Cytochemical and Immunotypic Features of Childhood Non-Hodgkin's Lymphoma

	Lymphoblastic	Burkitt's
Imprint cytology, Wright's stain	FAB L1 or FAB L2 blasts	FAB L3 blasts
Nuclear size	Smaller than macrophage nucleus	Approximates macrophage nucleus; nuclear monotony
Nuclear chromatin	Delicate	Coarsely reticulated
Nucleoli	Small, inconspicuous	Prominent
Mitotic index	High	High
Cytoplasm	Scant	Moderate
Cytoplasmic vacuoles	Inconspicuous	Prominent
Periodic acid–Schiff stain	Occasionally positive	Negative
Methyl green pyronine stain	Negative or focal positive	Strongly positive
Terminal deoxynucleotidyl transferase	Positive	Negative
Immunologic markers	T-cell, pre–B-cell or non–B-cell, non–T-cell	B-cell

NOTE: FAB, French–American–British classification of acute lymphoblastic leukemia

especially in the ileocecal region, retroperitoneum, or ovaries. One of the most common presentations is intestinal obstruction. A leukemic phase is unusual. Burkitt's lymphoma is most commonly seen in children but may also afflict adults.

Lymphoblastic lymphoma is most frequently seen in children and adolescents, but may also occur in adults. Mediastinal tumors are seen in at least 50% of patients, and the disease rapidly spreads to involve bone marrow, peripheral blood, and the central nervous system. Immunologic studies have revealed that most lymphoblastic

Non-Burkitt's	Large Cell (Histiocytic)
FAB L3 blasts	Variable, large transformed lymphocytes
Approximates macrophage nucleus; nuclear variability	Larger than macrophage nucleus
Coarsely reticulated	Clumped, vesicular
Prominent	Variable, often prominent
High	Variable
Moderate	Moderate to abundant
Prominent	Inconspicuous
Negative	Occasionally positive
Strongly positive	Variable, usually positive
Negative	Negative
Usually B-cell; may be non–B-cell, non–T-cell; rarely T-cell	Usually B-cell; may be non–B-cell; non–T-cell; T-cell occasionally; histiocytic rarely

lymphoma is composed of T-lymphocytes and contains TdT. Also, in contrast to the small noncleaved cell lymphomas, the cells stain only weakly positive, or even negative, with methyl green pyronine stain (Table 36–7).

The malignant cells in lymphoblastic lymphoma consist of a uniform population of cells similar to those seen in acute lymphoblastic leukemia. The nuclei may be convoluted (Figure 36–12) or nonconvoluted (Figure 36–13) and have a fine chromatin pattern. As with small noncleaved cell lymphomas, a high mitotic rate is a consistent finding. In the differential diagnosis, small noncleaved cell lymphoma and small lymphocytic lymphoma (in adults) should be considered. Because lymphoblastic lymphomas are usually treated differently than the other lymphomas described in this chapter, it is important that this diagnosis be made accurately.

Peripheral T-cell lymphoma refers to nonlymphoblastic, T-cell lymphomas other than mycosis fungoides and includes a wide spectrum of clinicopathologic disorders. A variety of other names, indicating the diversity of this entity, are used, including node-based T-cell lymphoma, T zone lymphoma, T-cell immunoblastic sarcoma, lymphoepithelioid (Lennert's) lymphoma, multilobated T-cell lymphoma, and T-cell lymphoma resembling immunoblastic lymphadenopathy.

Clinically, the majority of patients have stage III or IV disease with frequent involvement of the Waldeyer's ring, skin, liver, and lungs in addition to generalized lymphadenopathy. The majority of patients are adults. Survival rates are comparable to those for patients with aggressive B-cell lymphoma.

On histologic examination, all peripheral T-cell lymphomas have a diffuse pattern, and the most common cell types are mixed small and large cell (Figure 36–14) or large immunoblastic types. Peripheral T-cell lymphoma may be mistaken for Hodgkin's disease because Reed-Sternberg–like cells are not infrequently present (Figure 36–15). In contrast to Hodgkin's disease, however, there is an admixture of atypical-appearing small and medium-sized lymphocytes. It should be noted, however, that the distinction between peripheral T-cell lymphoma and Hodgkin's disease (mixed cellularity type) can be extremely difficult, even with the use of immunologic markers. Gene rearrangement studies may be useful in selected cases.

Nuclear multilobation was initially thought to be a reliable marker for certain T-cell lymphomas. It is now recognized that identical features may be seen in B-cell lymphomas (multilobated B-cell lymphomas). Lymphoepithelioid lymphoma or Lennert's lymphoma is characterized by the addition of a prominent epithelioid histiocyte component together with a mixed small and large cell population. Finally, a group of T-cell lymphomas closely resembles the entity called angioimmunoblastic lymphadenopathy (AILD). It is likely that many cases diagnosed as AILD in the past were, in fact, peripheral T-cell lymphomas.

Immunologic studies show that peripheral T-cell lymphomas have a mature T-cell phenotype and do not contain TdT, in contrast to the previously described lymphoblastic lymphoma. Most peripheral T-cell lymphomas have a helper cell phenotype.

Ki-1 lymphoma is the designation recently assigned to a pleomorphic large cell lymphoma that has been described in children and adults. Ki-1 is a monoclonal antibody raised against a Hodgkin's disease–derived cell line that reacts with Reed-Sternberg cells and activated lymphoid cells that are primarily of T-cell origin. The characteristic morphologic features of Ki-1 lymphoma include: a pleomorphic cellular infiltrate, sinus infiltration, fibrosis, partial lymph node involvement, sparing of follicles, and an abundance of plasma cells. The majority of cases have a T-helper phenotype. Most patients present with peripheral lymphadenopathy or skin lesions or both. The Ki-1 lymphoma may resemble malignant histiocytosis, Hodgkin's disease, nodular sclerosis, or metastatic carcinoma. This type of large cell lymphoma appears to be associated with a favorable prognosis in children.

Mycosis fungoides and Sézary's syndrome are closely related. Both are T-cell disorders (predominantly helper T-cell) primarily involving the skin; thus, the term cutaneous T-cell lymphoma has also been applied to these disorders. Clinically, mycosis fungoides presents as a scaly or eczematous lesion that progresses through a plaque stage to eventually form tumors in the skin. Sézary's syndrome is characterized by exfoliative erythroderma and malignant cells (Sézary cells) in the peripheral blood (see chapter 34). In fact, Sézary's syndrome may be considered a leukemic phase of mycosis fungoides. Biopsies of the skin reveal lymphocytic infiltrates in the upper dermis, frequently with infiltrates in the epidermis (Pautrier's abscesses) (Figure 36–16). The nuclei of malignant lymphocytes characteristically have deeply indented or convoluted contours.

The initial diagnosis of mycosis fungoides may be difficult to make. Frequently, several skin biopsies over a period of time are necessary. Special attention should be paid to the technical quality of the histopathologic sections. Because similar-appearing, atypical lymphocytes may be seen in a variety of benign inflammatory skin disorders, a diagnosis of mycosis fungoides should not be considered unless clusters or sheets of these atypical lymphocytes are present. In addition, the lymphoid infiltrates found in the skin in inflammatory disorders are also predominantly T-helper cells. Thus, demonstration of T-helper cells in the skin is not in itself diagnostic of mycosis fungoides.

As mycosis fungoides progresses, neoplastic cells may be seen in lymph nodes, lungs, liver, spleen, and other organs. Atypical lymphocytes with convoluted or cerebriform nuclei may be seen in the peripheral blood (so-called Sézary cell). A small number of similar-appearing lymphocytes may, however, also be seen in individuals who do not have mycosis fungoides. Therefore, usually >15% of the total lymphocytes in the peripheral blood smear should have cerebriform nuclei before a confident determination can be made that the cells are true Sézary cells. Blood smears for examination for Sézary cells should be made from fingersticks and should be technically "perfect." In mycosis fungoides, the presence of these cells in the peripheral blood is frequently associated with progressive disease.

Adult T-cell leukemia/lymphoma (ATLL) is a recently described, distinct clinicopathologic entity associated with a human retrovirus. The latter is referred to as the human T-cell leukemia/lymphoma virus (HTLV-1). Though it was initially described in Japan (where it is still most common) and later in the Caribbean, it probably has worldwide distribution. Clinically, this disorder is characterized by generalized lymphadenopathy, hepatosplenomegaly, skin lesions, peripheral blood involvement, and hypercalcemia. It is an aggressive disease with median survival to date <1 year.

A wide range of morphologic features have been described in ATLL. The most common are infiltrates of mature-appearing, medium-sized cells; mixed small, medium, and large cells; and large cell types analagous to the morphologic spectrum seen in B-cell lymphoma. Characteristically, the cells show pleomorphism with nuclear lobation, and condensed chromatin. The presence of cells with polylobated or "knobby" nuclei in the peripheral blood smear is probably the most diagnostic feature, although not all patients have blood involvement at the time of the initial diagnosis. The histologic subtype does not appear to influence the prognosis. The majority of patients are adults, but the disease has also been seen in adolescents.

"True" histiocytic malignancies comprise a heterogeneous group of disorders. They have been divided into histiocytosis X, malignant histiocytosis, and true histiocytic lymphoma. The histiocytosis X (Langerhans' cell histiocytosis) is thought by some to be an immune imbalance rather than a neoplasm and will not be discussed herein. Malignant histiocytosis is a rare disease usually characterized by rapid onset, fever, pancytopenia, hepatosplenomegaly, and lymphadenopathy. While they are more common in adults, they may also be seen in children, and are usually rapidly fatal. On histologic examination, atypical histiocytes proliferating within sinusoids of lymph nodes, liver, and spleen can be seen (Figure 36–8).

Malignant histiocytosis and so-called true histiocytic lymphoma may be closely related disorders, both being malignancies of the mononuclear phagocytic system. The histiocytic origin of the malignant cell may be difficult to document since the usual histiocytic markers (lysozyme, alpha-$_1$-antitrypsin) are often absent. The most reliable marker is the presence of nonspecific esterase. Recent studies, however, have shown that the constituent cells may have cytochemical and immunologic markers of a variety of histiocyte subtypes, T-lymphocytes (Ki-1), or B-lymphocytes. To make a diagnosis of malignant histiocytosis, the cells should cytologically exhibit

Table 36–8   Comparison of Non-Hodgkin's Lymphoma Features in Children and Adults

Children	Adults
Predominantly extranodal	Predominantly nodal
Rapidly proliferative	Often slowly proliferative
Rarely follicular	Often follicular
Often leukemic	Rarely leukemic

malignant features that differentiate them from those seen in benign hemophagocytic syndromes.

The pattern of tissue involvement is often a strong indicator of malignant histiocytosis. In addition to the infiltrate in the sinuses of the lymph node, the sinuses of the liver and the red pulp (cords and sinuses) of the spleen are frequently involved. Skin, bone, and soft tissues are also commonly involved sites.

The so-called true histiocytic lymphomas or the reticulum cell sarcomas can be divided into dendritic reticulum cell, interdigitating reticulum cell, fibroblastic reticulum cell, and histiocytic types (Figure 36–9). Only a limited number of such lymphomas have been described.

Non-Hodgkin's Lymphoma in Children

Malignant lymphoma in children differs in many ways from that in adults and deserves separate attention. Lymph node enlargement is a frequent finding in children, usually representing a transient response to localized infection. No single clinical feature allows one to predict whether one is dealing with a benign or malignant lymphadenopathy. When supraclavicular or generalized lymphadenopathy with systemic symptoms are present, however, a lymph node biopsy should be done immediately.

Children respond to antigenic stimuli with more pronounced lymph node hyperplasia than adults. Pathologists who have little experience evaluating lymph node biopsy specimens from children may mistake florid immunoblastic proliferations, often seen in viral infections (especially infectious mononucleosis), for large cell lymphoma.

In children, the non-Hodgkin's lymphomas are different than in adults in histologic type and the frequency of the lymphomas (Table 36–8). Lymphomas with a follicular pattern, which in adults account for about 50% of all non-Hodgkin's lymphomas, are very unusual

Table 36–9 Classification of Non-Hodgkin's Lymphoma in Children

Malignant lymphoma, lymphoblastic
Malignant lymphoma, Burkitt's
Malignant lymphoma, non-Burkitt's
Malignant lymphoma, large cell

SOURCE: Modified from Kjeldsberg CR, Wilson JW: Hum Path 1983; 14:612.

in children, and the majority (60% to 70%) of children have disseminated disease at the time of diagnosis. Small lymphocytic, small cleaved cell, and mixed cell lymphomas are rare in children. Childhood non-Hodgkin's lymphoma is generally limited to three major types: lymphoblastic lymphoma (35% to 47%), small noncleaved cell lymphoma (undifferentiated Burkitt's and non-Burkitt's types) (20% to 35%), and large cell lymphomas (30% to 35%) (Tables 36–7, 36–9).

There is a strong propensity for extranodal involvement in children and a close relationship between the histologic types and the anatomic sites of involvement. Thus, the lymphoblastic lymphomas are predominantly supradiaphragmatic, presenting with a mediastinal mass. The small noncleaved cell lymphomas usually occur in the abdomen, particularly in the ileocecal region. With present treatment regimens, it is crucial to distinguish lymphoblastic lymphoma from small noncleaved cell lymphoma and large cell lymphoma.

Approach to Diagnosis

There has recently been a significant improvement in treatment outcome of malignant lymphoma. Good management, however, requires a team approach, ie, good communication between the clinician, the oncologist, the radiotherapist, and the pathologist in planning the evaluation and management of the patient.

Following a clinical history and physical examination, the workup of a patient with possible malignant lymphoma should proceed in the following fashion:

1. A tissue biopsy, which is required to diagnose malignant lymphoma.

2. Complete blood count, including evaluation of a peripheral blood smear for circulating lymphoma cells.

Figure 36–17   Handling of a tissue biopsy specimen of suspected malignant lymphoma.

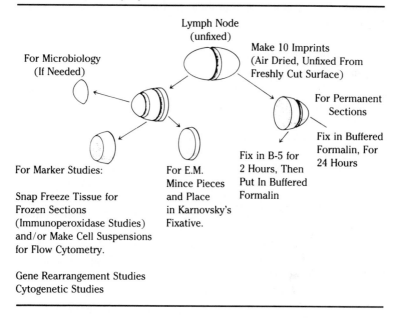

Lymph Node
(unfixed)

For Microbiology
(If Needed)

Make 10 Imprints
(Air Dried, Unfixed From
Freshly Cut Surface)

For Permanent
Sections

Fix in Buffered
Formalin, For
24 Hours

Fix in B-5 for
2 Hours, Then
Put In Buffered
Formalin

For E.M.
Mince Pieces
and Place
in Karnovsky's
Fixative.

For Marker Studies:

Snap Freeze Tissue for
Frozen Sections
(Immunoperoxidase Studies)
and/or Make Cell Suspensions
for Flow Cytometry.

Gene Rearrangement Studies
Cytogenetic Studies

3. Bone marrow aspirate and biopsy examination.
4. Radiological studies.
5. Liver and renal function assessment.

Tissue Biopsy

A tissue biopsy is essential for the diagnosis of non-Hodgkin's lymphoma (NHL), and is the most important part of the diagnostic evaluation; it is therefore discussed separately.

Histopathologic evaluation of a lymph node biopsy specimen is one of the most difficult problems in surgical pathology, and consultation from a hematopathologist is often desirable. The major reasons for difficulties in interpretation of lymph node biopsy specimens, however, are still technical in nature and result from improper handling of the biopsy specimen. Too frequently, a wrong lymph node is biopsied or an inadequate specimen is obtained. The lymph node must be delivered to the pathologist intact immediately following removal. Before fixation, the tissue is divided into multiple sections, as outlined in Figure 36–17, allowing a variety of studies to be performed. Not all of the procedures indicated in Figure 36–17 may be necessary to make a correct diagnosis; however, samples for immunologic and cytochemical studies should be obtained routinely. A section of the tissue should be snap-frozen routinely for possible immunologic studies using immunoperoxidase techniques.

When immunologic procedures cannot be performed in the hospital where the biopsy is being performed, the specimen can be sent considerable distances to reference laboratories without compromising the immunologic and cytochemical investigations. Frozen tissue may be sent in dry ice, or sections of frozen tissue may be sent. Another method that is simpler, but that may not work for all tumors, is to send tissue left intact in refrigerated saline solution. One day after the permanent sections have been reviewed, and it is apparent that marker studies may be helpful in the diagnosis, the tissue in saline solution can be placed into a styrofoam container with cold packs and sent to the reference laboratory.

A diagnosis should never be made on the basis of the immunologic or cytochemical studies alone but should always be correlated with clinical and histopathologic features of the biopsy specimen. To provide the best morphologic features, the specimen to be used for histopathologic studies should be fixed in a mercury-containing fixative, such as B-5, and not only in the usual 10% buffered formalin (if formalin is used, the tissue should be fixed for 24 hours). Postfixation in B-5 after the tissue has been fixed in formalin also gives satisfactory results. The sections of the biopsy specimen must be thin (one-cell thickness) and well stained. Plastic-embedded tissue sections give optimal morphologic features, which is especially helpful in small biopsy specimens, eg, skin, bone marrow, and gastrointestinal tract, and in needle biopsies. It can also be used to salvage lymph node biopsy material that is paraffin-embedded and poorly fixed.

The diagnosis and subclassification of malignant lymphoma should be made on the basis of the histopathologic features in a lymph node biopsy before any treatment is initiated. The initial diagnosis should not be made on the basis of a bone marrow or liver biopsy specimen alone. In true extranodal lymphomas, the diagnosis will, of course, have to be made from a biopsy of the organ involved; however, every attempt should be made to find a lymph node that can be biopsied.

Fine-needle aspiration or true-cut needle biopsy or both are proven methods for obtaining samples of malignant tissue in the appropriate clinical setting. These techniques may be used in the initial and follow-up diagnoses.

Cytologic examination of any effusion is mandatory to establish the presence of malignant cells in pleural or peritoneal cavity or in the cerebrospinal fluid. Good cytocentrifuge preparations should be made, and B-5–fixed material of concentrated pleural or peritoneal fluid may be useful for the diagnosis. Air-dried cytocentrifuge slides or a suspension of the cells may also be used for cytochemical and immunologic studies. A liver biopsy may be used to document the relatively common involvement of non-Hodgkin's lymphoma of the liver.

Hematologic Findings

The hematologic findings in malignant lymphoma are quite variable and depend on the type of lymphoma present. As described above, in certain types of lymphomas, the peripheral blood or the bone marrow or both are rarely involved (eg, large cell lymphomas). In other lymphomas, such as small lymphocytic and small cleaved cell lymphomas, blood and bone marrow involvement is frequently present.

Blood Cell Measurements. The majority of patients who present with non-Hodgkin's lymphoma have normal blood counts. Anemia develops during the course of the disease in about 50% of patients. One or several of the following may be the cause of anemia: bone marrow insufficiency caused by bone marrow replacement by lymphoma; therapy-induced bone marrow hypoplasia; hypersplenism; autoimmune hemolytic anemia; and bleeding from lymphoma in the gastrointestinal tract or from low platelet count.

Peripheral Blood Smear Morphology. Circulating lymphoma cells have been referred to as lymphosarcoma cell leukemia (chapter 34). This is not a specific clinicopathologic entity and may be seen in any of the subtypes of lymphoma. In follicular small cleaved cell lymphoma, a leukemic phase may be observed in 5% to 15% of patients. The leukemic cells have scant cytoplasm with a characteristic notched or clefted nucleus. Using more sensitive techniques, such as the flow cytometer, circulating malignant cells can be identified in the peripheral blood in a much higher percentage of patients.

Bone Marrow Examination. Bone marrow aspiration and a bone marrow biopsy should be done routinely in the disease staging of a patient with malignant lymphoma. A bilateral, posterior iliac crest biopsy will increase the chance of detecting lymphoma. A positive biopsy, which indicates stage IV disease, eliminates much of the remainder of the staging evaluation.

The bone marrow is involved at the time of diagnosis in 70%

to 80% of patients with follicular, small cleaved cell lymphoma, and in approximately 50% of patients with diffuse, small cleaved lymphoma and mixed cell type (Figure 36–18). The large cell lymphomas are much less frequently associated with bone marrow involvement. On the other hand, the bone marrow is frequently involved in lymphoblastic lymphoma.

The pattern of bone marrow involvement is usually focal or nodular rather than diffuse. No good correlation exists between the pattern of involvement (ie, diffuse or follicular) in lymph nodes and in the bone marrow. Nodules of lymphoma in the bone marrow must be differentiated from benign lymphoid nodules, which are commonly seen in older individuals. Nodules of malignant lymphoma are less well circumscribed than benign lymphoid nodules; in lymphoma, the infiltrate is frequently located adjacent to bone trabeculae (paratrabecular position). Furthermore, in benign lymphoid nodules, the lymphocytes are usually small and normal-appearing, and germinal centers may be seen. In general, a diagnosis of malignant lymphoma in the bone marrow should not be made if the infiltrate is made up of small, normal-appearing lymphocytes and the patient does not have biopsy-proven lymphoma in other sites.

Other Laboratory Tests

36.1   Radiologic Studies

Purpose.   In addition to establishing the specific diagnosis, the anatomic extent of the disease must be determined. Various radiologic techniques are used to detect disease in the mediastinum, retroperitoneum, and bones. Mediastinal and hilar lymph nodes are demonstrated primarily by standard postero-anterior and lateral chest films. For detecting disease below the diaphragm, a computed tomographic scan and a bilateral lower-extremity lymphangiogram are used. Splenic hilar, celiac, porta hepatis, and mesenteric nodes, however, are not demonstrated by lymphangiography. An inferior venacavogram is useful in demonstrating enlarged lymph nodes high in the para-aortic chain. The inferior venacavogram, when positive, is thought to be accurate in 90% of cases. The lymphangiogram, when positive, is considered to be accurate in 80% of cases. Liver and spleen scans, when positive, are considered accurate in 50% and 75%, respectively. An intravenous pyelogram can be used to demonstrate ureteral obstruction.

36.2   Renal and Liver Function Tests

Purpose.   Evaluation of renal and liver function by routine serum chemistries and urinalysis should be done in every patient. The results may help detect disease in those organs and must be done as part of the workup before giving the patient chemotherapy or radiotherapy or both.

36.3   Laparotomy

Purpose.   Controversy still exists about the need for exploratory laparotomy with splenectomy in staging of non-Hodgkin's lymphomas. Its use is probably rarely necessary, except in patients with diffuse, large cell lymphoma. In such cases, it may be used to determine if there is limited disease that may be cured by radiotherapy. If a laparotomy is to be performed, a preoperative lymphangiogram should be done as a guide to direct surgical sampling of the lymph nodes. In addition, a wedge biopsy specimen of the liver should be obtained.

36.4   Cytology of Effusions

Purpose.   Pleural or peritoneal effusions are not uncommon in malignant lymphomas, and cytological examination of fluid specimens is an essential part of the clinical evaluation in such situations. Immunologic marker studies done on cells from the effusion may be helpful in differentiating reactive from malignant effusions and in making the diagnosis. Such studies are especially useful in peritoneal effusions in a patient who may have Burkitt's lymphoma, or in a pleural effusion in a patient with lymphoblastic lymphoma involving the mediastinum.

Ancillary Tests

Immunologic Phenotype.   In addition to the histologic examination of the tissue biopsy specimen, immunologic phenotyping may, as mentioned above, be helpful in the subclassification of malignant lymphomas. To accomplish such studies, the tissue must be submitted to the laboratory in a fresh, unfixed state. Cell surface markers on cell suspensions made from tissue biopsy specimens

Table 36-10   Clinical Application of Immunophenotyping

Disease	Antibody Panel
Reactive lymphoid hyperplasia v malignant lymphoma	Light chains
Lymphoma v nonhematopoietic neoplasms (eg carcinoma)	Immunoglobulins Pan–B-cell and pan–T-cell Cytokeratin
Subclassification of malignant lymphoma	Immunoglobulins Pan–B-cell and pan–T-cell TdT, CALLA T subset antibodies LCA, Leu M1 (Hodgkin's disease)
Subclassification of leukemias	TdT, CALLA, Pan–B-cell and pan–T-cell, Antimyeloid Immunoglobulins

ABBREVIATIONS: LCA = leukocyte common antigen; TdT = terminal deoxynucleotidyl transferase; CALLA = common acute lymphoblastic leukemia antigen.

may be used to separate the malignant lymphocytes into B- and T-lymphocytes and subsets thereof. Immunocytochemical studies on frozen tissue specimens, such as the immunoperoxidase technique, may be very helpful in the diagnosis. These techniques may be useful in the correct classification of malignant lymphoma and in separating malignant lymphoma from reactive hyperplasia or poorly differentiated carcinoma (Table 36–10).

Cytochemistry.   Cytochemical studies, such as using the specific esterase stain, may be helpful in identifying immature granulocytic cells in granulocytic sarcomas (chloromas) to differentiate such tumors from malignant lymphoma or undifferentiated carcinoma. The identification of TdT (see chapter 32) is useful in diagnosing lymphoblastic lymphomas, as this enzyme is not present in other malignant lymphomas. TdT testing can be done on imprints of tissue biopsy specimens, on cytocentrifuge preparations made from cell suspensions of a biopsy, or on frozen sections using an immunofluorescent method or the immunoperoxidase procedure. The PAS and methyl green pyronine stains are helpful in separating lymphoblastic lymphoma from small noncleaved cell lymphoma (Table 36–7).

Gene Rearrangement.   Southern blot analysis may be used to study the immunoglobulin heavy and light chain genes and the gene for the T-cell receptor beta chain in genomic DNA derived from the lymphoma cells. While not yet in wide use, it may offer additional proof of clonality in many B- and T-cell lymphoproliferative disorders. Such studies may be indicated in selected cases where a definitive diagnosis cannot be made with other methods.

Cytogenetics.   Cytogenetic studies suggest that several discrete genomic defects may govern the evolution of malignant lymphoma. Recent studies suggest that chromosomal defects may serve as objective markers to assist in histopathologic classification and prognostic and therapeutic considerations. The chromosomal defect t(14;18) is strongly associated with low-grade lymphomas and follicular patterns; and t(8;14) and t(8;22) are associated with high-grade lymphomas, especially small noncleaved cell lymphomas. Other studies have shown that follicular small cleaved cell lymphomas with a single defect of t(14;18) have an initially indolent course. In contrast, the same type of lymphoma with t(14;18) and deletion 13q32 has an accelerated disease process. For cytogenetic studies, a portion of the fresh biopsy material is minced into a cell suspension. Chromosomes are harvested from direct preparations and short-term cultures.

Serum and Urine Protein Electrophoresis and Immuno-electrophoresis.   The non-Hodgkin's lymphomas may sometimes be associated with polyclonal or monoclonal gammopathy (usually IgM), or occasionally hypogammaglobulinemia.

Serum Biochemistry.   Serum calcium levels may be elevated in malignant lymphoma, and uric acid levels may increase dramatically during treatment. The latter is particularly common in fast-growing lymphomas such as Burkitt's lymphoma. The serum lactic dehydrogenase level is frequently elevated and may correlate with tumor burden.

Diseases Simulating Malignant Lymphoma

A variety of disorders other than malignant lymphomas may not only cause enlargement of lymph nodes but may also be mistaken on histologic examination for lymphoma (Table 36–11). Such conditions include: viral infections (infectious mononucleosis, herpes simplex, etc), toxoplasmosis, giant lymph node hyperplasia (Castleman's disease), sinus histiocytosis with massive lymphadenop-

Table 36–11 Causes of Lymph Node Enlargement Simulating Malignant Lymphoma

Nonspecific reactive follicular hyperplasia
Infectious mononucleosis
Toxoplasmosis
Viral lymphadenitis (herpes, cytomegalovirus, etc)
Acquired immune deficiency syndrome
Cat scratch disease
Syphilis
Dilantin lymph node hyperplasia
Rheumatoid arthritis
Dermatopathic lymphadenopathy
Giant lymph node hyperplasia (Castleman's disease)
Sinus histiocytosis with massive lymphadenopathy
Leukemia
Metastatic carcinoma and melanoma

athy, postvaccinal lymphadenitis, certain drug (hydantoin) reactions, cat-scratch disease, metastatic undifferentiated carcinoma, and acquired immunodeficiency syndrome (AIDS). Rheumatoid arthritis, lupus erythematosus, and secondary syphilis may also be associated with lymphadenopathy. It is therefore important that the pathologist have an accurate clinical history and strong familiarity with the lymph node changes produced by these lymphomalike disorders.

Lymphadenopathy associated with AIDS may be grouped into three patterns: type I shows florid atypical, follicular hyperplasia, often with plasmacytosis; type II shows diffuse lymphoid hyperplasia with breaking up or loss of germinal centers; and type III is characterized by lymphocyte depletion. The latter pattern represents the end-stage lymph node seen in fatal AIDS. The histologic changes observed, however, are not specific for AIDS. AIDS patients have an increased risk of developing non-Hodgkin's lymphoma, Hodgkin's disease, and Kaposi's sarcoma.

So-called pseudolymphoma is a lymphoreticular proliferation that forms tumors that have been considered benign or reactive. The most common sites are the skin, stomach, intestine, and lung. Immunologic studies, however, have shown that in most cases the so-called pseudolymphomas are low-grade malignant lymphomas.

Course and Treatment

Most patients with follicular low-grade lymphomas survive for more than 5 years, and many patients live more than 10 years after the diagnosis. The optimal method of treatment for advanced low-grade non-Hodgkin's lymphoma is not clear. Several effective treatment regimens are available, but none can yet be considered potentially curative.

Localized presentation of diffuse lymphomas are considerably more common than localized follicular lymphomas. This is also true of primary extranodal lymphomas. For pathologic stage I or II disease, radiation therapy yields 50% to 75% long-term, disease-free survival. In pathologic stage III and IV disease, radiation therapy alone is not satisfactory and must be combined with multidrug chemotherapy (sometimes chemotherapy alone may be effective).

It is paradoxical that patients with stage III and/or IV diffuse, large cell lymphoma, the most naturally aggressive lymphoma, may have the best chance of cure. Using multiagent chemotherapy, 60% of these patients may be curable.

Lymphoblastic lymphoma is treated with intensive multiagent chemotherapy, similar to acute lymphoblastic leukemia. Small non-cleaved cell lymphoma is treated with surgical debulking of abdominal tumors, combination chemotherapy, and intensive metabolic support. Approximately 50% of children with lymphoblastic lymphoma or small non-cleaved cell lymphoma are now potentially curable.

References

1. Beard C, Nabers K, Bowling MC, et al: Achieving technical excellence in lymph node specimens: An update. *Lab Med* 1985; 16:468–475.

2. Berard CW, Dorfman RF, Kaufman N (eds): *Malignant Lymphoma.* Int Acad Path Monograph, 1987

3. Colgan JP, Haberman TM: Hodgkin's disease and non-Hodgkin's lymphoma, in Fairbanks V (ed): *Current Hematology and Oncology,* vol 5. Chicago, Year Book Medical Publishers, 1987, pp 77–120.

4. Cossman J, Uppenkamp M, Sundeen J, et al: Molecular genetics and the diagnosis of lymphoma. *Arch Pathol Lab Med* 1988; 112:117–127.

5. Ioachim HL: *Lymph Node Biopsy.* Philadelphia, JB Lippincott, 1982.

6. Jaffe ES: *Surgical Pathology of the Lymph Nodes and Related Organs.* Philadelphia, WB Saunders Co, 1985.

7. Kjeldsberg CR, Wilson JF: Malignant lymphoma in children, in Finegold M (ed): *Pathology of Neoplasia in Children and Adolescents.* Philadelphia, WB Saunders Co, 1986.

8. National Cancer Institute sponsored study of classification of non-Hodgkin's lymphomas: Summary and description of a working formulation for clinical usage. The Non-Hodgkin's Lymphoma Pathologic Classification Project. *Cancer* 1982; 49:2112–2135.

9. Picker LJ, Weiss LM, Medeiros LJ, et al: Immunophenotyping criteria for the diagnosis of non-Hodgkin's lymphoma. *Am J Pathol* 1987; 128:181–201.

10. Sommers SC, Rosen PP: *Malignant Lymphomas: A Pathology Annual Monograph.* Appleton-Century-Crofts, 1983.

11. Yunis JJ, Frizzera G, Oken MM: Multiple recurrent genomic defects follicular lymphoma: A possible model for cancer. *New Engl J Med* 1987; 316:79–84.

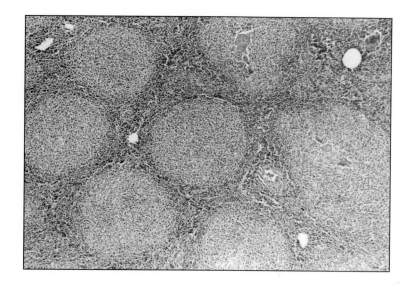

Figure 36-1 Low-power view of malignant lymphoma with follicular pattern.

Figure 36-2 Malignant lymphoma, small lymphocytic type. There is a diffuse infiltrate composed of small normal-appearing lymphocytes.

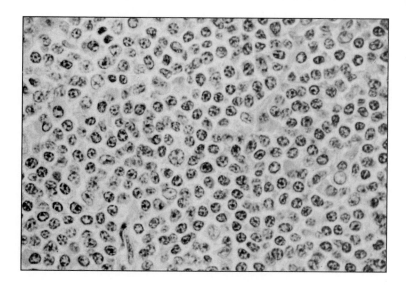

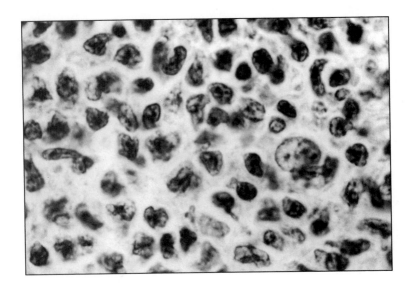

Figure 36–3 Malignant lymphoma, small cleaved cell type. There is a diffuse infiltrate composed predominantly of small lymphocytes with twisted and cleaved nuclei.

Figure 36–4 Malignant lymphoma, mixed small and large cell type. There is a diffuse infiltrate composed of atypical small lymphocytes and large lymphocytes.

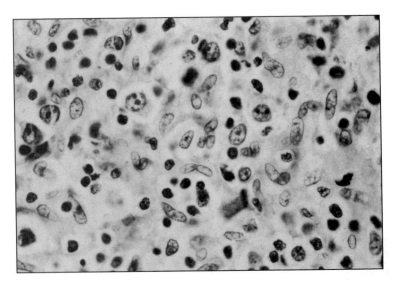

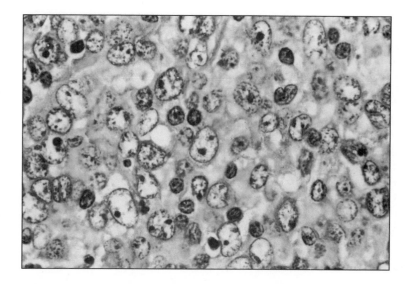

Figure 36–5   Malignant lymphoma, large noncleaved cell type. There is a diffuse infiltrate composed of large lymphocytes with round to ovoid nuclei and small, irregularly distributed nucleoli. Cytoplasm is scant to moderate.

Figure 36–6   Malignant lymphoma, large cleaved cell type. This is the least common of the large cell lymphomas and consists predominantly of large lymphocytes having irregular cleaved nuclear contours.

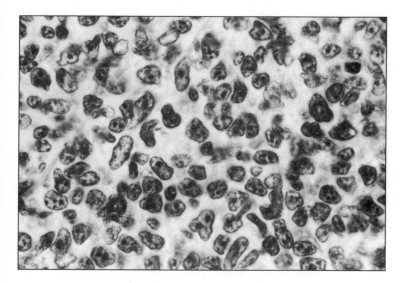

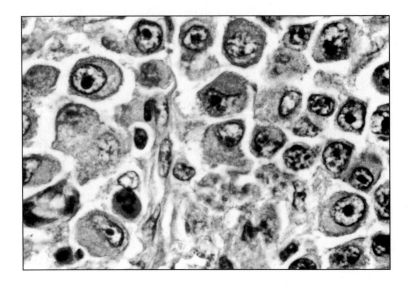

Figure 36–7   Malignant lymphoma, immunoblastic type. The immunoblasts have characteristically abundant cytoplasm and a round to ovoid nucleus containing a centrally placed, prominent nucleolus. The cells often have plasmacytic features.

Figure 36–8   Malignant histiocytosis. A large cell infiltrate is seen within a sinusoid.

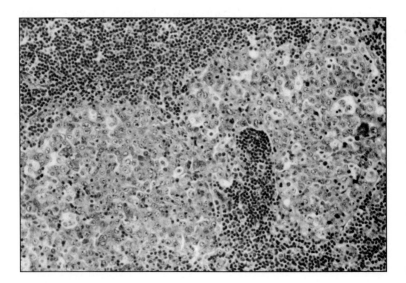

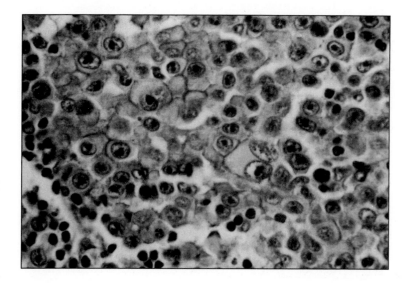

Figure 36–9   Malignant lymphoma, true histiocytic type. The tumor cells are large with abundant cytoplasm and distinct cytoplasmic membranes.

Figure 36–10   Malignant lymphoma, small noncleaved cell type (Burkitt's lymphoma). The medium-sized lymphocytes have moderate cytoplasm and a round to ovoid nucleus with a fairly prominent nucleolus or nucleoli.

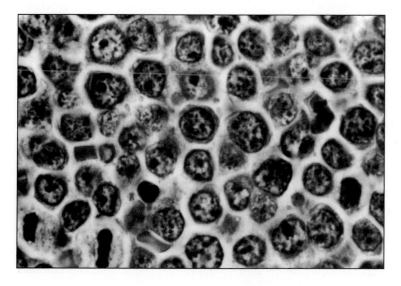

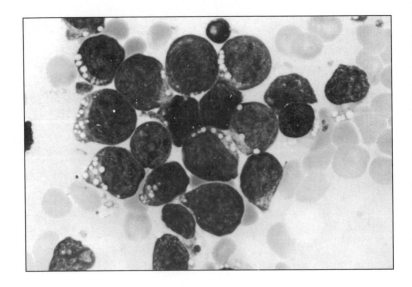

Figure 36–11   Malignant lymphoma, small noncleaved cell type (Burkitt's lymphoma). Imprint of lymph node showing sheets of cells characterized by prominent cytoplasmic vacuoles.

Figure 36–12   Malignant lymphoma, lymphoblastic, convoluted type. Sheets of lymphoblasts have fine chromatin pattern, indistinct nucleoli, convoluted nuclei, and scant cytoplasm.

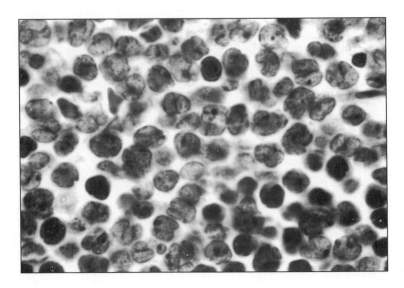

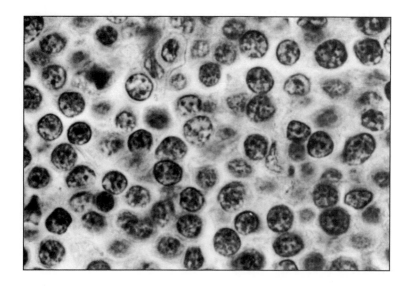

Figure 36–13   Malignant lymphoma, lymphoblastic, nonconvoluted type. In contrast to Figure 35–12, the blasts are predominantly round to ovoid and do not show distinct nuclear convolutions. Also, the nuclear chromatin is less delicate.

Figure 36–14   Malignant lymphoma, peripheral T-cell type. There is a diffuse infiltrate composed of atypical small, medium-sized, and large lymphocytes.

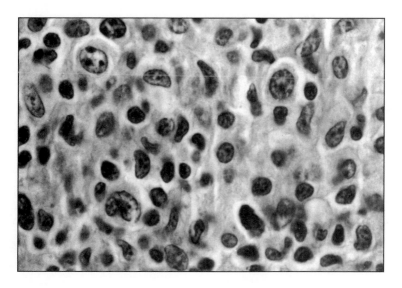

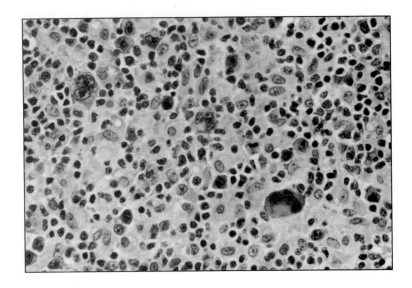

Figure 36–15   Malignant lymphoma, peripheral T-cell type. There is a diffuse infiltrate composed of atypical small, medium-sized, and large cell types, including Reed-Sternberg–like cells.

Figure 36–16   Mycosis fungoides. This skin biopsy shows a dermal lymphocytic infiltrate and characteristic infiltrates in the epidermis called Pautrier's abscesses.

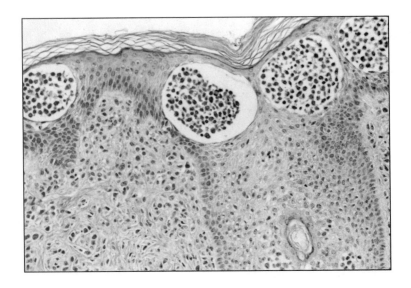

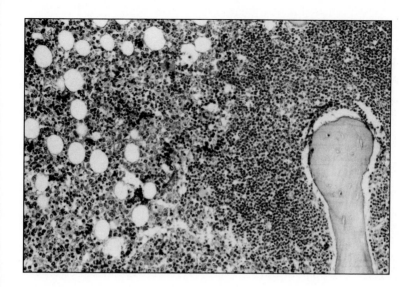

Figure 36–18   Bone marrow biopsy specimen showing malignant lymphoma. There is focal involvement composed of sheets of small lymphocytes adjacent to a bone trabecula.

37

Hodgkin's Disease

The malignant lymphomas are a group of diseases divided into Hodgkin's disease and non-Hodgkin's lymphoma. In both disorders, normal lymphoid architecture is replaced by collections of one or several cell types. Hodgkin's disease is characterized by the presence of multinucleate giant cells called Reed-Sternberg cells and mononuclear variants.

Pathophysiology

Hodgkin's disease is a complex disorder of the immune system composed of neoplastic mononuclear cells that are admixed with variable numbers of presumably reactive small lymphocytes, plasma cells, eosinophils, and histiocytes. The exact nature of the malignant cell population is still unknown. Controversy exists as to whether the neoplastic cells are transformed lymphocytes or histiocytes. The different histologic types vary both in clinical findings and in the cell line involved. Thus, the lymphocyte predominant type of Hodgkin's disease may be a B-cell, germinal center cell proliferation, while mixed cellularity Hodgkin's disease may involve primarily T-lymphocytes. Gene rearrangement analyses in Hodgkin's disease have been contradictory. Some studies have shown immunoglobulin gene rearrangement, others have shown a pattern consistent with polyclonal or monoclonal T-cells, and still others have shown only a germline pattern. Hodgkin's disease may be a clinical syndrome rather than a specific disease. The etiology of the disease is still unknown.

Clinical Findings

The annual incidence of Hodgkin's disease in the United States is approximately 35 per 1 million population for white males and 26 per 1 million population for white females; nonwhites have a slightly lower incidence. Hodgkin's disease has a bimodal age specific incidence curve with one mode in the 15- to 45-year age group and another after the age of 50 years.

The clinical presentation of Hodgkin's disease is usually a progressive, painless enlargement of one or more lymph nodes in the neck. Occasional patients present with a mediastinal mass that may be discovered on a routine chest film or on a film taken because of respiratory symptoms. Hodgkin's disease is more frequently associated with constitutional symptoms (so-called B symptoms), such as fever, night sweats, pruritus, and weight loss, than is non-Hodgkin's lymphoma. Physical examination may reveal, in addition to enlarged lymph nodes, splenomegaly and hepatomegaly. In contrast to non-Hodgkin's lymphoma, primary extranodal disease is very unusual.

Classification of Hodgkin's Disease

In contrast to the non-Hodgkin's lymphomas, one histopathologic classification is generally accepted, ie, the one proposed by Lukes and Butler and modified at the Rye symposium into four subcategories (Table 37–1). Three of the types (lymphocyte predominance, mixed cellularity, and lymphocyte depletion) differ mainly in the relative proportions of malignant mononuclear and Reed-Sternberg cells to the presumed reactive cells. Correlation is good between the ratio of reactive lymphocytes to neoplastic cells in the lymph node biopsy and the biologic behavior of the tumor. Thus, when lymphocyte proliferation is prominent, Reed-Sternberg cells are rare, the disease is more likely to be localized, and the prognosis is better. It should be recognized, however, that with the marked improvement in therapy for Hodgkin's disease, the prognosis is mainly dependent on the stage of the disease and is becoming independent of the histologic subclassification. The pathologist must be able to accurately make the initial diagnosis and be able to identify Hodgkin's disease in laparotomy specimens and biopsy specimens should relapse occur.

Table 37-1   Classification Schema for Hodgkin's Disease

Lukes and Butler	Rye Modification
Lymphocyte and/or histiocyte predominance	Lymphocyte predominance
Nodular	
Diffuse	
Nodular sclerosis	Nodular sclerosis
Mixed cellularity	Mixed cellularity
Lymphocyte depletion	Lymphocyte depletion
Diffuse fibrosis	
Reticular type	

The Reed-Sternberg cell, which is required for the pathologic diagnosis of Hodgkin's disease, is a large binucleated or multinucleated cell. It has moderately abundant cytoplasm with a characteristic clear halo around a large, prominent eosinophilic or amphophilic nucleolus. Mononuclear variants with the nuclear features of Reed-Sternberg cells, thought to be the actively proliferating component, are called Hodgkin's cells. Even though the presence of Reed-Sternberg cells are required for a pathologic diagnosis of Hodgkin's disease, similar, if not identical, cells may be observed in a variety of other disorders, including non-Hodgkin's peripheral T-cell lymphoma, infectious mononucleosis, and metastatic carcinoma. Therefore, to make a diagnosis of Hodgkin's disease, both the appropriate architectural and cellular environment and the presence of Reed-Sternberg cells are necessary.

Lymphocyte predominance type is characterized by complete or partial obliteration of the lymph node by small, mature-appearing lymphocytes and varying numbers of histiocytes. The pattern is usually vaguely nodular (Figure 37-1). Classical Reed-Sternberg cells (Figure 37-2) are few, and multiple sections may have to be examined to find any. Reed-Sternberg cell variants, called L&H cells, that feature lobated nuclei and small nucleoli are, however, often plentiful (Figure 37-3). The main differential diagnoses are atypical lymphoid hyperplasia and non-Hodgkin's lymphoma, small lymphocytic type. The nodular variant may also be mistaken for non-Hodgkin's lymphoma, follicular, mixed cell type. Progressive transformation of germinal centers may be mistaken for the nodular variant of this disease. Most patients with this type of Hodgkin's disease are young, have clinical stage I or II disease, and are asymptomatic.

Recent studies have suggested that the nodular lymphocyte predominance type of Hodgkin's disease is a germinal center cell proliferation, and questions have been raised whether this is a benign, premalignant, or malignant condition.

Mixed cellularity type is characterized by a greater number of abnormal mononuclear cells and readily found Reed-Sternberg cells (Figure 37–4). A variable number of eosinophils, plasma cells, and histiocytes are usually present. This type of Hodgkin's disease must be differentiated from various reactive lymphadenopathies (eg, infectious mononucleosis) and from certain types of non-Hodgkin's lymphoma, particularly the peripheral or node-based T-cell lymphomas (including so-called Lennert's lymphoma). As mentioned in chapter 36, it may sometimes be extremely difficult, even with immunologic markers, to distinguish certain T-cell lymphomas from this type of Hodgkin's disease. Patients with mixed cellularity Hodgkin's disease usually have stage III or IV disease and are symptomatic.

Lymphocyte depletion type, which is rare in the United States and Europe, reveals a paucity of lymphocytes with increased numbers of abnormal mononuclear cells. Reed-Sternberg cells are often numerous. Fibrosis and necrosis may be prominent. The patient is usually older, has stage III or IV disease, and is symptomatic. There is now, however, considerable doubt as to whether this entity exists. Most of the cases reported as lymphocyte depletion appear to have been non-Hodgkin's lymphoma (especially peripheral T-cell lymphoma), malignant histiocytosis, or nodular sclerosis Hodgkin's disease.

Nodular sclerosis Hodgkin's disease has two distinctive histologic features: the lymph node is divided into nodules by thick bands of collagen, and Reed-Sternberg cell variants are present in lacunar spaces (so-called lacunar cells) (Figures 37–5, 37–6). Extensive sheets of lacunar cells and atypical mononuclear cells are frequently present. Necrosis is not uncommon. A variant of nodular sclerosis, called syncytial, sarcomatous, or monomorphic type, is characterized by sheets of lacunar cells and atypical mononuclear cells (Figure 36–7). When a small biopsy specimen is obtained and little fibrosis is evident, it may be extremely difficult to differentiate this type of Hodgkin's disease from non-Hodgkin's large cell lymphoma, metastatic carcinoma, melanoma, or seminoma. Immunologic markers may be helpful in such instances; one must recognize, however, that at this time we have no specific marker for Hodgkin's disease.

Nodular sclerosis Hodgkin's disease is by far the most common type of Hodgkin's disease in the United States and Europe and occurs with equal frequency in both sexes, while in all the other types, males predominate. It is unusual in patients >50 years of

Table 37-2   Staging Procedures in Hodgkin's Disease

1. Clinical history and physical examination

2. Lymph node biopsy

3. Radiologic studies; chest x-ray; metastatic bone survey; whole lung tomography scan (optional); computed tomography scan of abdomen; lower limb lymphangiography

4. Laboratory tests: complete blood count, liver and renal function tests, urinalysis, erythrocyte sedimentation

5. Liver and spleen isotope scan

6. Bilateral iliac crest bone marrow biopsy

7. Laparotomy and splenectomy, liver biopsies, and intraabdominal lymph node biopsy (celiac, porta hepatis, mesenteric, paraaortic, iliac nodes), if information is likely to affect therapy

age. Nodular sclerosis is usually associated with lower cervical, supraclavicular, and mediastinal lymph node involvement. It is the type most commonly affecting the lungs. The majority of patients have clinical stage II disease.

Approach to Diagnosis

Successful treatment of Hodgkin's disease depends on accurate identification of all disease-bearing sites in the body. Compared to non-Hodgkin's disease, patients with Hodgkin's disease have less frequent involvement of Waldeyer's ring, the gastrointestinal tract, mesenteric lymph nodes, bone marrow, and skin. Generally, Hodgkin's disease is in a less advanced stage when initially detected. In addition, patients with Hodgkin's disease have more frequent involvement of the mediastinal lymph nodes than patients with non-Hodgkin's disease. The procedures required to stage Hodgkin's disease are outlined in Table 37–2. Once all these pretreatment evaluation data are collected, the patient's disease is assigned a Roman numeral stage according to the criteria in Table 37–3. The stage is also assigned a substage designation depending on the presence (B) or absence (A) of significant systemic symptoms.

Following a clinical history and physical examination, the workup of a patient with possible Hodgkin's disease proceeds in the following fashion:

1. Tissue biopsy—the diagnosis and subclassification of Hodgkin's disease should be made on the basis of histopathologic features in a lymph node biopsy specimen before initating therapy. The initial diagnosis should not be made on the basis of a bone

Table 37-3   Ann Arbor Modification of Rye Staging System

Stage I	Involvement of 1 lymph node region (I) or of a single extralymphatic organ or site (I_E)
Stage II	Involvement of 2 or more lymph node regions on the same side of diaphragm (II) or localized involvement of extralymphatic organ or site and 1 or more lymph node regions on the same side of diaphragm (II_E)
Stage III	Involvement of lymph node regions on both sides of diaphragm (III), which may also be accompanied by localized involvement of extralymphatic organ or site (III_E) or by involvement of the spleen (III_S), or both (III_{SE})
Stage IV	Diffuse or disseminated involvement of 1 or more extralymphatic organs or tissues with or without associated lymph node enlargement

ABBREVIATIONS: E = extranodal; S = spleen.

marrow biopsy or liver biopsy specimen alone. The histologic interpretation of a lymph node biopsy specimen is considered one of the most difficult areas of surgical pathology. The major reason for difficulties in the interpretation of lymph node biopsy specimens is improper handling of the biopsy specimen. (For a discussion on this subject, see chapter 36.)

2. Complete blood count.
3. Bone marrow aspirate and biopsy examination.
4. Radiological studies.
5. Liver and renal function studies.
6. Laparotomy—staging laparotomy is of value in distinguishing patients eligible for treatment with radiation therapy alone from those requiring combination chemotherapy. Clinical staging of abdominal disease is inaccurate in approximately 25% of patients.

Hematologic Findings

In contrast to the non-Hodgkin's lymphomas, abnormal hematologic findings are uncommon in Hodgkin's disease. Despite this fact, examination of the peripheral blood and bone marrow should be done routinely as part of the staging procedure.

Blood Cell Measurements.   A mild-to-moderate anemia is frequently present in patients with Hodgkin's disease. It is usually normochromic, normocytic, with low or normal reticulocyte count. In a small percentage of patients, autoimmune hemolytic anemia develops. One third of the patients have leukocytosis caused by neutrophilia. The platelet count is normal or increased. Rarely, severe anemia or pancytopenia resulting from extensive involvement of the bone marrow or hypersplenism may be observed.

Peripheral Blood Smear Morphology. Monocytosis or eosinophilia or both are seen in 10% to 20% of patients, and lymphopenia may be present in patients with extensive disease.

Bone Marrow. A bilateral posterior iliac crest bone marrow biopsy should be performed routinely in the staging procedure in patients with Hodgkin's disease. Bone marrow involvement is unusual (less than 10% of patients) at time of diagnosis, especially in lymphocyte predominant type and nodular sclerosis. When the marrow is involved, the lesion is usually focal, is often associated with fibrosis, and may resemble a granuloma. Reed-Sternberg cells may be difficult to identify. The presence of mononuclear cells, with nuclear features of Reed-Sternberg cells, in the characteristic cellular environment of Hodgkin's disease should be regarded as consistent with marrow involvement provided that a diagnosis of Hodgkin's disease has been made from a lymph node biopsy specimen.

Other Laboratory Tests

37.1 Radiologic Studies

The radiologic evaluation plays a crucial role in determining the extent of disease. It should start with routine chest films. If any abnormalities are found, computed tomography (CT) is performed. The latter procedure better indicates the extent of mediastinal lymphadenopathy.

A bilateral lower-extremity lymphangiogram is essential in detecting disease in the retroperitoneal lymph nodes. It should be noted that splenic, hilar, celiac, porta hepatis, and mesenteric nodes are not demonstrated by lymphangiography. The CT scan is particularly useful in the delineation of lymphadenopathy, which is not revealed on lymphangiography. Skeletal surveys or bone scans may be included in search of lytic or, less commonly, osteoblastic lesions. A gallium citrate scan may be helpful in detecting disease in a variety of sites and may be used in patients unable to undergo lymphangiography. A CT scan may also reveal tumor nodules in the spleen.

37.2 Laparotomy

Exploratory laparotomy with splenectomy and open liver biopsy is used in patients considered to have stage I or II disease after clinical examination and radiologic tests. At surgery, the surgeon should biopsy all major lymph node groups regardless of the size and gross appearance of the nodes. Application of radiopaque clips at biopsy sites will later assist the radiotherapist in port design. The spleen and splenic hilar lymph nodes should be removed, and a wedge biopsy specimen should be taken from the liver.

The pathologist must carefully examine the removed spleen because excellent correlation exists between splenic involvement and the probability of hepatic involvement. It is extremely rare to have Hodgkin's disease in the liver without splenic involvement. The spleen must be cut into thin sections and carefully inspected; multiple sections should be examined microscopically.

Approximately 30% of patients thought to have stage I or II disease will be reclassified as having stage III disease after laparotomy.

Course and Treatment

Because of improvements in diagnostic techniques and therapy, 75% of patients with Hodgkin's disease can now be cured. Factors that adversely affect the prognosis include: stage III disease with involvement of lower abdominal lymph nodes, stage IV disease, old age, constitutional B symptoms, bulky disease, and extensive splenic involvement (>4 nodules).

The primary treatment of Hodgkin's disease that is confined to lymph nodes is extended-field radiotherapy. Patients with stage III or IV disease are treated with combination chemotherapy. Selected patients may be treated with combined radiotherapy and chemotherapy.

References

1. Bennet JM (ed): *Lymphomas, Including Hodgkin's Disease.* The Hague, the Netherlands, Martinus Nijhoff Publishers, 1981.

2. Colby TV: Pitfalls in the diagnosis and classification of Hodgkin's disease: Surgical pathology and classification for the 1980s: Is the Lukes-Butler classification relevant? In Bennet JM (ed): *Controversies in the*

Management of Lymphomas. The Hague, the Netherlands, Martinus Nijhoff Publishers, 1984, pp 19–52.

3. Colgan JP, Haberman TM: Hodgkin's disease and non-Hodgkin's lymphoma, in Fairbank V (ed): *Current Hematology and Oncology.* vol 5. Chicago, Year Book Medical Publishers, 1987, pp 77–120.

4. Grogan TM: Hodgkin's disease, Jaffe, EB (ed): in *Surgical Pathology of the Lymph Nodes and Related Organs.* Philadelphia, WB Saunders Co, 1985, pp 86–134.

5. Kaplan HS: *Hodgkin's Disease,* ed 2. Cambridge, Mass, Harvard University Press, 1980.

6. Timens W, Visser L, Poppema S: Nodular lymphocyte predominant type of Hodgkin's disease is a germinal center lymphoma. *Lab Invest* 1986; 54:457–461.

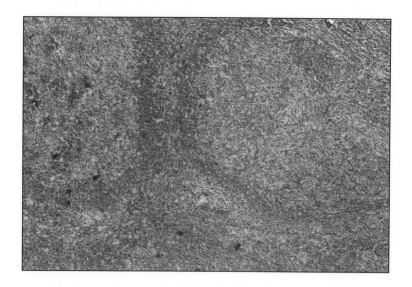

Figure 37–1　L&H nodular lymphocyte predominance Hodgkin's disease. Low-power view illustrating the vague nodules in this disorder.

Figure 37–2　A classic Reed-Sternberg cell surrounded by small lymphocytes, occasional plasma cells, and histiocytes.

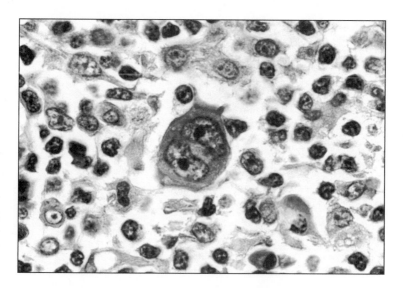

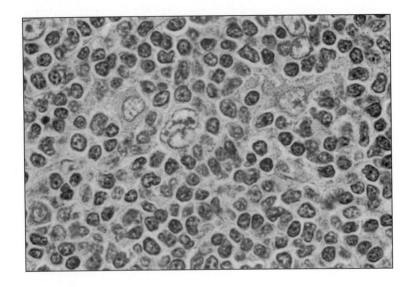

Figure 37–3   Lymphocyte predominance Hodgkin's disease. A so-called L&H cell (a Reed-Sternberg cell variant) is seen in the center.

Figure 37–4   Mixed cellularity Hodgkin's disease. Several Reed-Sternberg cells and mononuclear variants thereof are seen admixed with multiple small lymphocytes and scattered plasma cells.

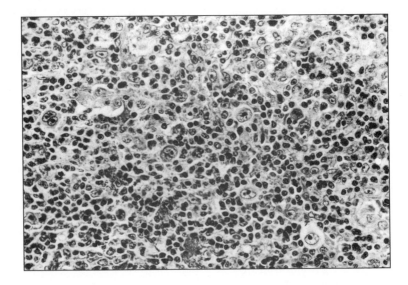

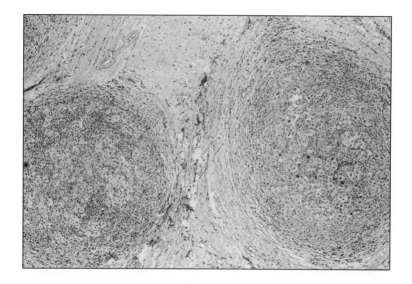

Figure 37-5 Nodular sclerosis Hodgkin's disease. Two distinct nodules separated by broad bands of collagen are seen. The nodules contain numerous lacunar cells.

Figure 37-6 Nodular sclerosis Hodgkin's disease. A high-power view of lacunar cells.

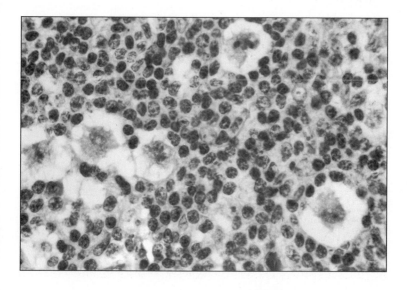

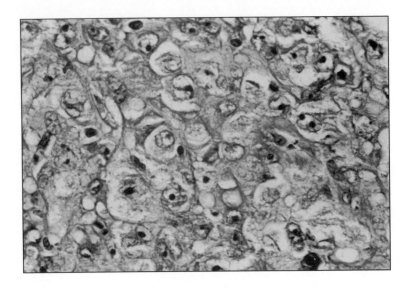

Figure 37–7   Syncytial or sarcomatous variant of nodular sclerosis Hodgkin's disease. Sheets of lacunar cells and large atypical mononuclear cells are seen.

PART 11

Immunoproliferative
Disorders

38

Multiple Myeloma
and Related Disorders

Malignant immunoproliferative disorders are defined as neoplastic clonal proliferation of plasma cells, pre–B-lymphocytes, or B-lymphocytes resulting in abnormal production of immunoglobulins (Igs). The immunoglobulin abnormality is used to classify the disease. The malignant immunoproliferative disorders are multiple myeloma, macroglobulinemia, light-chain myeloma, and heavy-chain disease. Multiple myeloma is associated with IgG or IgA paraproteins, rarely IgD or IgE; light-chain myeloma with kappa or lambda light-chain paraproteins; macroglobulinemia with IgM paraprotein; heavy-chain disease with γ, α or μ heavy-chain paraproteins.

Pathophysiology

Immunoglobulins are composed of 2 heavy and 2 light chains linked by disulfide bonds (Figure 38-1). The sequence of amino acids in the heavy chains, molecular weight (MW) 55000, is specific for the immunoglobulin class, annotated gamma for IgG, mu for IgM, alpha for IgA, delta for IgD, and epsilon for IgE. IgG has 4 subtypes IgG_1, G_2, G_3, and G_4, and IgA, 2 subtypes, IgA_1 and IgA_2. The shorter sequence of amino acids in the light chains (MW, 22000) is specific for lambda or kappa chains. The light chains can link to any set of heavy chains, but both light chains are the same on any single

Figure 38–1 Schematic diagram of immunoglobulin monomer. The shaded area (Fab) is variable in amino acid constitution consistent with multiple gene products. The clear area is the crystallizable fragment (Fc), which is relatively constant, consistent with a product of a smaller family of genes.

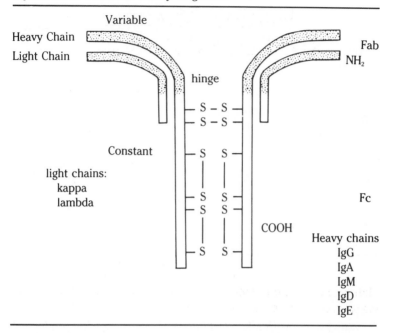

molecule. Partial hydrolysis of a globulin molecule with papain separates it into a crystallizable fraction (Fc) and the heavy-light-chain residue responsible for antibody activity (Fab).

Each immunoglobulin class has a characteristic structure that determines molecular size. Immunoglobulin G, IgD, and IgE are monomeric (ie, they have 1 set of heavy and light chains), whereas IgM is pentameric with 5 sets, and IgA varies as monomer, dimer, or trimer, or in secretions where it has an additional secretory piece, J. The size of the molecule and its sequence of amino acids determine its electrical charge, and, therefore, its migration by electrophoresis, as well as other physicochemical characteristics, including viscosity or solubility (Table 38–1).

In general, 1 plasma cell produces 1 type of immunoglobulin. Thus, proliferations of a single cell clone will yield a monotonous population of immunoglobulin molecules, defined by a single light-chain type, and migrating to a single narrow zone on electrophoresis, seen as a monoclonal spike. These abnormal molecules are known as M-proteins (for myeloma or monoclonal) or paraproteins.

Table 38–1   Characteristics of Normal Immunoglobulins

Class	Heavy Chain	Subtypes	MW
IgG	γ	4	150,000
IgA	α	2	170,000
With secretory piece			390,000
With J piece			
IgM	μ	2	900,000
IgD	δ	1	150,000
IgE	ε	1	196,000
	Fc		53,000

Paraproteins may be abnormal in amount, structure, or configuration.

Multiple myeloma is a proliferation of plasma cells producing, in most cases, either IgG or IgA paraproteins of either light-chain type. In a few cases, IgD is the abnormal protein and, very rarely, IgE is produced. Light-chain disease is a myeloma variant; the light chains conjugate to form dimers, the Bence-Jones (BJ) protein, in serum and urine. The dimers form the fibrillar polymers of amyloid, and early renal failure is common. Waldenström's macroglobulinemia is associated with lymphoma-producing IgM paraproteins. The heavy-chain diseases produce pathologic proteins with amino acid deletions in the hinge region, site of usual conjugation to light chains; thus the heavy chain circulates without light chains (Table 38–2).

Clinical Findings

Because the pathologic cell types are related, a similarity can be seen in the signs, symptoms, and laboratory findings for multiple myeloma (MM) and the related disorders of light-chain myeloma, macroglobulinemia, and heavy-chain diseases as summarized in Tables 38–2 and 38–3. Immunoproliferative disorders usually come

Configuration	Function	Normal Serum Concentration (mg/dL)
Monomer	2° phase antibody	800–1800
Monomer	Secretory antibodies	180–490
Dimer		
Trimer		
Pentamer	1° phase antibody complement fixing	50–180
Monomer	? Precursor to IgM, IgG; ? receptor on lymphocyte	3
Monomer	Reaginic antibody	0.3

to attention because of moderate normochromic anemia of undetermined origin and/or one of the following reasons: (1) an abnormal band seen on routine electrophoresis, (2) nephrotic syndrome or renal insufficiency of undetermined origin, (3) back pain or radiographic evidence of unsuspected fractures of ribs or vertebrae, (4) acute spinal cord compression from vertebral collapse, or (5) hypercalcemia. Myeloma is usually found in patients over 40 years old, commonly presenting with fatigue, bone pain if a fracture has occurred, and pallor due to anemia. Hepatosplenomegaly and lymphadenopathy are unusual in IgG and IgA myeloma. The pathologic protein usually proliferates at the expense of normal immunoglobulins; because these proteins are antibodies, their loss leads to serious recurring infection. IgD myeloma and light-chain disease are associated with amyloidosis and early renal failure more frequently than other types of myeloma. Lambda light-chain disease is more severe than kappa, possibly because of more rapid deterioration of renal function or amyloidosis or both. IgD myeloma is more frequently associated with lymphadenopathy, hepatosplenomegaly, extra-medullary tumors, and amyloidosis than the more common IgG and IgA myelomas. Macroglobulinemia is usually associated with lymphocytic lymphoma and may present with lymphadenopathy, and, in late stages, hepatosplenomegaly. Each heavy-chain type produces a different clinical picture: gamma, lym-

Table 38–2 Clinical and Laboratory Findings in Immunoproliferative Disease

| Disease | Immunoglobulin | | Electrophoretic Pattern |
	Heavy Chain	Light Chain	
Myelomas			
IgG (75%)	γ	κ or λ	Narrow spike
IgA (15%)	α	κ or λ	Broader spike
IgD (1%-2%)	δ	Usually λ	Hypogamma
IgE (2 cases)	ε	κ or λ	Narrow spike
Light-chain myeloma (10%)	None	κ or λ	Hypogamma
Macroglobulinemia	μ	κ or λ	Small spike beta
Heavy-chain disease			
Gamma (70)[a]		None	Broad-band polyclonal
Alpha (120)[a]		None	Broad-band alpha$_2$-beta
Mu (15)[a]		None	None
Delta (1)[a]		None	Narrow peak

NOTE: Characteristic findings in classical or well-advanced disease. Complications are not limited to the specific immunoglobulin class but are more likely for each type.

ABBREVIATIONS: BJ = Bence-Jones protein; CLL = chronic lymphocytic leukemia.

[a] Number of cases

Urine BJ	Bone X-Ray	Cell Type	Complications
60%	Osteolytic lesions	Plasma cell	Infection
70%	Osteolytic lesions	Plasma cell	Infection
100%		Plasma cell	Amyloidosis
Unknown		Plasma cell	Plasma cell leukemia
100%	Diffuse osteoporosis	Plasma cell Lymphocyte, mixed	Amyloid kidney Hypercalcemia
30%–40%	Minimal	Lymphocyte, Plasma cell	Hyperviscosity Bleeding Cold agglutinin hemolytic anemia
γ chain	Normal	Lymphocyte	Palatal edema
None	Normal	Plasma cell	GI lymphoma Malabsorption
κ chain, BJ	Osteoporosis	Lymphocyte (CLL)	Amyloidosis
	Osteolytic lesions	Plasma cell	

Table 38–3 Hematologic Characteristics of Immunoproliferative Disorders

Disease	Blood
Myeloma	Normochromic anemia
	Rouleaux
	Plasma cell leukemia (IgE)
Macroglobulinemia	Normochromic anemia
	Lymphocytosis
	Neutropenia, eosinophilia
Light-chain myeloma	Anemia
	Rouleaux
Heavy-chain disease	
Gamma	Lymphocytosis
Mu	CLL
Alpha	Normal
Delta	Normal

ABBREVIATIONS: CLL = chronic lymphocytic leukemia.

phocytic lymphoma; mu, CLL; and alpha, gastrointestinal lymphoma, which is more common in the young and of increased frequency in the Mediterranean area. One reported case of delta heavy-chain disease presented as myeloma. Epsilon heavy-chain disease is presumed to exist, but has not been found as yet. Hepatosplenomegaly and lymphadenopathy are seen in lymphomas associated with macroglobulinemia or gamma heavy-chain disease. The gastrointestinal lymphoma of alpha chain disease may produce malabsorption.

Bones are involved focally in some myelomas (Figure 38–2), and more diffusely in others, seen as osteoporosis. Osteolytic lesions are due in part to osteoclast-activating factor. Extramedullary plasmacytomas may occur in the nasopharynx or, rarely, in the breast. The majority are followed by disseminated myeloma within a few years. Solitary plasmacytomas of bone are rare, but may also disseminate within a few years.

Marrow	Liver/ Spleen	Bone X-Ray
Plasma cells	No increase	Osteolytic lesions
Lymphocytes, plasma cells	Enlarged	Rare abnormality
Plasma cells	No increase	Osteoporosis
Lymphocytes, plasma cells, eosinophils	Enlarged	No abnormality
Lymphocytes	Enlarged	Osteoporosis
Moderate plasma cells	No increase	No abnormality
Plasmacytosis		Osteolytic lesions

Approach to Diagnosis

Since malignant immunoproliferative diseases are defined by the abnormal protein, diagnosis depends on detection of an abnormal globulin, identification of it as monoclonal, and characterization of its heavy and light chains. The pathologic cell type is confirmed by bone marrow or tissue examination.

1. Hematologic findings include a modest normochromic anemia, and the peripheral smear should be examined for plasma cells and lymphocytosis. Bone marrow aspirate is necessary to determine the significance of abnormal protein electrophoresis, the pathologic cell type, and the extent of the disease. Sedimentation rate is a nonspecific test of limited usefulness and is abnormal in anemia or in the presence of increased globulin.

2. Serum protein electrophoresis is used to detect monoclonal spikes or hypogammaglobulinemia. Protein electrophoresis has

supplanted the albumin:globulin ratio and is a very accurate way of quantitating albumin. Any abnormality of globulins may be seen on the scan pattern. Albumin:globulin ratio, frequently obtained as part of an automated chemistry panel, is unreliable, since hypogammaglobulinemia and small abnormal spikes less than 2 g/dL may neither reverse the ratio nor cause significant elevations of total globulin.

3. Immunoelectrophoresis (IEP) is performed when any clonal peaks or hypogammaglobulinemia are found on routine protein electrophoresis. With hypogammaglobulinemia, specific tests should be performed for urinary light chains. Immunoglobulin quantitation is correlative, but not diagnostic. Immunofixation is useful if IEP does not clearly show a monoclonal protein.

4. Urine protein electrophoresis and immunoelectrophoresis are performed whenever a monoclonal serum protein or hypogammaglobulinemia is found. Urine immunoelectrophoresis is absolutely necessary to diagnose heavy-chain diseases.

5. Radiographic studies of the long bones, ribs, vertebrae, and skull help discern lytic lesions, generalized osteoporosis caused by plasma cell proliferation, or pathologic fractures.

6. Serum viscosity is of prognostic and therapeutic value, particularly when the paraprotein is IgM.

7. Coagulation screening tests can be performed on patients who are bleeding to categorize the diathesis as a guide to treatment with blood components. Bleeding diatheses occur most often with IgM paraproteins.

8. Renal function is screened by serum creatinine, particularly in light-chain disease where renal amyloidosis is common. Clinical studies that involve dehydration (eg, intravenous pyelogram) should be avoided to prevent inspissating the abnormal proteins in renal tubules, further compromising renal function.

9. Radiographic studies of the small intestine are helpful in diagnosis of alpha heavy-chain disease.

10. Serum calcium may rise significantly in myeloma, causing lethargy and cardiac arrhythmia. Hypercalcemia appears to be closely related to Bence-Jones proteinuria.

11. Serum Beta-2-microglobulin may be helpful in determining tumor burden and, therefore, prognosis. Plasma cell labeling index may also be helpful, but is not generally available.

12. Immunofluorescent or immunoperoxidase studies may be useful in identifying monoclonal cell populations. These studies may be especially useful in diagnosis of nonsecretory myeloma. In selected cases, gene rearrangement study may be useful.

Hematologic Findings

Multiple myeloma is a multifocal nodular proliferation of plasma cells associated with a paraprotein in all but a few rare cases (less than 1%). In almost all immunoproliferative diseases, mild-to-moderate anemia is present. Leukopenia and thrombocytopenia are uncommon but may result from chemotherapy. Hepatosplenomegaly and lymphadenopathy are unusual in myeloma, although they are seen in lymphomas associated with macroglobulinemia or gamma heavy-chain disease.

Blood Cell Measurements. Moderate normochromic anemia (Hb 80 to 110 g/L or 8 to 11 g/dl) is present. Rarely, there is a macrocytic anemia unresponsive to vitamin B_{12} or folic acid therapy. Hypochromic anemia results from significant gastrointestinal bleeding. The white cell count is normal, but if marrow replacement is extensive, leukopenia and thrombocytopenia may be present. In terminal disease or IgE myeloma, plasma cell leukemia can result in white cell counts of 50 to 100 $\times$ 10^9/L (50 to 100 $\times$ 10^3/μl).

Platelets are of normal appearance and numbers unless the patient is undergoing chemotherapy. Abnormal function results from coating with paraprotein, most commonly with IgM.

Peripheral Blood Smear Morphology. Peripheral blood smears may show rouleaux formation and a background of gray stain representing the paraprotein (Figure 38–3). Nucleated red cells are seen even early in the disease, but become more numerous with progressive anemia resulting from bone marrow involvement.

Plasmacytoid lymphocytes may be found late in the course of myeloma. True plasma cell leukemia is rare, appearing late in myeloma, although it may be an initial feature of IgE myeloma. This diagnosis is difficult to make on morphologic grounds unless abnormal plasma cells or plasmablasts are circulating.

Bone Marrow Examination. A bone marrow aspirate and biopsy should be done. The bone marrow cellularity varies from normal to total replacement by plasma cells. Sampling error is critical in the nodular proliferations of myeloma. Increases in plasma cells (>0.10 or 10%), lymphocytes (>0.20 or 20%), or both are usually present. Infiltrates may be nodular or diffuse, and there is no morphologic characteristic that will be diagnostic of the associated paraprotein. Nevertheless, some generalizations can be made. In IgG myeloma monotonous sheets of plasma cells are usually found that are mostly mature with few plasmablasts (Figure 38–4). A patient with IgA myeloma may have diffuse infiltration of other marrow elements by immature plasma cells and variable numbers of lymphocytes. Occasionally, flamelike discoloration of plasma cell cytoplasm (thesaurocytes) is seen. In light-chain myeloma, plasma cells and lymphocytes diffusely infiltrate the marrow. In macroglobulinemia there is diffuse replacement of marrow by plasmacytoid lymphocytes.

Although liver disease and chronic infection may be associated with moderate plasmacytosis, those plasma cells are usually mature, do not appear in aggregates, and, combined with lymphocytes, comprise less than 20% of the total number of cells. Plasmablasts and multinucleated plasma cells are usually pathologic. Very rarely, plasma cell myeloma has no circulating paraprotein. Immunofluorescent studies of air-dried unstained smears or immunoperoxidase staining of bone marrow may help determine whether the plasma cells are monoclonal or not (Figure 38–5).

Other Laboratory Tests

38.1   Serum Protein Electrophoresis

Purpose.   Serum protein electrophoresis is a screening test for monoclonal spikes or hypogammaglobulinemia (Figure 38–6).

Principle.   Proteins, being amphoteric, migrate in an electrical field. A pathologic protein with a monotonous population of similarly charged molecules migrates to one single location creating a dense band, or spike, of paraprotein. In light-chain disease, the small molecules are excreted rapidly in the urine, depleting serum gamma globulin (seen as hypogammaglobulinemia).

Specimen.   One milliliter of serum or plasma is adequate and may be stored refrigerated or frozen. Electrophoretic patterns of plasma yield an additional band between beta and gamma representing fibrinogen.

Procedure.   Serum is inoculated most commonly on transparent cellulose acetate membranes and electrophoresis is performed at a pH of 8.6, separating the proteins into albumin and the four globulins (alpha$_1$, alpha$_2$, beta, and gamma). The proteins are precipitated on the membrane with glacial acetic acid and stained with Ponceau S, a red dye, or amido black. The amount of dye absorbed to each band is proportional to the amount of protein. The patterns can be evaluated visually for abnormal

Figure 38–6 Schematic comparison of protein electrophoretic pattern and immunoelectrophoresis. ↑ = inoculation point for protein electrophoresis. Inoculation point for IEP is the antigen well. Electrophoretic separation appears as immunoprecipitate point sources along the path of migration indicated by dotted circles. Distance of migration varies with size of the protein molecule. G, A, and M indicate IgG, IgA, and IgM, respectively.

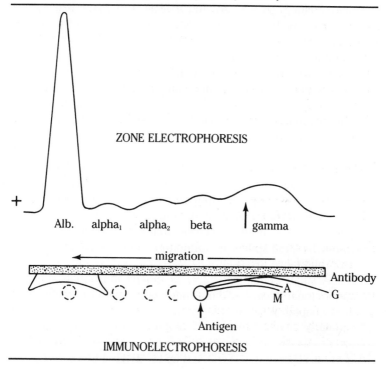

bands or quantitated by densitometry. The latter method utilizes the total protein, determined by refractometry or chemically, and divides this value in proportion to the dye absorbance of each protein band. The proportion is translated onto paper as a series of peaks. The area under each peak is calculated and converted to grams per deciliter and is reported alone or with the paper pattern in most institutions. In some cases the cellulose pattern may be attached to the report as well.

Interpretation. Normal ranges are: albumin, 35 to 60 g/L (3.5 to 6 g/dl); alpha$_1$, 1 to 4 g/L (0.1 to 0.4 g/dl); alpha$_2$, 4 to 12 g/L (0.4 to 1.2 g/dl); beta, 5 to 11 g/L (0.5 to 1.1 g/dl); and gamma, 5 to 16 g/L (0.5 to 1.6 g/dl).

Abnormal bands are found most often in the beta or gamma zone and may vary from 10 to 120 g/L (1.0 to 12.0 g/dl) or higher. Quantitated values may be misleading since small, abnormal bands that are seen easily by inspection of the patterns may not change the gamma per deciliter significantly. Since quantitation depends on the relative dye staining of the different zones, high levels of paraprotein result in falsely low levels of albumin, and albumin/globulin ratios may be inaccurate. Although the course of the disease or treatment can be estimated by repeating protein electrophoresis patterns every 2 to 3 months, a wide latitude (±3 g/L or 0.3 g/dl) must be allowed for quantitation; changes of 5 g/L (0.5 g/dl) are probably significant.

Characteristic patterns in neoplastic disorders are hypogammaglobulinemia—light-chain disease, IgD myeloma; spikes in beta or gamma zones—IgG or IgE myeloma, IgM macroglobulinemia; broad-based spikes—IgA myeloma, heavy-chain disease; minimonoclonal spikes (<2 g/L or 0.2 g/dl)—metastatic carcinoma of the stomach, prostate, breast, or colon, or other lymphomas. The size, shape, and location of spikes are suggestive but not diagnostic of the paraprotein type. Identification requires immunoelectrophoresis. The small spikes seen with metastatic tumors may be caused by reactive plasmacytosis around necrotic tumor or tumor metastases. Rarely biclonal spikes are found in immunoproliferative or myeloproliferative disease.

A small percentage (3%) of elderly individuals produce monoclonal spikes without immunoproliferative malignancy (see chapter 39).

38.2 Urine Electrophoresis and Tests for Bence-Jones Protein

Purpose.   Monoclonal spikes in unconcentrated urine are diagnostic of immunoproliferative malignancy and confirm the significance of monoclonal spikes or hypogammaglobulinemia seen on serum protein electrophoresis. Classic heat precipitation tests for Bence-Jones protein are not reliable and should be abandoned.

Principle.   As in serum, a monolithic population of similarly charged protein molecules migrate as a band on zone electrophoresis and can be quantitated. Excretion of abnormal proteins may damage the kidney, and electrophoresis detects a nephrotic pattern of protein loss in addition to the monoclonal spikes.

Specimen. The first voided morning specimen is refrigerated but not frozen to avoid disruption of light-chain dimers. Specimens may require 50 or 100 times the concentration before electrophoresis is performed, in order to detect minute amounts of protein in early disease. Twenty-four-hour urine samples are difficult to collect and are generally unnecessary.

Procedure. Urine is inoculated on cellulose membranes and electrophoresis is performed at a pH of 8.6. Proteins are quantitated by densitometry and reported as grams or milligrams per deciliter. The pattern should be attached to the report.

Interpretation. Monoclonal bands seen on electrophoresis are significant regardless of the amount and should be characterized by immunoelectrophoresis. Small amounts of protein (0.02 to 0.1 g/L or 2 to 10 mg/dl) may be seen in urine, particularly in elderly patients. Fifty percent of IgG or IgA myelomas are associated with Bence-Jones proteinuria, while 100% of light-chain myelomas have Bence-Jones proteins. Standard electrophoresis shows a monoclonal band in the same zone as seen on serum. Immunoelectrophoresis usually identifies abnormal heavy chains and light chains, reflecting the serum pattern. Only the pathologic light chain appears in urine, which proves helpful in interpreting the serum proteins. Light chains polymerize as amyloid fibrils in renal tubular epithelium and can be seen on renal biopsy by electron microscopy or with immunofluorescence.

38.3 Serum and Urine Immunoelectrophoresis

Purpose. Immunoelectrophoresis characterizes protein (as monoclonal, ie, of one light-chain type) and identifies its specific heavy chain in order to classify the underlying disease. Absence of light chains is diagnostic for heavy-chain disease.

Principle. An initial protein electrophoretic migration on agar or cellulose membranes is followed by application of antiserum along the path of migration. Individual protein molecules diffuse toward the antibody, forming immune precipitin arcs wherever antigen meets specific antibody.

Specimen. Aliquots of serum or random urine should be refrigerated rather than frozen to avoid dissociation of trimers or pentamers common to IgA and IgM or dissociation of light and heavy chains. Once paraproteins are identified, specimens may be frozen. Urine specimens frequently require 20 to 50 times the original concentration to detect minute amounts of light chain. Serums with large amounts of abnormal globulin require dilution to avoid antigen excess, which hinders identification. Saline-diluted specimens should not be frozen.

Procedure. Immunoelectrophoresis is available in large hospital laboratories and most local reference laboratories. The test requires 24 to 48 hours to complete and experience in interpretation. Immunoelectrophoresis is primarily a qualitative procedure that uses agar gel or cellulose as the support medium. It is semiquantitative in that protein arcs may be high, low, or absent. Urine or serum is inoculated into a well and electrophoresed for 40 to 60 minutes at a pH of 8.6 to separate component proteins. Antiserum from rabbits or goats is then inoculated along the path of migration. The electrophoretically separated albumin and many globulins diffuse toward the antiserum. Wherever antigen and antibody specificity correspond, a precipitin arc is deposited (Figure 38–6). Antisera to whole human serum or specific sera for each heavy chain and both light chains are available. Specific antiserum for IgD or IgE is in short supply and is not routinely used. The precipitin arcs are denatured with glacial acetic acid, and the agar is evaporated to a film and stained to provide a permanent record. Reports are usually interpretive and may be accompanied by photographs of the precipitin arcs.

Interpretation. Paraproteins have characteristic skewing of precipitin arcs rather than the smooth symmetric appearance of a heterogeneous population of molecules. The abnormal immunoglobulin is usually present to the exclusion of the normal, and the presence of a single light-chain type identifies it as monoclonal, as summarized in Table 38–2. A heavy-chain paraprotein without light chains defines heavy-chain disease. Monoclonal light chains without heavy chain is seen in light-chain myeloma. The association of serum paraproteins with urinary Bence-Jones protein is seen in Table 38–4. Seventy-five percent of paraproteins are IgG, 15% IgA, 10% light-chain only, <1% IgD, and rarely, IgE. Approximately 70% of IgG myelomas are G-kappa and 30% are G-lambda, which does not appear to be of clinical significance in prognosis. Kappa and lambda chains are equally divided in other classes. In light-chain myeloma, however, the lambda-chain variant has a worse prognosis leading to early renal failure.

Table 38–4   Patterns of Abnormal Serum and Urine Proteins in Immunoproliferative Disorders

Disease	Occurrence of Serum Protein Constituents	Occurrence Urine BJ Protein in Pattern Category
Multiple myeloma		
Myeloma globulin only	50%	No BJ protein
Myeloma globulin + BJ protein	20%	60% in IgG myeloma 70% in IgA myeloma 100% in IgD myeloma
BJ protein only	20%–30%	100% in light chain
No myeloma globulin	<1%	No BJ protein
Macroglobulinemia	10%	40%

ABBREVIATION: BJ = Bence-Jones.

Notes and Precautions.   Antigen excess produces prozones with antibody that are soluble and may wash away during processing, producing false-negative results.

Immunoelectrophoresis should not be performed without concurrent standard electrophoresis as a guide to amount and location of the abnormal protein. Routine electrophoresis serves as a guide to specimen dilution needed for testing to avoid prozones.

38.4   Serum Immunoglobulin Quantitation

Purpose.   Immunoglobulin quantitation alone has limited usefulness in immunoproliferative malignancy, as opposed to immunodeficiency disorders. It may be confirmatory in interpretation of immunoelectrophoresis.

Principle.   Usually quantitated in serum only, measurement of immunoglobulins G, A, M, and D is widely available by rate nephelometry. Soluble immune complexes formed by specific antisera with the immunoglobulin (antigen) in a dilute solution scatters incident light at 450 to 550 nm. The amount of light scatter is dependent on the size of the complex and time. Early in the reaction complexes are too small to scatter light, but as the reaction proceeds the antiserum is consumed, the rate of increase in scatter slows, and the amount of light scatter is maximal. The scatter at this point is proportional to antigen concentration. Protein range of measurement is 10 to 200 g/L (1 mg/dl to 20 g/dl). IgE is present in such small amounts that it is measured by RIA. Quantitation of light chains is not currently available. Older techniques of immunodiffusion are slow and less accurate.

Specimen. Five microliters of serum are used.

Procedure. Specific antisera are mixed with serum or urine at a series of fixed dilutions. A background measurement is taken when the patient's specimen is added, and the rate of increase in light scatter is measured. A microprocessor calculates the concentration of immunoglobulin. If the rate of complex formation is outside the measuring range, the next dilution is assayed automatically. At the end of reaction calibrator serum is added to detect antigen excess and thus avoid falsely low results due to prozone effect.

Interpretation. Immunoglobulin concentration is age dependent but, since immunoproliferative malignancies are diseases of adults, normal values are:

Immunoglobulin	Normal Range
IgG	8 to 12 g/L (800 to 1200 mg/dl) + 2 SD
IgA	1.8 to 4.8 g/L (180 to 480 mg/dl)
IgM	0.5 to 1.5 g/L (50 to 150 mg/dl)
IgD	.03 g/L (3 mg/dl)
IgE	.003 g/L (.3 mg/dl)

In multiple myeloma, one globulin will be 5 to 10 times the normal concentration with characteristic decreases in the others. Quantitation with abnormal electrophoretic pattern is partial evidence of paraprotein, but quantitation cannot establish the protein as monoclonal.

Notes and Precautions. Immunodiffusion of saline-diluted specimens, particularly for IgM, is often not linear with concentration and may give extraordinary values beyond those quantitated on electrophoresis. For this reason nephelometric techniques are preferred over immunodiffusion.

38.5   Serum Immunofixation

Purpose.   In some cases the monoclonal protein is associated with large amounts of residual normal protein which may obscure the expected abnormal arc in IEP. This is particularly true for light chains. Immunofixation may clarify the pattern.

Principle.   The patient's serum sample is subjected to electrophoresis to separate protein zones. The migration path is overlaid with membranes soaked in specific antibody to each immunoglobulin. The test can be applied to CSF and to urine concentrates as well.

Specimen.   Serum may be diluted so that the protein of interest is approximately 0.5 g/L (50 mg/dl).

Procedure.   Serum is inoculated into a series of wells in a supporting thin-layer gel or a cellulose acetate membrane and electrophoresed for 1 hour. Strips of cellulose acetate soaked in anti-IgG, -IgA, -IgM, -kappa, and -lambda are applied over the separate migration paths and allowed to diffuse for 1 hour. Antigen-antibody recognition results in immune precipitates on the supporting membrane. These are rinsed of excess reactants, fixed in glacial acetic acid, and stained. Prepared kits are available, and the test is not difficult to perform.

Interpretation.   A sharp narrow band indicates a monoclonal population, whereas a broad blurred band is consistent with polyclonality. Oligoclonal protein bands are more obvious than on standard electrophoresis, even in the presence of residual normal polyclonal immunoglobulin.

Notes and Precautions.   The concentration of antigen to antibody is much more critical in this technique. Complexes with antibody excess may be lost with the rinse procedure, and abnormal bands may not always be detected.

38.6   Sedimentation Rate

The sedimentation rate is retarded if anemia is severe, and increased when fibrinogen or immunoglobulins are increased. Corrected sedimentation rates are not helpful. The normal range is 0 to 20 mm/h for females and 0 to 10 mm/h for males. Sedimentation rates greater than 100 mm/h are rarely seen in any disease except myeloma. Light-chain myeloma may have a normal sedimentation rate.

38.7   Serum Viscosity

Purpose.   Tests for serum viscosity are used to estimate clinical risk of thrombosis or bleeding in IgM or IgA paraproteinemia and to assess the need for plasmapheresis. It is used to evaluate therapy as well. It should be ordered whenever a patient with paraproteinemia exhibits visual or CNS symptoms, or has a bleeding diathesis.

Principle.   Normal serum or plasma has a viscosity only slightly greater than water. With marked paraproteinemia of large molecules, such as IgM, or of molecules that conjugate easily with others, such as IgA, marked increases may be seen in serum viscosity. Such increases are often temperature dependent, with cryoglobulins or cryofibrinogens causing gelling of plasma or serum at room temperature or below. Increased viscosity leads to dilatation and sludging of retinal vessels with resultant blindness. Larger vessel thrombosis in limbs leads to Raynaud's phenomenon or cutaneous gangrene; coating of platelets is associated with bleeding. When viscosity is increased markedly it can be relieved by mechanical removal of the plasma by plasmapheresis.

Specimen.   Blood is obtained at 37° C and plasma or serum or both are removed. Serum can be stored in a refrigerator once separated from red cells. Whole blood should not be refrigerated since it may gel in the presence of cryoglobulins or cryofibrinogens.

Procedure.   Serum or plasma is allowed to flow through glass tubes of narrow diameter, Ostwald viscometers, and the flow between 2 etched lines is timed. Flow rate is compared with that of water, and a serum:water ratio is calculated. Ratios are obtained at 37° C, room temperature, and 4° C.

Interpretation.   The normal serum:water ratio is 1.0 to 1.7. Significant elevations are ratios greater than 8 at 37° C. The increase in ratio at room temperature or at 4° C for serum indicates that cryoglobulins are present, and increased ratios with plasma indicate that cryofibrinogen, and possibly cryoglobulin, are present as well. The presence of cryoproteins is of significance in plasmapheresis, which may use a cold centrifuge. Although hyperviscosity is characteristic of IgM, it is also seen with IgA paraproteins, which tend to polymerize easily.

38.8   Tests of Renal Function

Purpose.   Tests of renal function that document decreasing renal function suggest myeloma kidney or amyloid. Light chains that circulate as polymers are more likely to cause amyloid deposition. Deposition in glomerular mesangium and in renal tubular epithelium leads to renal failure, which is the cause of death in 30% of cases. Serum creatinine is an accurate measure of glomerular function, so tests for serum creatinine and creatinine clearance are performed.

Interpretation.   Serum creatinine may be mildly elevated (260 μmol/L or 3.0 mg/dl), an unfavorable prognostic sign. With decreased renal clearance, Bence-Jones protein is retained and appears as small spikes in serum electrophoresis.

38.9   Serum Calcium Quantitation

Purpose.   Tests for serum calcium are of therapeutic interest in myeloma, since hypercalcemia can be related to lethargy or cardiac arrhythmias. Hypercalcemia occurs in 30% of patients with myeloma, possibly because of osteoclast-activating factor. Occasionally hypercalcemia provokes no clinical symptoms because ionized calcium remains normal due to binding of calcium to the variable region of the monoclonal protein. Because myeloma bone disease is osteolytic, tests for increased bone formation, eg, alkaline phosphatase, are not helpful.

Interpretation.   The normal range for serum calcium is 9 to 11 mg/dl (2.24 to 2.74 mmol/L). Hypercalcemia is usually associated with BJ proteinuria. Clinical symptoms of lethargy or arrhythmia appear above values of 3.5 mmol/L.

38.10   Beta-2-Microglobulin

Purpose.   The level of beta-2-microglobulin increases in proportion to the tumor burden and may be helpful in prognosis and in evaluating disease progression.

Principle.   Beta-2-microglobulinemia (MW 12000) is synthesized by all nucleated cells and is normally found unbound in plasma in low concentrations (2 μg/mL). It is elevated in lymphoproliferative disorders when the tumor burden is increased or there is rapid cell multiplication.

Specimen.   The specimen consists of serum.

Procedure.   Beta-2-microglobulin is measured by RIA or ELISA techniques and is available from many reference laboratories.

Interpretation.   Values above 6 μg/mL in multiple myeloma indicate a poor prognosis. The correlation with other lymphoproliferative disorders has not been well established as yet. Since beta-2-microglobulin excretion depends on renal function, plasma levels may be elevated in renal failure of any cause, and clinical prognosis should then be made with caution.

38.11   Bone Roentgenograms

Bone roentgenograms show osteolytic lesions in the skull, ribs, vertebrae, and long bones in IgG or IgA myeloma. Early disease may show osteoporosis initially, and light-chain myeloma is often associated with diffuse osteoporosis. Other imaging techniques and scintiscans do not demonstrate lytic lesions well, but computed tomographic (CT) scans may identify myeloma infiltrates when roentgenograms are normal in patients with severe bone pain.

38.12   Chromosome Analysis

Pre–B-cell malignancies and plasma cell dyscrasias are frequently associated with translocation, involving chromosome t(11;14)(q13; q32). Finding such a marker supports the diagnosis of a neoplastic monoclonal protein. The analyses are available at reference laboratories and in some large hospitals.

38.13   Gene Rearrangement

In the absence of secreted monoclonal protein or membrane phenotypic markers, one can document monoclonicity by gene rearrangement. The test is available in a few reference laboratories.

Special Diagnostic Considerations

Of the related plasma cell dyscrasias, macroglobulinemia is much less common, and heavy-chain disease is rare. The initial diagnostic approach is as outlined earlier for myeloma. A few specific comments can be made regarding these less common diseases. Clinical findings are outlined in Tables 38–4 and 38–5.

Macroglobulinemia

Waldenström's macroglobulinemia is a lymphoplasmacytic infiltrate of marrow and lymph nodes with production of an IgM paraprotein. Bone roentgenograms usually show osteoporosis. There is a normochromic anemia with marked rouleaux formation. Late in the disease lymphoma cells appear in the peripheral blood. The bone marrow is hypercellular and often replaced by lymphocytes. Serum proteins show modest spikes in the beta or beta-gamma zone. The IgM paraproteins are often cold agglutinins of anti-I specificity, and there is associated cold AIHA. Cryoglobulin or cryofibrinogen may also be present, and the paraprotein may have rheumatoid factor activity. Because of its molecular size, IgM paraprotein does not usually appear in the urine, although its unconjugated light chains appear in 30% to 40% of cases.

Macroglobulinemia is associated frequently with hyperviscosity producing retinal vein thrombosis and central nervous system symptoms. Coagulation studies indicate defects in platelet function, possibly as a result of coating by paraprotein, inhibition of coagulation Factors II, V, VII, or VIII, and abnormalities in fibrin monomer polymerization. The resulting bleeding diathesis may be seen as purpura, mucosal bleeding, or retinal hemorrhages.

Treatment is directed at correcting hyperviscosity symptoms and treating the underlying lymphoproliferative disorder. Plasmapheresis is helpful in removing IgM paraprotein.

Heavy-Chain Disease

Heavy-chain diseases are a varied group manifesting a paraprotein of heavy chain only, due to deletions at the hinge region that intererfere with light-chain attachment or to a failure in light-chain synthesis or both. There are four variants of heavy-chain disease; gamma HCD, alpha HCD, mu HCD, and delta HCD. Epsilon HCD, although postulated, has not been found as yet.

Gamma HCD may end in lymphoma; 60% of patients have hepatosplenomegaly and lymphadenopathy. Lymph node histologic

Table 38–5   Characteristics of Heavy-Chain Disease

Class[a]	Serum Electrophoresis	Urine BJ
γ Heavy Chain Disease (70)	Broad-based, fast γ or β, IgA, IgM not decreased	IEP mirror image of serum IEP
μ Heavy Chain Disease (15)	May be normal or small beta spike; μ and κ chains separate	κ chain
α Heavy Chain Disease (120)	Smudged broad α₂-β band	No α chain
δ Heavy Chain Disease (1)	β-γ peak	None

ABBREVIATIONS: IEP = immunoelectrophoresis; CLL = chronic lymphocytic leukemia; BJ = Bence-Jones protein.

[a]Number of cases appear in parentheses

findings may be extremely variable. The serum protein electrophoresis may not show any abnormality and the paraprotein may only be seen on immunoelectrophoresis (IEP). Alpha HCD disease appears in younger individuals of the Mediterranean area, and is manifested by lymphomatous mucosal infiltrates in the small intestine and severe malabsorption syndrome. Respiratory lymphoplasmacytosis has appeared in some cases in Europe and the United States. A few patients have entered remission on antibiotic therapy with and without chemotherapy. Mu HCD rarely shows an abnormal electrophoretigram although the IEP is abnormal. Bence-Jones proteinuria is common. Clinical disease resembles chronic lymphocytic leukemia (CLL). Delta HCD was similar to myeloma with osteolytic bone lesions in the only case reported.

Course and Treatment

Plasma Cell Leukemia.   Plasma cell leukemia can occur de novo or as the terminal event in a patient with previously diagnosed multiple myeloma. The diagnostic criteria include: the presence of

Blood	Bone Marrow	Other Tissue
Atypical lymphs, pancytopenia, eosinophilia	Nondiagnostic, pleomorphic with lymphoplasmacytosis	Lymphadenopathy of nonspecific histology
CLL	70%–80% lymphocytes; few plasma cells	Amyloid
—	Slight decrease in plasma cells	Small intestine lymphoma Respiratory lymphoplasmacytosis
—	Plasmacytosis	Osteolytic lesions

>20% plasma cells in the peripheral blood or an absolute lymphocytosis exceeding 2000/μL; evidence of cellular monoclonality; and radiographic evidence of skeletal disease or bone marrow involvement. Incidence of plasma cell leukemia is approximately 2%. Patients with plasma cell leukemia have a greater degree of tissue infiltration, an advanced stage of disease, and a poor survival. The patients are more likely to have hypercalsemia or renal failure, or both.

Clinical course is dependent on tumor cell mass and associated systemic symptoms, eg, fever, weight loss, azotemia. Survival in cases with fever in the absence of infection or greater than 10% weight loss may be less than 1 year. Survival is also dependent on immunoglobulin class, shortest in IgD myeloma or lambda light-chain disease (<1 year) to 3 or 4 years in IgM macroglobulinemia and IgG myeloma. A small proportion of patients develop AML following chemotherapy for the myeloma. Death is usually due to infection or renal failure.

Treatment has remained unchanged in recent years and consists of chemotherapy with melphelan or prednisone. Supportive therapy includes antibiotic therapy, dialysis, and plasmapheresis. The latter is most successful for monoclonal proteins that remain intravascular due to their larger molecular configuration, eg, IgM macroglobulinemia and IgA myeloma.

References

1. Bataille R, Grenier J, Sanej J: Beta$_2$-microglobulin in myeloma: Optimal use for staging, prognosis, and treatment: A prospective study of 160 patients. *Blood* 1984; 63:468–476.

2. Check I, Piper M: Quantitation of immunoglobulins, in Rose NR, Friedman H, Fahey JL (eds): *Manual of Clinical Immunology,* ed 3. Washington, DC, American Society of Microbiology, 1986, pp 138–151.

3. Davey FR, Kurec AS: Multiple myeloma, in Gambino SR (ed): American Society of Clinical Pathologists Check Sample No. H85-1, 1985.

4. Dick FR: Plasma cell myeloma and related disorders with monoclonal gammopathy, in Koepke JA (ed) *Laboratory Hematology.* New York, Churchill Livingstone, 1984, pp 445–481.

5. Johnson AM: Immunoprecipitation in gels, in Rose NR, Friedman H, Fahey JL (eds): *Manual of Clinical Immunology,* ed 3. Washington, DC, American Society of Microbiology, 1986, pp 21–24.

6. Kyle RA, Greip PR: Multiple myeloma and the monoclonal gammopathies, in Fairbanks VF (ed): *Current Hematology.* New York, John Wiley & Sons, 1981, pp 470–522.

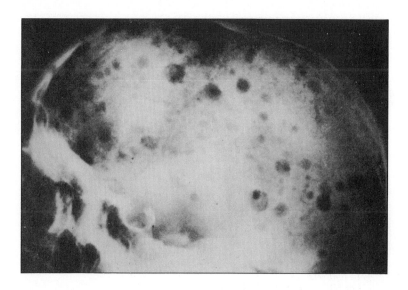

Figure 38–2   Osteolytic lesions in a skull x-ray seen most frequently in IgG and IgA myeloma.

Figure 38–3   Peripheral smear rouleaux formation in patient with myeloma.

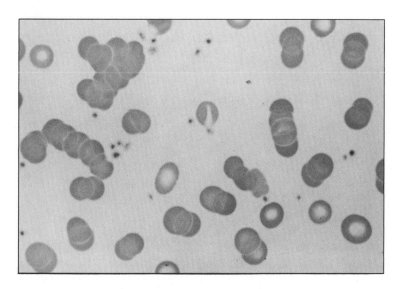

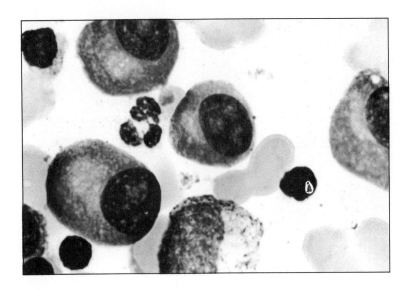

Figure 38–4   Immature plasma cells in bone marrow aspirate. Reverse pinocytosis is seen at cell edge and abnormal protein is deposited in the background.

Figure 38–5   Bone marrow aspirate showing plasma cells labeled with fluorescein-conjugated anti-kappa.

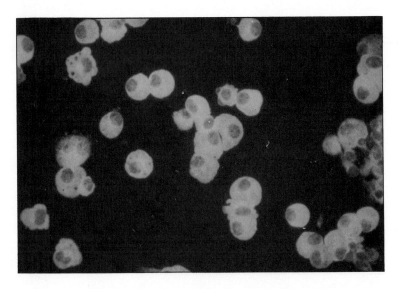

39

Other Disorders Associated with Monoclonal Gammopathy

Several disorders (other than those discussed in chapter 38) may be associated with monoclonal gammopathy. These include benign monoclonal gammopathy, secondary monoclonal gammopathies, cryoglobulinemia, and amyloidosis (Table 39–1).

Pathophysiology

Normal immune mechanisms involve interaction between monocytes or macrophages and subpopulations of lymphocytes; B-lymphocytes undergo blast transformation and mitotic division to produce clones of plasma cells producing a spectrum of immunoglobulins (Igs), both monoclonal and polyclonal. Immunoglobulin production begins in the endoplasmic reticulum with cytoplasmic production of IgM and IgD. As the cell matures to a B-lymphocyte, membrane IgD is lost and the cell secretes IgM. With antigenic stimulation, lymphocytes make a transition to mature plasma cells with secretion of IgG, IgA, or IgM.

In benign monoclonal gammopathy there is secretion of a paraprotein without evidence of plasma cell dyscrasia or other specific clinical disorder. The protein is produced by a clone of plasma cells reaching finite size, but remaining stable for as many as 10 years. Benign monoclonal gammopathy is seen increasingly with age, present in 1% of patients over 50 years of age, 3% of patients 70

Table 39–1   Immunoproliferative Disorders

Benign monoclonal gammopathy

Secondary monoclonal gammopathy

  Metastatic cancer

    Breast
    Prostate
    Colon
    Lung
    Biliary tract

  Collagen-vascular disease

    Rheumatoid arthritis
    Systemic lupus erythematosus

  Infectious disease

    Tuberculosis
    Osteomyelitis
    Pyelonephritis
    Cytomegalovirus

  Liver disease

    Cirrhosis
    Hepatitis

  Hematologic disease

    Autoimmune hemolytic anemia
    Spherocytosis
    Pernicious anemia
    Hodgkin's disease

  Metabolic disease

    Gaucher's disease
    Osteoporosis

  Skin disease

    Pyoderma gangrenosum
    Familial xanthomatosis

  Amyloidosis

    Primary (idiopathic)
    Secondary
    Myeloma-associated
    Familial

  Cryoglobulinemia

    Type I–III

years of age, and up to 10% of patients 80 years of age and older. The paraprotein is usually IgG but may be IgA or IgM, or very rarely, kappa or lambda chains. Benign monoclonal gammopathy is characterized by a monoclonal spike less than 3.0 g/dL without Bence-Jones proteinuria. Though no morphologic mass lesion is seen, monoclonal plasma cells may be identified in the bone marrow. There is also a mild increase in plasma cells, and multiple myeloma occurs in 5% to 10% of cases. Thus benign monoclonal gammopathy may be a premyelomatous process analogous to preleukemia.

Secondary monoclonal gammopathy is associated with chronic infection or inflammation, and with certain tumors, and is most often associated with rheumatoid arthritis. The cause of the paraprotein is unknown, but antibody to tumor antigens or product of cancer cells has been suggested. The protein may be merely coincidental in elderly patients.

Amyloidosis is the tissue deposition of linear, nonbranching, hollow fibrils. Although the chemical composition of these fibrils may vary, their ultrastructure is the same. Amyloid fibers composed of immunoglobulin light chains, or, more commonly, their amino terminal fragments, are designated AL, and those composed of amyloid A, protein AA. The latter circulates in serum complexed to high-density lipoprotein and is a degraded form of an acute phase-reactant protein produced in the liver in response to inflammatory cytokines. Its level fluctuates with chronic inflammation or infection. Only occasionally is the serum AA deposited in tissue as amyloid. AL protein is produced in association with multiple myeloma. In some familial forms and senile cardiac amyloid, the precursor may be prealbumin.

Amyloidosis can be classified as primary (idiopathic) or secondary (associated with chronic inflammation or infection), and a type associated with myeloma that is similar to the primary type. Secondary-type amyloidosis, unlike the idiopathic or myeloma type, is not associated with an M-protein.

Cryoglobulins may be either cryofibrinogen or cryoglobulin with cryoglobulin the more common and clinically important. They are associated with chronic inflammation and lymphoplasmacytic disorders. They should not be confused with cold agglutinins, which, by definition, have red cell antibody activity.

Clinical Findings

Patients with benign monoclonal gammopathy are asymptomatic. Patients with secondary monoclonal proteins have symptoms of the underlying disorder (Table 39–2). Twenty percent of patients with

Table 39–2   Classification and Localization of Amyloidosis

Classification	Major Protein Component	Organ Involvement	Laboratory Finding
Primary amyloidosis	AL	Renal tubules, heart, tongue, skeletal muscle, GI tract, ligaments, nerve, skin	BJ proteinuria
Amyloidosis with myeloma	AL	Kidney, heart, GI tract	BJ proteinuria, other paraproteinuria
Secondary amyloidosis	AA	Renal glomeruli spleen, liver, adrenals	No BJ proteinuria
Familial amyloidosis	AFp		
Localized amyloidosis	AL	Lung, bladder, skin, larynx	No BJ proteinuria

ABBREVIATIONS: AL = amyloid light chain; AA = amyloid protein A; AFp = amyloid familial pre-albumin; BJ = Bence-Jones.

benign monoclonal gammopathy progress to myeloma after 8 to 10 years.

Primary amyloidosis has no evidence of preceding disease, whereas amyloidosis with multiple myeloma appears at approximately the same time as the myeloma, although it can precede the disease by several months. Clinical symptoms in primary and myeloma-associated amyloidoses vary with the specific organ involved: tongue (macroglossia), heart (congestive heart failure), kidney (renal failure), skin (purpura), ligaments (carpal tunnel syndrome), gastrointestinal tract (bleeding). Secondary amyloidosis is seen in chronic inflammation eg, tuberculosis, osteomyelitis, and is frequently associated with rheumatoid arthritis (10% to 15%). In secondary amyloidosis no monoclonal protein is found in either serum or urine, although there is usually proteinuria. Amyloid infiltrates liver, spleen, kidney, and adrenal glands causing enlargement, pressure atrophy, and organ failure. There may be nephrotic syndrome, malabsorption, or peripheral neuropathy.

Cryoglobulins are created by antibody complexes (IgG and IgM) and may produce ischemic symptoms when the protein gels in response to lowered body temperature. Occlusion of vessels in the extremities may cause Raynaud's phenomenon (50%), vascular purpura (60%) or cold urticaria, arthralgia or arthritis (20%). Cryofibrinogen is not clinically significant, and proteins that gel serum with heat (pyroglobulins) are also of no significance. Single component monoclonal cryoglobulinemia (type I) is either idiopathic or linked to a clonal immunoglobulin disorder (multiple myeloma, Waldenström's macroglobulinemia). Mixed monoclonal cryoglobulinemia (type II) and mixed polyclonal cryoglobulinemia (type III) are found in association with autoimmune disorders and connective tissue disorders.

Approach to Diagnosis

Benign monoclonal gammopathy is a diagnosis of exclusion of myeloma. Amyloidosis should be considered and excluded when myeloma is associated with early renal failure, when IgD or light-chain myeloma is present, and when multiorgan failure or cardiomyopathy are present in patients with a history of chronic inflammatory disease.

1. Hematologic measurements may be normal or may show mild to moderate normochromic anemia.

2. Bone marrow aspiration is necessary to exclude myeloma when a paraprotein is present. A plasma cell infiltrate supports the diagnosis of myeloma and possibly myeloma-associated amyloidosis.

3. Protein and urine electrophoresis screens for monoclonal bands confirmed as to immunoglobulin class by IEP.

4. Urinary IEP is used to identify Bence-Jones protein which is supportive of malignant immunoproliferative disorders or myeloma amyloidosis. No Bence-Jones protein is found in secondary amyloidosis or in benign monoclonal gammopathy.

5. Screening tests are performed for cryoglobulin, which can be roughly quantitated by cryocrit.

6. Radiolabeling index, gene rearrangement studies and chromosome analysis may be useful in differentiating benign monoclonal gammopathy and myeloma (Table 39–3).

7. Tissue biopsy with Congo red staining for amyloid is needed to document the disease. Electron microscopic study will identify the characteristic fibrils.

Table 39–3 Laboratory Findings in Malignant v Benign
Monoclonal Gammopathy

	Malignant	Benign
Anemia	2+	0
Bone marrow plasma cells	3+	<5%
Plasma cell morphology	Normal to abnormal	Normal
Bone lesions	Osteolytic or osteoporosis	None
M protein concentration	>3.0 g/dL	<2.0 g/dL
M protein concentration stability	Increase	Stable >5 years
Concentration of uninvolved Igs	Strong decrease	Normal or slight decrease
Serum albumin	Decrease	Normal
Urine monoclonal protein	+ in 75% of cases	None
Plasma cell labeling index H³	Increase	Normal
Gene rearrangement	Monoclonal	Normal
Chromosome analysis	t 11;14	Normal

Hematologic Findings

Hepatosplenomegaly is seen in both idiopathic and myeloma associated amyloidosis. Lymphadenopathy is uncommon. Benign monoclonal gammopathy is not associated with lymphadenopathy or hepatosplenomegaly. Benign monoclonal gammopathy is characterized by monoclonal spikes <3.0 g/dL, without proteinuria. Cryoglobulinemia may be associated with anemia in association with myeloma or macroglobulinemia.

Blood Cell Measurements. Mild normochromic anemia is present in cryoglobulinemia and amyloidosis. Leukocyte counts are normal as are platelet counts. Thrombocytopenia may be due to hypersplenism in amyloidosis.

Peripheral Blood Cell Morphology.   No morphologic abnormalities.

Bone Marrow Examination.   There may be mild plasmacytosis with cryoglobulinemia. In MGUS plasma cells are scattered and less than 5%.

Bone X-Rays.   No abnormalities except those due to primary disease in secondary amyloidosis. Amyloidosis itself can involve bone.

Other Laboratory Tests

39.1   Urine and Serum Protein Electrophoresis

Purpose.   Protein electrophoresis is a screening procedure used to detect monoclonal bands. The clinical significance and course of the disease depends more on the presence of urine paraproteins.

Principle, Specimen, and Procedure.   See Tests 38.1 and 38.2.

Interpretation.   Serum paraprotein in benign monoclonal gammopathy is <3.0 g/dL. The level should remain stable over 5 to 10 years. Urine monoclonal proteins are very unlikely to be present in benign monoclonal gammopathy. Bence-Jones proteinuria is present in renal amyloidosis in primary or myeloma-associated disease.

39.2   Urine and Serum Immunoelectrophoresis

Purpose.   Characterization of paraproteins is helpful in determining the significance and course of paraproteins found on serum or urine protein electrophoresis. Cryoglobulins can be removed from serum and studied.

Specimen.   Cryoglobulins are allowed to gel in serum at 4° C, removed, rinsed free of other serum proteins in saline, and redissolved at 37° C.

Procedure. The dissolved cryoglobulin is treated as serum in a standard IEP procedure (see Test 38.3).

Interpretation. Characterization of cryoglobulin as monoclonal or polyclonal may be helpful in the diagnosis of the underlying disease, but has little influence on the clinical course or treatment in and of itself.

Light-chain proteinuria, particularly lambda light chain is strong support for clinically suspected renal amyloidosis. The presence of paraproteinuria or paraproteinemia is evidence against secondary amyloidosis. Benign monoclonal gammopathy does not have paraproteinuria; the presence of paraproteinuria indicates further studies should be done to exclude myeloma.

39.3   Evaluation of Cryoprecipitable Proteins

Purpose. The presence of cryoproteins may support the diagnosis of benign or malignant disease.

Principle. Serum or plasma is separated from specimens that have been maintained at 37° C. The cryoprecipitated protein can be removed from serum (cryoglobulin) or from plasma (cryofibrinogen), redissolved by warming, and then identified by immunoelectrophoresis as is done for paraproteins. The cryoprotein is categorized as type I, II, or III depending on whether it is polyclonal or monoclonal, and whether it appears as more than one immunoglobulin class. The cryoprecipitable protein can be roughly quantitated by cryocrit.

Specimen. Serum or plasma is separated from a clot or EDTA blood sample maintained at 37° C.

Procedure. For a cryocrit an aliquot of serum or plasma is placed in a Westergren tube as for a sedimentation rate, chilled in an ice water bath, and kept refrigerated for 8 to 12 hours. The cryoprecipitate is measured in millimeters. The tube is then warmed to 37° C; a true cryoprecipitate should return to solution. The cryoprecipitate can be removed from the serum or plasma with orange sticks or the supernatant normal serum/plasma aspirated and discarded. The precipitate can be rinsed in iced saline to remove nonprecipitating proteins and the separately redissolved precipitate inoculated as for serum in immunoelectrophoresis. The protein is tested against anti-IgM,

-IgA, -IgG, -kappa, -lambda, and -fibrinogen. The cryoprotein can be tested for rheumatoid factor (RF) activity.

Interpretation.   Cryoglobulins >3 mm may be clinically significant. Normal patients may have transient cryoglobulins in trace amounts associated with infection.

Type I cryoglobulinemia is monoclonal: only one light chain is present; it is associated with lymphoproliferative disorders and multiple myeloma.

Type II cryoglobulinemia is mixed: monoclonal IgM having RF activity, usually IgM-kappa, and polyclonal IgG. This type is seen in Waldenström's macroglobulinemia, chronic active hepatitis, or essential mixed cryoglobulinemia.

Type III cryoglobulinemia is mixed: polyclonal IgM with RF activity is present with polyclonal IgG. This is the most common type, and is seen in autoimmune disease and infectious disease such as latent syphilis.

Types II and III cryoproteins that contain antigen-antibody complexes are seen in systemic lupus erythematosus (SLE).

Ancillary Procedures

Tissue Biopsy for Amyloid.   In suspected amyloidosis it is useful to document the tissue infiltration by amyloid.

Amyloid fibrils refract light in a characteristic pattern. In addition, the P component can be demonstrated with stains for glycoprotein eg, PAS, crystal violet, methyl violet.

Rectal biopsy material is the easiest to obtain, but must be fairly deep to include submucosa. Although the liver can be biopsied when hepatomegaly is present, there is risk of infection and bleeding. Renal biopsy also has attendant risks of bleeding, but may be necessary in renal failure. A bone marrow biopsy may be useful for detecting amyloid.

Surgical specimens from release of carpal tunnel syndrome should be submitted for amyloid stains.

Biopsy specimens may be fixed in formalin.

Hematoxylin-eosin staining shows amorphous eosinophilic deposits in biopsy tissue. Confirmation studies are performed by Congo red stain, which yields a greenish birefringence under polarized light. Crystal or methyl violet also stain para-amyloids a brilliant purple color with normal light.

Amyloid is usually seen in blood vessel walls of the rectal biopsy. In AL amyloid renal tubules may show amyloid whereas in AA the glomerular mesangium is more often involved.

Negative studies do not exclude the diagnosis of amyloidosis.

Course and Treatment

Benign monoclonal gammopathy progresses to myeloma in 8 to 10 years in 10% of cases. The remaining cases remain stable. Follow-up studies in stable patients should be performed annually to quantitate their proteins, and more frequently if clinical symptoms appear. In those patients with myeloma, the standard treatment is melphelan and prednisone.

Amyloidosis associated with myeloma greatly shortens the course of that disease to less than 6 months. Primary amyloidosis produces progressive irreversible deposition of amyloid with death from renal failure or cardiac failure in less than 18 months. Secondary amyloidosis has a clinical course determined by the underlying disease; in chronic infection it has, on rare occasions, been partially reversible with successful treatment of the infection.

Cryoglobulinemia is usually not progressive, the underlying disease determining the course. In some cases, however, ischemic ulceration of skin or gangrene occurs requiring surgical intervention. Plasmapheresis is occasionally successful in altering clinical symptoms; success of the procedure is monitored by measuring the cryocrit.

References

1. Buxbaum J. The amyloidoses: I. Biochemistry of the amyloid proteins. *Lab Management* 1987; 18:38–42.

2. Glenner GC: Amyloid deposits and amyloidosis: The fibrilloses, parts 1 and 2. *N Engl J Med* 1980; 302:1283–1292, 1333–1343.

3. Lichtman M: Classification of lymphocyte and plasma disorders, in Williams W, Beutler E, Erslev AJ, et al (eds): *Hematology*, ed 3. New York, McGraw-Hill International Book Co, 1983, pp 934–935.

4. Lichtman M: Benign monoclonal gammopathy, in Williams W, Beutler E, Erslev AJ, et al (eds): *Hematology*, ed 3. New York, McGraw-Hill International Book Co, 1983, pp 966–969.

5. Osserman EF, Merlini G, Butler VP Jr: Multiple myeloma and related plasma cell dyscrasias. *JAMA* 1987; 258:2930–2937.

6. Salmon SE (ed): Myeloma and related disorders. *Clinics in Hematology*, vol 11, no 1. London, WB Saunders Co Ltd, 1982.

7. Winfield JB: Cryoglobulinemia. *Hum Pathol* 1983; 14:350–354.

PART 12

Bleeding Disorders

40

Diagnosis of Bleeding Disorders

Some bleeding disorders, whether acquired or congenital, can be so severe as to be incapacitating and others are so mild that excessive bleeding is manifested only following surgery or trauma; the majority fall between these two extremes. As a general rule, the more severe disorders are almost invariably more of a therapeutic than a diagnostic problem, while the reverse is true of the milder cases.

Pathophysiology

The initial or primary events that stop bleeding from a very small wound are the formation of a platelet plug, which seals the hole in the vessel wall, and arteriolar vasoconstriction. The plug is subsequently fortified by fibrin strands. Exposure to subendothelial components and collagen is believed to be the stimulus that causes the platelets to aggregate and form the primary plug. Aggregation is probably dependent on the von Willebrand factor and other plasma factors, such as ADP released from lysed red cells or platelets after exposure to collagen. A defect in one of these plasma factors, a qualitative defect in platelets, thrombocytopenia, or a defect in the vascular wall can result in failure of the primary hemostatic mechanism, causing spontaneous bleeding or purpura.

The formation of fibrin proceeds in a stepwise manner referred

Figure 40–1   Modified cascade or waterfall mechanism of blood coagulation. Bypass and inhibitory mechanisms are not shown for the sake of simplicity. PL indicates phospholipid; HMW-K, high-molecular-weight kininogen.

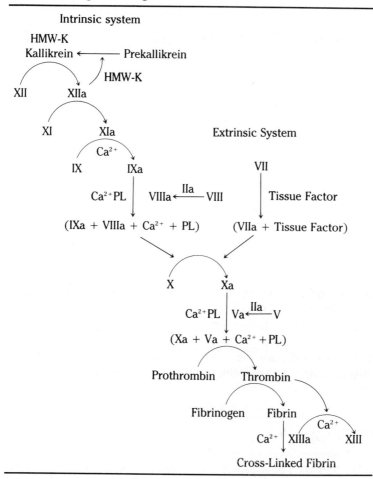

to as a cascade or waterfall (Figure 40–1). Blood clotting in vitro is initiated by contact of the blood with a foreign surface, such as glass or kaolin. The factors involved in this early contact phase are factors XII and XI, high–molecular-weight kininogen (HMW-K), and Fletcher factor (Table 40–1). Even patients with severe deficiencies of these factors, however, with the exception of some patients with factor XI deficiency, are completely asymptomatic. There are several possible explanations for this. For example, the complex of activated factor VII and tissue factor can activate factor IX, thereby bypassing the contact phase, but the physiological significance of this and other bypass mechanisms is unclear.

Table 40-1   The Contact Factors

Preferred Term	Synonyms
XII	Hageman factor
XI	Plasma thromboplastin antecedent
Prekallikrein	Fletcher factor
HMW-K	High molecular weight kininogen; Fitzgerald, Williams, Flaujeac factors

Table 40-2   The Vitamin K–Dependent Clotting Factors

Preferred Term	Synonyms
Prothrombin	II
VII	Proconvertin
IX	Christmas factor, plasma thromboplastin component
X	Stuart, Prower factors

Table 40-3   The Thrombin-Sensitive Factors

Preferred Term	Synonyms
Fibrinogen	I
V	Proaccelerin, accelerator globulin
VIII	Antihemophilic factor, VIIIc, antihemophilic globulin
XIII	Fibrin stabilizing factor, Laki-Lorand factor

Defective synthesis of any of the other factors shown in Tables 40-2 and 40-3 may give rise to a bleeding disorder, the two most common of which are hemophilias A and B, which are attributable to a deficiency of factors VIII and IX, respectively.

Clinical Findings

Purpura is not directly attributable to trauma and is characterized by the type of bleeding seen in severe thrombocytopenia. Such bleeding differs from that resulting from defective fibrin formation, which is referred to as the coagulation or hemophilioid type. The main clinical characteristics of the two types of bleeding are shown in Table 40-4.

It is not unusual to find severe acquired or hereditary abnormalities in clotting tests of patients who have never bled excessively, even after challenges such as major surgery. More rarely, some patients clearly have a bleeding tendency, yet the abnormality cannot be detected by currently available tests.

Approach to Diagnosis

Congenital bleeding disorders can characteristically be distinguished from acquired disorders by family history, age, circumstance of onset, and the presence or absence of an underlying disorder. Hemophilia A and B are both sex-linked recessive diseases of males. In almost 50% of patients, a clear-cut sex-linked history is obtained. The clinical manifestations of the milder forms of hemophilia A and B resemble von Willebrand's disease (see chapters 42 and 43). This disease, however, is transmitted as an autosomal dominant or recessive trait. Hereditary deficiencies of the coagulation factors other than factor VIII or IX are usually transmitted in an autosomal recessive manner and are very rare. In moderately severe congenital hemorrhagic states, the bleeding manifestations begin at a very early age. Long remissions may occur, however, and mild cases of hemophilia may present for the first time in the second or third decade of life or later. The absence of excessive bleeding following lacerations of the skin or tongue or after relatively minor operations, such as tonsillectomy and dental surgery, especially extraction of wisdom teeth, is strong evidence against a congenital hemorrhagic state. On the other hand, excessive bleeding that necessitates blood transfusion is strongly suggestive of this condition.

A secondary bleeding tendency may be a sequela of a systemic disease, such as leukemia, acute infection, uremia, and liver disease, or may be drug induced. Scurvy is still seen from time to time. Particulars of dietary history may point to this diagnosis.

The approach to diagnosis usually begins with the following:

1. Hematologic evaluation to detect anemia and thrombocytopenia.
2. Screening tests for bleeding abnormalities. In patients with no personal or family history of bleeding who are to undergo surgery, the tests should include examination of the peripheral blood smear to screen for number of platelets (or a platelet count) and a determination of bleeding time, activated partial thromboplastin time (APTT), and prothrombin time (PT) (Table 40–5). If all of these tests produce normal results, no further tests are carried out and surgery may be performed. If an abnormality, however mild, is found, more specialized tests are required. When there is a personal or family history of bleeding, a similar group of

Table 40–4 Differentiation of Hemophilioid States
and Purpuric States

Clinical Characteristic	Hemophilioid States
Bleeding source	Usually small artery
Bruises	Often intramuscular, deep and large
Preceding trauma	Frequent
Venipuncture	No superficial ecchymosis but massive hemorrhage may occur if firm pressure is not maintained long enough
Epistaxis	Seldom a predominant symptom
Gastrointestinal bleeding	Rarely a major symptom unless peptic ulceration is also present
Hematuria	Common
Menorrhagia	Uncommon, most patients are males
Dental bleeding	Starts hours or even days later and may last several days; not controlled by pressure
Onset of bleeding after trauma	Usually late (1–4 hours after event)
Postoperative bleeding	Late bleeding with wound hematomas
Symptoms of mildly affected patients	Large hematomas after injury; persistent and often dangerous bleeding after trauma
Hemarthroses	Occur in severe cases
Inheritance	Often sex linked
Sex incidence	Rare in females
Bleeding time	Normal

Source: Modified with permission from Biggs R, Macfarlane RG: *Treatment of Hemophilia and Other Coagulation Disorders.* Oxford, Blackwell Scientific Publications, Ltd, 1966.

Purpuras

Usually capillary

Cutaneous and mucosal petechiae and/or ecchymoses, usually small

Unusual

Superficial ecchymoses around venipuncture site despite clean venipuncture

Often a major source of bleeding

Often a major source of bleeding

Uncommon

Common

Starts immediately, lasts several hours, and is often controlled by pressure

Usually immediate

Bleeding mainly at the time of operation

Mucous membrane bleeding, eg, epistaxis and menorrhagia

Absent

No sex-linked hereditary history

Common in females

Usually prolonged

Table 40–5   Routine Coagulation Screening Tests

Disease	APTT
von Willebrand's disease	Normal or Increased
Hemophilia A and B	Increased[a]
Thrombocytopenic purpura	Normal
Liver disease or vitamin K-deficient state	Normal or Increased

[a]A normal APTT does not exclude a mild form of hemophilia A and B

screening procedures are carried out; if these yield normal results, additional tests to exclude von Willebrand's disease (see chapter 42), factor XIII deficiency, alpha$_2$-antiplasmin deficiency, and fibrinogen abnormality are indicated.

3. Specific factor assays and tests for inhibitors are performed if the APTT and PT are prolonged. Assays for Fletcher factor and HMW-K are costly because the deficient plasmas are scarce. These tests should be performed only when deficiencies of the other factors have been excluded.

4. Tests for qualitative platelet abnormalities are performed when the bleeding time is borderline or prolonged despite a normal platelet count, or if all the other blood coagulation tests produce normal results.

5. Evaluation of von Willebrand's factor may be performed when factor VIII is decreased or the bleeding time is prolonged or both, including determination of von Willebrand's antigen and the quantitative ristocetin aggregation test (see chapter 42).

6. If all of the above tests yield normal results in a patient with a clear-cut bleeding tendency, a deficiency of alpha$_2$-antiplasmin or an abnormality in fibrinogen should be considered. The thrombin time is usually adequate for the latter purpose while alpha$_2$-antiplasmin may be quantitated using a synthetic substrate (see chapter 45).

Hematologic Findings

Hematologic abnormalities are found primarily in association with thrombocytopenia. Bleeding disorders are also seen in diseases such as polycythemia vera that are associated with thrombocytosis.

Blood Cell Measurements.   A representative normal range for the platelet count is 150 to 440 $\times$ 10^9/L (150 to 440 $\times$ 10^3/μl).

Prothrombin Time	Bleeding Time	Platelet Count
Normal	Normal or Increased	Normal
Normal	Normal	Normal
Normal	Increased	Decreased
Increased	Normal or Increased	Normal or Decreased

In blood smears made from blood collected in EDTA, platelets are discrete, and a rough estimate of platelet numbers can be made by comparative counts of the red cells and platelets in representative fields.

Peripheral Blood Smear Morphology. Characteristic white cell morphology is seen in thrombocytopenias associated with such disorders as infectious mononucleosis and leukemia. Characteristic red cell changes are often associated with disseminated intravascular coagulation, including fragmented red cells or schistocytes (helmet cells).

Bone Marrow Examination. Bone marrow study helps to distinguish immune thrombocytopenias from hypoplastic and infiltrate disorders. In the immune thrombocytopenias, megakaryocytes are adequate or increased in number, whereas they are absent or decreased in hypoplastic or replaced marrows.

Other Laboratory Tests

40.1 Bleeding Time Test

Purpose. The bleeding time is used as a screening test for abnormalities of the primary hemostatic mechanism, particularly disorders of platelet function and von Willebrand's disease. It is independent of the coagulation mechanism.

Principle. The bleeding time is the length of time it takes for bleeding to cease from a small superficial wound made with a sharp blade under standardized conditions. It is a rough function of the efficacy of the primary hemostatic mechanism. The bleeding time is measured as the interval between puncture of the skin and cessation of bleeding.

Procedure. The best standardized and most reproducible techniques are based on Ivy's method. A blood pressure cuff is placed around the patient's upper arm and the pressure is raised to 40 mm Hg. Two small punctures are made along the outer surface of the patient's forearm. The drops of blood issuing from the bleeding points are absorbed at intervals of 30 sec into two filter paper disks, one for each puncture wound, until bleeding ceases. The average of the times required for bleeding to stop from the puncture wounds is taken as the bleeding time.

Several modifications of this technique have been devised in attempts to standardize the skin puncture. Perhaps the best and least traumatic of these is a sterile disposable device (Simplate, General Diagnostics, Division of Warner-Lambert Pharmaceuticals Co, Morris Plains, NJ) that makes two uniform incisions 5 mm in length by 1 mm in depth by means of spring-loaded blades contained in a plastic housing. The device is placed firmly on the nonhairy part of the skin of the forearm without pressure and positioned so that the incision will be either parallel or perpendicular to the fold of the elbow, with care taken to avoid superficial veins, scars, and bruises; the blade is then released by depression of the triggering device. The normal bleeding time with this method making the parallel incision is <8 minutes.

Interpretation. There is a fairly good correlation between platelet count and bleeding time. If the platelets are qualitatively normal, the platelet count usually has to drop to $<80 \times 10^9/L$ $(80 \times 10^3/\mu l)$ before an abnormality in the bleeding time becomes apparent. The prolongation does not become pronounced until the count falls to $<40 \times 10^9/L$ $(40 \times 10^3/\mu l)$. A prolongation is also seen in some patients with qualitative platelet abnormalities or myeloproliferative disorders. The bleeding time is prolonged in about one third of all patients with von Willebrand's disease if the mild cases are included. Occasionally, a prolonged bleeding time is the sole abnormality that can be found, despite exhaustive tests, in a patient with a lifelong history of bleeding.

Notes and Precautions. By far the most common cause of a prolonged bleeding time that has been performed by an experienced technologist is the ingestion of a drug that interferes with platelet function. As little as 600 mg of acetylsalicylate (aspirin) taken seven days before can result in a significantly prolonged bleeding time. Aspirin is not considered to be a drug or medication by many patients and is present in a large number of proprietary preparations (Table 40–6). If the patient has taken aspirin, and bleeding time is normal, the result is significant and valid; if the bleeding time is prolonged, the test must be repeated at a later time.

The Simplate method may leave two small scars, and the patient should be so warned. There is no purpose in performing the bleeding time test on a patient with a platelet count $<40 \times 10^9/L$ ($40 \times 10^3/\mu l$).

40.2 Whole Blood Coagulation Time and Clot Observation and Retraction

Purpose.   The test of whole blood coagulation time and clot observation and retraction monitors heparin therapy and screens for abnormalities in fibrinolysis. It is a very insensitive index of clotting function and of little value for the detection of mild-to-moderate bleeding disorders.

Specimen.   Whole blood is used.

Principle.   The time required for blood to clot in a test tube is a crude measure of intrinsic clotting. Failure of the clot to retract may result from a qualitative or quantitative platelet defect. A weak clot or one that breaks down indicates abnormal fibrinolysis, which is usually secondary to disseminated intravascular coagulation.

Procedure.   Venous blood obtained by a clean venipuncture is withdrawn into a plastic syringe. To minimize contamination with tissue juice, some coagulation laboratories prefer a two-syringe technique. After 1 to 2 mL of blood has been withdrawn into the first syringe, it is disconnected from the needle, and only blood collected into the second syringe is used. One-milliliter aliquots of the blood are immediately transferred into 3 12×77-mm glass tubes, which are placed in a heating block at 37° C and tilted gently every 30 sec until a clot is seen in one of the tubes. The stopwatch is then stopped and the clotting time recorded. The clotting times of the remaining 2 tubes need not be determined. If no clot is present in any of the tubes after 10 minutes, the clotting time should be recorded as abnormal. The tubes are inspected at the end of 1 hour and again on the following morning. In the original Lee and White clotting test,

Table 40–6   Compounds Containing Aspirin

ACA capsules and ACA no. 2

Acetidine capsules

Alka-Seltzer

Allylgesic[a]

Amytal with ASA[a]

Anacin

Anahist

APC

ASA

ASA compound

ASA compound with codeine

Aspirbar

Aspodyne

Bayer aspirin

Buff-A

Buffacetin

Bufferin

Buffinol

Colrex

Coricidin

Darvon with ASA[a]

Darvon-N with ASA[a]

Empiral[a]

Empirin

Excedrin

P-A-C compound[a]

Percodan[a]

Persistin

Phenaphen[a]

Phenergan compound[a]

Robaxisal[a]

Sedagesic

Sine-Off tablets

St. Joseph aspirin

SOURCE: Adapted with permission from Leist ER, Banwell JG: Products containing aspirin. N Engl J Med 291:710, 1974. For complete list consult Leist ER, Banwell JG: N Engl J Med 291:710, 1974, and Selner J: N Engl J Med 292:372, 1975.

[a]Available through prescription only

the first tube was tilted at intervals of 30 sec until a solid clot formed. The second and third tubes were then treated similarly in sequence. The clotting time was the time required for a solid clot to form in the third tube.

Interpretation.　　When performed in the manner described previously, normal blood clots appear within 7 minutes. If no clot has formed by 10 minutes, a defect in intrinsic coagulation is present and there is no point in determining the exact time of clotting. The test is prolonged when a severe deficiency ($< 6\%$) of a clotting factor (other than factor VII or XIII) or a circulating anticoagulant, including heparin, is present.

At the end of 1 hour, the degree of clot retraction and the general size of the clot is noted. It should be firm and occupy a volume approximately equal to half the total volume of the blood. If it occupies a volume more than this or if it has not retracted at all, the result is considered abnormal. The test is not very sensitive, however, and a normal result does not exclude a platelet abnormality. By freeing the clot from the tube and tilting the tube up and down so the clot impinges on the bottom of the tube, some idea of its weight can be gauged. Sometimes the clot will show signs of breaking up, indicating that it is weak and defective, and on inspection the following morning it may appear to have completely disintegrated. In a few patients with severe intravascular coagulation and secondary fibrinolysis, the clot may have very ragged margins and be soft and flabby. As it disintegrates red cells form a clearly demarcated layer in the bottom of the tube. When the concentration of fibrinogen is low, the clot may initially be normal in size but after retraction may be so small as to be overlooked. Rapid lysis of a firm clot may be seen in alpha$_2$-antiplasmin deficiency but there are several other causes and the finding is usually of no clinical significance. In the past, the whole blood clotting time was the test used most often to monitor heparin therapy. It is cumbersome and time-consuming, however, and the same information can be obtained more conveniently by the use of the APTT.

Notes and Precautions.　　Tubes that have been siliconized some time in the past may extend clotting times, and only disposable tubes or new tubes that have been washed with acid should be used. The whole blood clotting time may be normal in moderately severe cases of hemophilia. It cannot be overemphasized that this test can never be used as the sole screening test for disorders of coagulation.

40.3 Activated Partial Thromboplastin Time (APTT)

Purpose. The APTT is used as a screening test for deficiencies of plasma coagulation factors other than factors VII and XIII. The test is also used to monitor heparin therapy.

Principle. Platelet-poor plasma contains all the coagulation factors necessary for the formation of intrinsic prothrombinase or plasma thromboplastin with the exception of calcium ions and phospholipid. In the APTT test, phospholipid and CA^{++} are added to the plasma, and, therefore, the clotting time is a function of intrinsic prothrombinase formation. The extent of exposure of the plasma to glass surfaces is controlled by exposing the plasma to optimal surface activation by addition of an activating agent, such as kaolin, ellagic acid, celite, or silica. Factor VII is not measured, as it is involved in the extrinsic pathway only, nor is factor XIII, as it is involved only in clot stabilization. As platelet-poor plasma is used, the test is not influenced by quantitative or qualitative abnormalities in the platelets.

Specimen. Blood is collected by clean venipuncture using a plastic syringe. Nine parts of the whole blood are mixed with one part anticoagulant, but an adjustment in the ratio of anticoagulant to whole blood may be made in cases where the hemotocrit value is very high. The anticoagulant is 3.2% or 3.8% trisodium citrate. Most specialized coagulation laboratories use a 3.8% (0.1 M) buffered citrate solution; EDTA or heparin should not be used. The blood is best collected in a plastic tube, and plastic pipettes are used to process the plasma. Most general laboratories use plain or silicone-coated glass tubes; the latter are available commercially (Becton and Dickenson, Rutherford, NJ).

Procedure. The test is performed by mixing the platelet-poor plasma from the patient or healthy subject with phospholipid and an activating agent to achieve optimal contact activation. An optimal amount of calcium is then added, and the clotting times are recorded.

Interpretation. The normal range for the APTT is dependent on a large number of variables. Semiautomated instruments with photoelectric devices for the determination of the end point give shorter values than when the clotting time is determined

Table 40–7   Factors Measured by Activated Partial Thromboplastin Time and Prothrombin Time Tests

APTT	PT	Both Tests
XII	VII	
HMW-K (Fitzgerald)		
Fletcher (prekallikrein)		
XI		
IX		
VIII		
V	V	V
X	X	X
Prothrombin	Prothrombin	Prothrombin
Fibrinogen	Fibrinogen	Fibrinogen

ABBREVIATIONS: APTT = activated partial thromboplastin time; PT = prothrombin time.

visually; however, variability is found from instrument to instrument even of the same type and manufacturer. It is therefore important to know the normal range for the particular laboratory performing the test. Using an automated device (MLA Model 700, American Scientific Products, Mount Vernon, NY: preincubation period is at least 5 minutes), APTT reagent (manufactured by General Diagnostics, Division of Warner-Lambert Pharmaceuticals Co, Morris Plains, NJ), and buffered citrate, the normal range in the University of California Hospital laboratory, San Diego, has usually been between 25 and 28 secs, varying somewhat with the particular batch of reagent used.

The APTT is prolonged when one or more of any of the factors necessary for the formation of intrinsic prothrombinase is deficient. These include: factors XII, HMW-K, prekallikrein, XI, X, IX, VIII, and V, and also prothrombin and fibrinogen (Table 40–7). If the period of contact activation is greater than 2 or 3 minutes, the test may become insensitive to prekallikrein. The sensitivity of the test to deficiencies of the other factors varies from factor to factor. As a general rule, the level has to decrease to below 40% before the APTT becomes significantly prolonged.

Specific inhibitors of clotting factors may also result in a prolongation of the APTT. The most frequently encountered of these is an antibody against factor VIII. The so-called lupuslike anticoagulant, which is an antibody that appears to act non-specifically, is one of the most frequent causes of a prolonged APTT found on routine preoperative screening. In monitoring heparin therapy, when heparin is given continuously by intravenous drip for the treatment of venous thromboembolism, the APTT should be prolonged to 1.5 to 2.0 times the patient's APTT determined before heparin therapy. However, the sensitivity of the method to heparin depends on the type and concentration of the activator and the phospholipid used. The results are not always reliable, particularly when the blood sample has been withdrawn through an intravenous catheter used to infuse the heparin. The test is more helpful than the Lee and White clotting test for the monitoring of heparin therapy, as it is more convenient and less time-consuming. Whether such therapy needs to be monitored at all, however, remains an unsettled question.

Notes and Precautions. The normal range is sometimes not included on the report, although a normal control value is given. This is because the range tends to vary from time to time depending on variations in the batch of APTT reagents used and whether the end point is determined by machine through changes in the sensitivity of the instrument. The normal range is quite narrow, however, when individuals with low levels of factors XI or XII or those with the lupuslike anticoagulants are excluded. Such subjects are encountered quite frequently in the healthy population of individuals with no family or personal history of a bleeding tendency. If the plasma is very turbid or icteric, the change of optical density caused by fibrin formation may be too small to trigger the clot timing device of instruments that use photoelectric devices. The value of the APTT (and PT) printed by the machine will then be the highest value the instrument is capable of recording; whenever these values are obtained on such an instrument, the test should be repeated using a manual method.

40.4   One-Stage Prothrombin Time (PT)

Purpose. The one-stage PT test (sometimes referred to as the Quick test, named for its discoverer) is used to screen for abnormalities of those factors that are involved in the extrinsic pathway (factors V, VII, and X, and prothrombin and fibrinogen). It is used to monitor the effects of the coumarin anticoagulants and to study patients with hereditary and acquired disorders of clotting.

Principle. When tissue extract, loosely referred to as thrombo-plastin, is added to plasma in the presence of calcium, it reacts with the factor VII to form a product that converts factor X to its activated form, factor Xa; this, in turn, reacts with the factor V and phospholipid present in the tissue extract to form ex-trinsic prothrombinase, which converts prothrombin to throm-bin. Thrombin then converts fibrinogen to fibrin. The rate of fibrin formation is therefore a function of the concentration of factors V, VII, and X and prothrombin and fibrinogen; the test measures the overall activities of these factors (Table 40–7).

Specimen. Tests may be performed on the same specimen of plasma used for the APTT test. It is important to collect the normal control plasma in the same manner as the patient's plasma at approximately the same time.

Procedure. One volume of tissue extract is added to an equal volume of plasma. The mixture is then recalcified by the ad-dition of an optimal amount of calcium chloride, and the clot-ting time is recorded. Both the patient's and the healthy control subject's values are reported.

Interpretation. The normal range for the PT varies with the tissue extract and techniques, but most commercial thromboplastins are adjusted to give mean PTs of 12 ± 0.5 sec with normal plasmas. The normal range is very narrow, and a difference >1.5 sec between the patient's time and the normal control time is probably significant. The use of the PT as the control of anticoagulant therapy is discussed in detail in chapter 46. For this purpose, the ratio of the patient's PT to that of the healthy control subject is often employed, and for each throm-boplastin there is an optimal ratio range. Accordingly, in inter-preting the results for this purpose, the type and source of the thromboplastin should be known as well as the relative sen-sitivity of the reagent compared to the World Health Organi-zation standard. A prolongation of the PT usually indicates de-fective or decreased synthesis of the vitamin K–dependent clotting factors, with the exception of factor IX, which is also depressed but not measured by this test. The test is also sen-sitive to a decrease in factor V concentration, which is some-times seen in cirrhosis of the liver and chronic hepatitis.

A hereditary deficiency of one of the factors affecting the PT test is very rare. The PT is sometimes prolonged when a very potent lupus-type anticoagulant or an inhibitor of factor V is present. It may also be slightly prolonged in disseminated intravascular coagulation associated with decreases in factor V and fibrinogen. Factors measured by the APTT and PT are compared in Table 40–7.

Notes and Precautions.   If normal plasma is left at cold temperatures for several hours, the PT of normal and pathologic plasmas may shorten significantly; it is believed that the contact factors are involved in this process. Thus, if the patient's blood is drawn in the afternoon while the control plasma was collected in the morning and kept in the refrigerator, the patient's time, although normal, may be significantly longer than that of the control subject. Thus, it is important that the control plasma be drawn approximately at the same time as that of the test specimen. To obviate the need for fresh normal controls, it is common practice to use commercial standards or aliquots of freshly frozen normal pooled plasma.

The test should not be performed if a small clot is present within the specimen. As discussed earlier, the clot timing devices of photoelectric instruments may fail to detect fibrin formation in very turbid or icteric specimens and a manual technique must then be employed.

40.5   Thrombin Time

Purpose.   The thrombin time is used to screen for abnormalities in the conversion of fibrinogen to fibrin. These may be caused by qualitative or quantitative abnormalities of fibrinogen or by inhibitors, such as heparin or fibrin/fibrinogen split products.

Principle.   The addition of thrombin to plasma converts fibrinogen to fibrin and bypasses both the intrinsic and extrinsic pathways. The time taken for plasma to clot on addition of thrombin, referred to as the thrombin time, is a function of fibrinogen concentration.

Procedure.   One part of a solution of thrombin is added to a mixture of 1 part of the patient's citrated plasma and 1 part of normal saline, and the clotting time is recorded. Two strengths of thrombin should be used. One strength (approximately 1 U/mL) should give a normal clotting time of 9 to 11 sec and the other a time of 25 to 35 sec with normal pooled plasma.

Interpretation.   A prolongation over the normal time of ≥3 sec with the stronger solution and ≥5 sec with the weaker is considered abnormal. If the plasma does not clot with either strength in 5 min, either the concentration of fibrinogen is <5 mg/100 mL or, far more likely, a potent antithrombic substance, almost invariably heparin, is present. A moderate prolongation is also likely to be caused by heparin but occasionally may result from fibrin or fibrinogen split products, hypofibrinogenemia, hyperfibrinogenemia, the presence of certain paraproteins, or dysfibrinogenemia. When a significant abnormality is found, the test must be repeated using the stronger thrombin solution on a mixture consisting of equal parts of patient and normal plasma. If the thrombin time of the mixture is ≥3 sec longer than the control's, an inhibitor is present. If the thrombin time is corrected to within 2 sec of the control, hypofibrinogenemia or dysfibrinogenemia is likely.

Notes and Precautions. A slight prolongation with the weaker strength and a normal value with the stronger is probably not significant. If a potent inhibitor is present, as demonstrated by little or no correction with normal plasma, the cause is almost always heparin medication. Occasionally, contamination with heparin occurs when the blood is withdrawn through a catheter through which heparin had previously been infused. If contamination of the specimen with heparin can be definitely excluded, however, a new specimen should be withdrawn and the test repeated. If an anticoagulant can still be demonstrated, a protamine titration test for heparin or a reptilase time test should be performed. The principle of the latter test is that reptilase, a snake venom that is available commercially, converts fibrinogen to fibrin directly, and its action is not inhibited by heparin. The test is performed similarly to the thrombin time, with reptilase substituted for thrombin. A normal reptilase time with a prolonged thrombin time in this setting is evidence that the patient has received heparin or that heparin contamination has occurred.

References

1. Lammle B, Griffin JH: Formation of the fibrin clot: The balance of procoagulant and inhibitory factors. *Clin Haematol* 1985; 14:281–342.

2. Ogston D, Bennett B: The blood coagulation cascade, in Poller L (ed): *Recent Advances in Blood Coagulation.* New York, Churchill-Livingstone Inc, vol 4, 1985, pp 1–10.

3. Rapaport SI: Preoperative hemostatic evaluation: Which tests, if any? *Blood* 1983; 61:229–233.

4. Triplett DA, Smith C: Routine testing in the coagulation laboratory, in Triplett DA (ed): *Laboratory Evaluation of Coagulation.* Chicago, American Society of Clinical Pathologists Press, 1982, pp 27–51.

41

Thrombocytopenic Purpura

The term "purpura" refers to spontaneous bleeding characterized by petechiae, superficial ecchymoses, bleeding from mucous membranes, and increased bleeding from small vessels. Purpura primarily attributable to a fall in the platelet count is referred to as "thrombocytopenic purpura." Purpura may also occur in the absence of thrombocytopenia, and thrombocytopenia is not necessarily associated with purpura.

Pathophysiology

Thrombocytopenia may be caused by decreased production or excessive destruction of platelets; a smaller number of cases result from redistribution of the platelets with splenic pooling (Table 41–1). Reduced production that occurs in hypoplastic or aplastic anemia is caused by leukemia, multiple myeloma, myelofibrosis, or infiltration of the bone marrow by carcinoma or lymphoma. It is also seen in vitamin B_{12} or folic acid deficiency, but in such cases the thrombocytopenia is rarely severe enough to result in significant bleeding.

Excessive destruction of platelets can usually be attributed to an autoantibody directed toward a platelet-associated antigen. Such antibodies are found in some patients with systemic lupus erythematosus (SLE) or lymphoma. Evidence of these diseases may not

Table 41–1   Causes of Thrombocytopenia

Decreased platelet production

Marrow injury
Drugs, chemicals, or radiation

Bone marrow infiltration
Carcinoma, leukemia, lymphoma
Myelofibrosis

Congenital abnormalities
Aldrich-Wiskott syndrome
Fanconi's syndrome

B_{12} or folic acid deficiency

Increased platelet destruction

Autoantibodies
Postinfectious fever
Lupus erythematosus
Lymphomas
Hemolytic anemia (Evans' syndrome)
Drugs
Idiopathic

Alloantibodies
Fetal maternal incombatibility
Post-transfusional purpura

Platelet injury
Viral or bacterial
Prosthesis

Disseminated intravascular coagulation

Sequestration of platelets in spleen

Thrombotic thrombocytopenic purpura

Dilution after massive transfusion

---

be apparent at the onset of bleeding. Rarely, an isoagglutinin develops in patients who have received multiple transfusions. Almost any drug can cause an antibody-mediated thrombocytopenia, the best known being the sulfonamides, quinine, quinidine, digitoxin, and heparin. The drug acts as a hapten, combining with a serum protein to form an immunogenic complex. Antibodies arise against this complex and, for reasons that are not entirely clear, the antigen-antibody complex binds to the platelet membrane through a part of the IgG molecule. The list of drugs that may induce immune thrombocytopenia is long, and while some drugs are more immunogenic than others, it appears that almost any drug can induce idiopathic thrombocytopenic purpura (ITP). Antibodies may develop after viral infections, such as rubella, measles, or infectious mononucleosis. The demonstration of an autoantibody had been difficult to achieve; however, the advent of monoclonal technology has resulted in the development of special techniques for their detection that are currently performed in a few research and reference laboratories. Even with the most sensitive of these techniques, antibodies can be demonstrated in only about 90% of cases. The platelet destruction occurs by IgG bound to the platelet surface interfacing with Fc receptors found on cells of the reticuloendothelial system, resulting in phagocytosis of the IgG bearing platelets. Platelet counts from the majority of patients with ITP have increased amounts of platelet-associated IgG, and while this IgG is not necessarily an autoantibody, the term "autoimmune thrombocytopenic purpura" is sometimes used for these cases, while the term "idiopathic thrombocytopenic purpura" is reserved for those cases in which no antibody has been demonstrated. The specificity of increased platelet-associated IgG for the diagnosis of autoimmune thrombocytopenic purpura is low, for increased amounts are found in some septicemic patients and in most patients with active SLE (without accompanying thrombocytopenia) and in some patients with other conditions. Some drugs, such as the thiazide diuretics, appear to cause thrombocytopenia by suppressing platelet production through a toxic effect on the megakaryocytes in sensitive persons. Viruses can cause thrombocytopenia by interfering with megakaryocytic maturation, but peripheral destruction of platelets by immune mechanisms also occurs with viral infections. Mild subclinical thrombocytopenia is frequent in infectious mononucleosis, AIDS, Rocky Mountain spotted fever, tuberculosis, malaria, and gram-negative infections. In some of these conditions, the thrombocytopenia may be attributable to disseminated intravascular coagulation (DIC), but other factors may be operative. Any condition associated with an enlargement of the spleen may cause thrombocytopenia by the sequestration of the platelets in splenic sinusoids.

Clinical Findings

Thrombocytopenia is the most common cause of major bleeding in children and adults and, with rare exceptions, it is an acquired disorder. The bleeding manifestations include: petechiae, spontaneous bruising, and mucosal bleeding; it can usually be distinguished from those seen in hemophilioid states (see chapter 40 and

Figure 41–1   Flow Diagram for Diagnosis of Thrombocytopenia

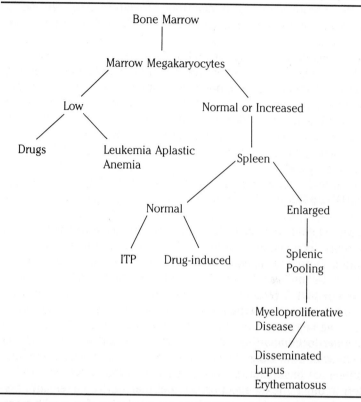

Table 40–4), in which petechiae are not seen and the hematomas tend to be deeper and more often related to trauma. In acute ITP, the onset is usually quite sudden, with severe manifestations, such as petechiae and bleeding from the mucous membranes. There is often a history of a viral infection, and young children are most often affected. In contrast, the onset of chronic ITP tends to be insidious, adults are more often affected, and the course tends to be protracted. Differentiation between the acute and chronic forms may be difficult, if not impossible, at the time the thrombocytopenia is first discovered. A history of a recent infection or ingestion of some drugs has special relevance. A complete review of systems may suggest other diseases that may be associated with thrombocytopenia such as a collagen disease, lymphoma, sarcoidosis, AIDS, or tuberculosis. Particular attention should be given to the type of bruising, whether of the capillary type seen with thrombocytopenia or the small arteriolar or hemophiloid type, and to the presence or absence of adenopathy and splenomegaly. The finding of an enlarged spleen virtually excludes the diagnosis of ITP.

Hereditary thrombocytopenic states are rare and include Fanconi's syndrome and thrombocytopenia with bilateral absence of radii. In both of these conditions, megakaryotic hypoplasia is present. Similar hypoplasia may be seen as a result of intrauterine infections with viral organisms such as rubella, or exposure of the fetus to drugs such as thiazide diuretics in the maternal circulation. Cyclic thrombocytopenia is a rare condition in which transfusion of normal platelet-free plasma results in the production of platelets in the patient. The Wiskott-Aldrich syndrome, which is inherited as a sex-linked recessive trait, is characterized by thrombocytopenia, recurrent infections, and eczema.

Approach to Diagnosis

With the general availability of reliable platelet counting methods, the diagnosis of thrombocytopenic purpura is simple. The normal platelet count is usually stated to be between 150 and 440 $\times$ 10^9/L (150 and 440 $\times$ 10^3/μl). Strictly speaking, thrombocytopenia should refer to any count significantly below the lower level of normal. However, slight and clinically unimportant depressions of the count occur so frequently that the term is rather arbitrarily used to refer to counts that are well below the normal range and are associated with excessive bleeding from raw surfaces. As a general rule, such bleeding does not occur unless the platelet count falls below 100 $\times$ 10^9/L (100 $\times$ 10^3/μl) or there is a concomitant qualitative disorder of the platelets or concomitant von Willebrand's disease. In these cases, the degree of reduction of the platelet count may not correlate with the severity of the bleeding. Purpura is common when the platelet count falls below 40 $\times$ 10^9/L (40 $\times$ 10^3/μl) and may reach quite severe proportions when the platelet count decreases to below 5 $\times$ 10^9/L (5 $\times$ 10^3/μl) with central nervous system and gastrointestinal tract bleeding. While the diagnosis of thrombocytopenic purpura presents no difficulty, the diagnosis of ITP or the primary form of the disease can be made only by a process of elimination and may be extremely difficult. Much depends on leads obtained from the history and clinical examination findings. Diagnostic evaluation proceeds as follows (Figure 41–1):

1. Hematologic evaluation to confirm thrombocytopenia and exclude thrombocytopenia secondary to leukemia, aplastic leukemia, infiltration of the bone marrow by metastatic carcinoma, multiple myeloma or lymphoma, DIC, and hemolytic anemia, including microangiopathic hemolytic anemia and associated states, such as thrombotic thrombocytopenic purpura and the hemolytic uremic syndrome.

2. Blood coagulation screening tests. A normal thromboplastin time (APTT) and prothrombin time (PT) excludes an associated co-agulation abnormality, such as a lupus anticoagulant. The bleeding time gives an assessment of the severity of the primary hemostatic defect, but this test is not necessary with severe thrombocytopenia or if purpura is present.

3. Special coagulation tests. A test for the detection of soluble fibrin monomers and fibrin split products should be performed when it is necessary to exclude DIC. In all patients with a normal platelet count and a prolonged bleeding time, platelet aggrega-tion studies should be performed. Study of ristocetin-induced aggregation is particularly valuable in suspected von Wille-brand's disease.

4. A Coombs' test is performed to exclude an associated autoim-mune hemolytic anemia.

5. Tests for SLE should be performed and repeated at least twice if the patient has an enlarged spleen. Sometimes during the course of ITP, the tests will become positive for SLE.

6. A test for heterophilic antibodies is carried out when atypical lymphocytes are seen on the peripheral blood smear.

7. Blood and viral cultures are performed whenever a bacterial or viral cause is suspected.

8. A test for platelet-associated IgG is often performed.

9. If the patient is receiving heparin or another drug suspected of causing the thrombocytopenia, an in vitro test using the drug, the patient's plasma or serum, and normal platelet-rich plasma is performed.

Hematologic Findings

In ITP, the peripheral blood is usually unremarkable, except for the sparsity or absence of platelets. The diagnosis of ITP is made by excluding all known causes of thrombocytopenia.

Peripheral Blood Smear Morphology. In thrombocyto-penia caused by leukemia, blast cells are almost invariably present in the peripheral blood, while in hypoplastic or aplastic anemia, neutropenia with no blast cells is present. Atypical lymphocytes suggest a viral cause, such as infectious mononucleosis. Frag-mented red cells or schistocytes (helmet cells), together with some spherocytes, are found in micoangiopathic hemolytic anemia and point to the diagnosis of DIC, thrombotic thrombocytopenic pur-pura, or the hemolytic uremic syndrome. Oval macrocytes and poi-kilocytosis with hypersegmented polymorphs are seen in folic acid or vitamin B_{12} deficiency. Spherocytosis and polychromatophilia and a high reticulocyte count suggest an associated immune hemolytic anemia. Heavy bleeding in a thrombocytopenic patient (eg, a patient with menorrhagia) may result in a normocytic or ultimately a hypochromic, microcytic anemia.

Platelet counts are diminished on the smear, and they may be larger than normal, reflecting a predominance of young forms. Large, bizarre platelets suggest an associated qualitative functional abnormality. Such abnormalities are discussed in the following chapter.

Accurate platelet counts are important in gauging the progress and severity of the disease. The most reliable counts are obtained using an electronic counter.

Bone Marrow Examination. In ITP, the bone marrow is usually normal except for quantitative and subtle qualitative changes in the megakaryocytes. Megakaryocytes are present in normal or increased numbers. They are less granular and more basophilic than normal megakaryocytes, indicating defective maturation or decreased production of platelets. Large megakaryocytes that have an increased number of nuclear divisions may be seen. In aplastic or myelophthisic anemia, megakaryocytes are decreased or absent. Bone marrow examination is necessary to exclude an otherwise unapparent primary bone marrow disease, such as leukemia.

Other Laboratory Tests

41.1 Bleeding Time Test

The bleeding time is almost invariably prolonged with platelet counts below $40 \times 10^9/L$ ($40 \times 10^3/\mu l$), and this test should not be performed when the patient is known to have a platelet count below this value.

41.2 Prothrombin Time (PT) and Activated Partial Thromboplastin Time (APTT)

The PT and APTT are normal in ITP. The APTT may be prolonged if the patient has systemic lupus erythematosus or if some other perhaps coincidental abnormality, such as von Willebrand's disease, is present. In DIC, the PT and APTT may be prolonged, and a test for fibrin split products and serial fibrinogen determinations help to exclude the condition.

41.3 Platelet Function Tests

If the platelet count is above $80 \times 10^9/L$ ($80 \times 10^3/\mu l$) platelet aggregation tests may be useful in excluding a qualitative platelet disorder associated with mild thrombocytopenia. In autoimmune thrombocytopenia, however, the platelets may be damaged by antibody and may fail to aggregate normally. Clot retraction is abnormal.

41.4 Detection of Antiplatelet Antibodies

(See Aster RH: Detection of antiplatelet antibodies: Inhibition of clot retraction, in Williams WJ, Beutler E, Erslev AJ (eds): *Hematology,* ed 3. New York, McGraw-Hill International Book Co, 1983, pp 1675–1677.)

Purpose. This test detects drug-induced or posttransfusional platelet antibodies.

Principle. In the presence of complement and the suspected drug, if relevant, platelets are damaged by the antibody, and clot retraction is impaired.

Specimen. Serum or citrated plasma is used, and no special precautions are required.

Procedure. The patient's and normal control serum or plasma are each incubated with freshly drawn compatible blood. If a drug is suspected as the cause, a very low concentration in distilled water is included in the mixture. The two tubes are incubated at 37° C. At the end of 1 hour, the degree of clot retraction is determined by inspection or by determining the amount of fluid in the tubes after removal of the clots. The test may be modified by substituting platelet-rich plasma for fresh whole blood and adding magnesium to permit complement activity; the mixture is clotted by addition of calcium.

Interpretation. The failure of the blood containing the patient's serum to retract as fully as that containing the control serum indicates the presence of a platelet antibody. If the purpura is caused by a drug-induced antibody, impairment of retraction may be seen at very low concentrations of the drug in the tube containing the patient's serum.

Notes and Precautions. Some drugs at certain concentrations inhibit clot retraction by a direct action, and no retraction will be seen in either tube.

41.5 Test for Heparin-Induced Thrombocytopenia

(See Sherican D, Carter C, Kelton JG: A diagnostic test for heparin-induced thrombocytopenia. *Blood* 1986; 67:27–30.)

Purpose. Thrombocytopenia may occur as a serious and diagnostically difficult complication of heparin therapy. Five percent to 10% of patients may be so affected, and a small portion of these have an associated arterial thrombosis. The thrombocytopenia that develops typically occurs 6 to 10 days after initiation of heparin therapy but may occur after only 2 days in patients who have previously received heparin therapy.

Principle. Sera from patients with heparin-induced thrombocytopenia will initiate carbon-14-serotonin platelet release at therapeutic concentrations of heparin but not at high concentrations of heparin.

Specimen. Citrated whole blood is obtained from patients after the development of thrombocytopenia.

Procedure. Platelet-rich plasma is prepared and incubated with carbon-14-serotonin, and the platelets then are washed. The platelet count is adjusted. Test serum is then mixed with one of two heparin concentrations (0.1 U/mL and 100 U/mL final concentration) and with an aliquot of carbon-14-serotonin–labeled platelets. After incubation and mixing, EDTA is added to terminate the release reaction. The mixture is then centrifuged, and an aliquot of the supernatant is counted in a scintillation counter. The percent serotonin release can then be calculated from the values for background radioactivity, test sample release, and total radioactivity.

Interpretation. A positive test result occurs when there is >20% release at 0.1 U/mL of heparin and <20% release at 100 U/mL of heparin.

41.6　Test for Platelet Associated Immunoglobulins

(See Rosse WF, Devine DV, Ware R: Reactions of immunoglobulin G-binding ligands with platelets and platelet-associated immunoglobulin G. *J Clin Invest* 1984; 73:489-496.)

Purpose.　The test is used to measure IgG and IgM bound to the patient platelets (direct test) or present in patient's serum (indirect test).

The direct test measures autoantibody on the surface of the platelet. It is useful in separating ITP from nonimmune causes. Although the presence of increased amounts of platelet-associated antibody is not specific for ITP, this does occur in nearly all such patients.

The indirect assay is helpful in detecting the presence of alloantibodies, which may be found in posttransfusion purpura and also may be involved in drug-induced thrombocytopenia.

Principle.　Monoclonal antibodies to antigenic determinants on IgG or IgM are produced. These will bind to their target antigen in a 1:1 ratio, and the amount of ligand may be determined by detection of a radiolabel, iodine-125, previously attached to the monoclonal antibody. Patients' platelets are used in the direct assay and are assayed for the amount of angi-IgG or anti-IgM bound. In the indirect assay, patient serum is first incubated with normal control platelets.

Specimen.　The minimum sample required is 35 mL of whole blood collected in EDTA.

Procedure.　The platelet count of the sample is determined, and platelet-rich plasma is prepared. A platelet pellet is isolated by centrifugation and then suspended in buffer. The platelets are washed by the same procedure 2 more times. The platelets are recentrifuged, taken up in a small aliquot of buffer, and counted. A measured quantity of platelets is then mixed with iodine-125 anti-IgG (or anti-IgM) monoclonal antibody and incubated with mixing at 37° C. A measured quantity of these platelets is then layered over a phthalate oil support and microcentrifuged. The platelet pellet produced is then isolated and counted in a gamma counter.

The number of IgG (or IgM) molecules on each platelet can then be determined from the known quantities of the specific activity of the antibody, the molecular weight of the targeted immunoglobulin, the number of platelets, and Avogadros number.

Interpretation. The results are reported as the number of immunoglobulin molecules per platelet. If the result shows only slight elevation, it suggests that an immunologic process might be involved but that other causes should be explored. Significantly elevated levels indicate involvement of an immunologic process.

Course and Treatment

Acute ITP is usually a self-limiting disease and most patients, who are usually children, recover without any treatment. If there is life-threatening bleeding, however, therapy with platelet transfusions and prednisone is usually administered. Acute ITP that does not respond to conservative measures and chronic ITP are treated with glucocorticoids. Predisone in doses from 1 mg/kg is often used, and this dose is increased if there is no response after a few days. If steroid therapy is unsuccessful after 3 or 4 weeks, splenectomy should then be considered. If the thrombocytopenia is refractory to these measures, short-term immunosuppressive therapy is often used. In recent years, intravenous immunoglobulin has been used as an alternative to splenectomy, but it is expensive, and the benefits are often temporary.

References

1. Bierling P, Divine M, Famet J-P, et al: Persistent remission of adult chronic autoimmune thrombocytopenic purpura after treatment with high doses of intravenous immunoglobulin. *Am J Hematol* 1987; 25:271–275.

2. Blockmans D, Bounameaux H, Vermylen J, et al: Heparin-induced thrombocytopenia: Platelet aggregation studies in the presence of heparin fractions or semi-synthetic analogues of various molecular weights and anticoagulant activities. *Thromb Haemost* 1986; 55:90–93.

3. Harrington WJ: Are platelet-antibody tests worthwhile? *N Engl J Med* 1987; 316:211–212.

4. Karpatkin S: Autoimmune thrombocytopenic purpura. *Semin Hematol* 1985; 22:260–288.

42

Functional Platelet Disorders

The term "functional platelet disorder" is used in this chapter to refer to a group of disorders characterized by purpura, small-vessel bleeding, and excessive bruising, in which there is an impairment of one or more platelet functions, with a normal platelet count and a prolonged bleeding time. In von Willebrand's disease, the defect in platelet function is attributable primarily to an abnormal plasma protein, while in the remainder of these disorders, a biochemical platelet abnormality usually exists.

Pathophysiology

When the platelets are exposed to damaged endothelial wall, the platelets adhere to the exposed collagen fragments of basement membrane and change their shape from smooth discs to spheres with pseudopods. They then secrete the contents of their granules, a process referred to as the "release reaction." Platelets then form aggregates on those platelets that have already adhered to the endothelium; this constitutes the primary hemostatic plug and arrests bleeding. Shape change and release are induced readily in vitro by a variety of stimuli that include pH and temperature changes and are reversible. Thrombin and adenosine diphosphate (ADP) are potent release and aggregating agents; the addition of relatively low concentrations of ADP to platelet-rich plasma induces release and primary aggregation of platelets that is reversible, while the release from the platelets of ADP derived from the dense bodies during the release reaction induces second-phase or irreversible aggregation. Arachidonic acid, a carbon-20 fatty acid and the principle component of the platelet membrane phospholipids, also induces aggregation and is a percursor of the prostaglandins that have an important role in aggregation. Arachidonic acid is formed from the phospholipids by the action of phospholipase whenever platelets are stimulated. The arachidonic acid, in turn, is converted by cyclo-oxygenase to labile endoperoxidase precursors (PGG_2 and PGH_2), which, in turn, are converted by thromboxane synthetase to thromboxane A_2. Thromboxane A_2, which has a very short half-life, is a powerful platelet-aggregating agent and vasoconstrictor and can induce a release reaction. An important controlling mechanism for the release reaction is the concentration of cyclic adenosine monophosphate (AMP), which is derived from ATP by adenylate cyclase and degraded by phosphodiesterase. The cyclic AMP activates a kinase that decreases the sensitivity of platelets to activating stimuli. Theophylline, which inhibits phosphodiesterase and dipyridamole (Persantine), which breaks down adenylate cyclase, both increase platelet cyclic AMP, thereby inhibiting the release reaction. Prostaglandin synthesis also occurs in the endothelial cells with formation of arachidonic acid and labile endoperoxidase, but there is no thromboxane synthetase in the endothelial cells, and prostaglandin I_2 (prostacyclin) is formed instead of thromboxane A_2. In contrast to thromboxane A_2, prostacyclin is an inhibitor of aggregation and a vasodilator; it acts by stimulating adenylate cyclase, thereby increasing the cyclic AMP concentration. Aspirin irreversibly acetylates and inactivates cyclo-oxygenase in the platelets, resulting in decreased synthesis of thromboxane A_2, with inhibition of the release reaction. In the endothelial cells, however, decrease of prostacyclin synthesis occurs and results in enhancement of the release reaction. As endothelial cells, unlike platelets, can synthesize more cyclo-oxygenase, the aspirin effect is relatively short-lived, while the effect on platelets is as long as the life span of the affected platelet. An ideal effective dosage scheme for aspirin should inhibit production of thromboxane A_2 but not prostacyclin.

The process by which platelets adhere to themselves or to damaged endothelium is not well understood. Both fibrinogen and von Willebrand's factor are essential for normal adhesion, which is defective in patients who have no fibrinogen or von Willebrand's disease. Fibronectin, collagen, and thrombospondin, which are present in the alpha granules of platelets, also have important roles. The binding site for fibrinogen on the platelet resides on a specific glycoprotein referred to as GP IIb-IIIa; in the rare hereditary bleeding disorder, thrombasthenia, this glycoprotein is lacking. The receptor for von Willebrand's factor is on a platelet-surface glycoprotein known as GP Ib, which is absent in the rare hereditary disorder Bernard-Soulier syndrome.

Von Willebrand's disease (vWd) is characterized by the deficiency or functional abnormality of the plasma protein essential for normal platelet function and is referred to as the von Willebrand's factor (vWf). This protein is a high-molecular-weight glycoprotein synthesized by endothelial cells and megakaryocytes and is present within the alpha granules of platelets as well as on the platelet membrane and in the subendothelium. It circulates in the blood as a noncovalently linked complex with the procoagulant protein, factor VIII (also known as factor VIIIC), which is present in only trace amounts. The vWf stabilizes factor VIII and plays an important role in the interaction of platelets with the injured vessel wall. Electrophoresis of normal plasma in agarose containing sodium dodecyl sulfate followed by incubation with an Iodine-125-labeled antibody to vWf reveals multiple bands with molecular weights ranging from 1×10^6 to 20×10^6, reflecting the presence of large circulating polymers of a single subunit protein (MW 230,000); this technique is known as multimeric analysis. The vWf, after modification by the antibiotic ristocetin, aggregates normal platelets. It has been shown that the larger multimers are the most effective in this regard.

Clinical Findings

Patients with hereditary qualitative platelet disorders or von Willebrand's disease usually have a mild-to-moderate bleeding disorder, in which there is excessive bleeding from the smallest cuts or wounds, a prolonged bleeding time, mucous membrane bleeding, and easy bruising, which occurs on trivial trauma or apparently spontaneously. The ecchymoses are almost invariably superficial, and the deep-tissue hematoma and hemarthroses of severe hemophilia are rarely seen. These disorders are all transmitted in an autosomal manner, but there is an apparent female sex predilection, because heavy menstrual bleeding focuses attention on the bleeding disorder. Normally, except in the rare severe cases, the easy bruising and excessive bleeding from cuts are not severe enough to cause patients of either sex to seek medical attention. Many of the cases are so mild that symptoms are manifested only when some precipitating factor, such as ingestion of aspirin or mild associated thrombocytopenia following an infection, is present. A careful history of recent medication is essential, with special attention to aspirin or over-the-counter pain relievers containing aspirin. Patients frequently deny ingestion of aspirin or any medicines containing aspirin, yet they, on repeated questioning, or after an abnormal result is obtained on platelet function testing, recall taking an over-the-counter aspirin preparation (see Table 40–6).

Many other drugs, such as antihistamines, interfere with platelet function; the more important of these are shown in Table 42–1. The thrombocytopenia that can accompany an infectious fever, such as infectious mononucleosis, may precipitate bleeding in a patient with a previously undiagnosed hereditary qualitative platelet disorder or von Willebrand's disease. If in such a case the first platelet count is performed a few days after the bleeding episode, the reduction in the platelet count may seem insignificant. Subsequent platelet counts, however, will show a progressive increase, suggesting that moderate thrombocytopenia may have existed at the time that bleeding occurred.

Approach to Diagnosis

Platelet aggregation studies are needed to delineate the platelet functional disorders and should be performed on patients suspected on clinical grounds of having a life-long disorder of this type. As mild forms of von Willebrand's disease are more frequently encountered than the other platelet functional disorders, a specific laboratory workup for von Willebrand's disease is also performed. Platelet aggregation studies are rarely needed in the acquired disorders of this type, especially when the cause is obvious; eg, aspirin ingestion, uremia, or a myeloproliferative disorder.

The hereditary qualitative platelet disorders may be classified on the basis of platelet aggregation tests (Table 42–2 and Figure 42–1). They fall into three main groups: Bernard-Soulier disease, thrombasthenia, and the thrombopathies. Bernard-Soulier disease is characterized by a failure of the platelets to aggregate with ristocetin in the presence of normal plasma; aggregation is normal with ADP, epinephrine, collagen, and thrombin. Moderate thrombocytopenia may be present, and the platelets tend to be very large. The basic defect is an abnormality of a membrane-specific glycoprotein, GPIb. Other, similar conditions have been termed "giant platelet syndromes." Bernard-Soulier disease is inherited in an autosomal recessive manner; it is very rare, and consanguinity is common among the parents of affected individuals. The hemorrhagic manifestations are severe.

Thrombasthenia, or Glanzmann's disease, is another very rare condition in which there is no aggregation with any concentration of ADP, epinephrine, or collagen. Clot retraction is poor or absent. The basic defect is an abnormality or absence of a platelet surface glycoprotein, GP IIb-IIIa. The platelets, while failing to aggregate, undergo most of the normal changes, including the release reaction

Table 42–1   Drugs that Affect Platelet Function

Anesthetics

    Cocaine (local)

    Procaine (local)

    Volatile general anesthetics

Antibiotics

    Ampicillin

    Carbenicillin

    Gentamicin

    Penicillin G

    Ticarcillin

Anticoagulants

    Dextran

    Heparin (?)

    Warfarin sodium

Anti-inflammatory and Analgesics

    Aspirin

    Colchicine

    Ibuprofen (Motrin)

    Indomethacin (Indocin)

    Mefenamic acid (Ponstel)

    Phenylbutazone (Butazolidin)

    Sulfinpyrazone (Anturane)

Cardiovascular Drugs (ie, vasodilators and antilipemic)

    Clofibrate

    Dipyridamole (Persantine)

    Nicotinic acid

    Papaverine (Myobid)

    Theophylline

Genitourinary Drugs

    Furosemide (Lasix)

    Nitrofurantoin (Furadantin)

(Continued.)

Table 42–1 *Continued.*

Psychiatric Drugs

Phenothiazines

Tricyclic antidepressants: imipramine (Tofranil), Triavil, amitriptyline, (Elavil)

Sympathetic Blocking Agents

Phenoxybenzamine hydrochloride (Dibenzyline)

Propranolol (Inderal)

Miscellaneous

Antihistamines (diphenhydramine hydrochloride)

Ethanol

Glyceryl guaiacolate ether (cough suppressant)

Hashish compounds

Hydroxychloroquine sulfate

Nitroprusside sodium

Vinblastine sulfate (Velban)

SOURCE: Reprinted with permission from Triplett DA, Harms OS, Newhouse P, et al: *Platelet Function. Laboratory Evaluation and Clinical Application.* Chicago, American Society of Clinical Pathologists, 1978.

when stimulated by collagen or thrombin. The platelets on the peripheral blood film are round and isolated but are otherwise unremarkable. Like Bernard-Soulier disease, the condition is associated with severe bleeding manifestations and is inherited in an autosomal recessive manner.

The thrombopathies, characterized by abnormalities in the release reaction, are quite common, in contrast to Bernard-Soulier and Glanzmann's diseases. They can be divided into two subgroups: storage pool disease, in which there is a deficiency of the specialized pool of ADP, and defects in the mechanism responsible for the release of the storage pool contents, which are normal. Both of these subgroups are characterized by the absence of a secondary wave of aggregation with epinephrine or ADP. Aggregation with ristocetin is normal. Differentiation of the two subgroups requires special tests or procedures not usually available in most coagulation laboratories. In storage pool disease, dense granules are decreased, as seen by electron microscopy. In the second subgroup, the storage

Figure 42–1   Flow diagram for diagnosis of qualitative platelet disorder. Single asterisk indicates may be decreased or normal in von Willebrand's disease; double asterisk, patient's plasma is used with normal platelets; and ADP, adenosine diphosphate.

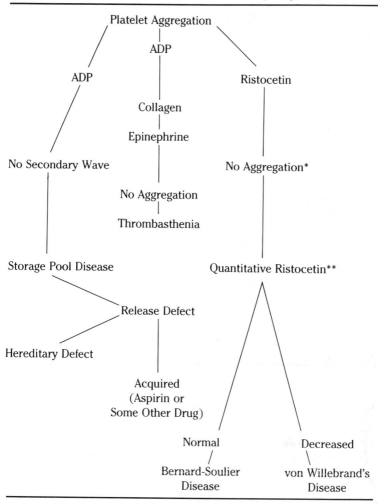

pool and dense granules appear normal but fail to release their constituents when the platelets are exposed to ADP, epinephrine, or collagen. This type is by far the most frequently encountered type of hereditary qualitative abnormality of platelets, and the platelet defects closely resemble those seen after ingestion of aspirin. It has been pointed out recently that many patients with this condition have normal or borderline results on bleeding times that are significantly prolonged after aspirin ingestion; this type of case has been

Table 42–2   Congenital Quantitative Abnormalities
of Platelet Function

| Giant Platelet Syndromes | Aggregation Response | |
| | ADP or Epinephrine | |
	Primary	Secondary
Bernard-Soulier disease	Normal or Decreased	Normal or Decreased
von Willebrand's disease	Normal	Normal
Thrombasthenia	Absent	Absent
Storage pool disease	Normal or Decreased	Absent
Release defect (aspirinlike disorder)	Normal or Decreased	Absent
Intermediate type	Normal	Decreased

ABBREVIATIONS: ADP = adenosine diphosphate; ATP = adenosine triphosphate.

referred to as an intermediate syndrome of platelet dysfunction. For convenience, however, this condition may be considered a very mild type of release defect. Its importance lies in the fact that postoperative bleeding can be avoided in these patients by abstinence from drugs known to interfere with platelet function. The condition may not be recognized with routine screening tests for hemostasis. Considerable heterogeneity is seen within the groups and subgroups, and forms exist with features of more than one group.

Qualitative platelet abnormalities have been reported in patients with glycogen storage disease, type I, and Wilson's disease, as well as in some patients with hereditary disorders of connective tissue, including Ehlers-Danlos and Marfan's syndromes (Table 42–3).

There are several variants of von Willebrand's disease. In the great majority of cases, quantitative deficiency of von Willebrand's factor exists. The activity of this protein, as determined by the quantitative ristocetin-induced platelet aggregation (RIPA) technique, is reduced in proportion to the protein (von Willebrand's factor antigen), as measured by immunological methods, usually by Laurell

Aggregation Response		
Collagen	Ristocetin	Special Features
Normal	Absent	Large platelets seen on smear, clinically severe
Normal	Absent or Decreased	Patient's platelets aggregate with ristocetin in presence of normal plasma
Absent	Normal	Clot retraction poor or absent; clinically severe
Normal or Decreased	Normal	Electron microscopy shows decreased or absent dense granules
Normal or Decreased	Normal	Platelet ATP:ADP ratio increased; ATP:ADP ratio in platelets normal
Normal or Decreased	Normal	Bleeding time abnormal after aspirin ingestion; very mild

immunoelectrophoresis. This is by far the most frequently encountered type of von Willebrand's disease and is referred to as type I. The bleeding time is usually prolonged while the level of factor VIII usually approximates to the von Willebrand's factor but may be higher or even normal. Asymptomatic or mild forms of this type of von Willebrand's disease are frequently found in which the level of the von Willebrand's factor falls between 40% and 60%, with an incidence that may be as high as 1 in 20 population; in these patients, the bleeding time is usually normal. The next most frequently encountered type is referred to as type IIA and is quite rare. In this form of the disease, a qualitative defect of von Willebrand's factor is seen, while the amount of protein synthesized may be normal. The defect appears to be a failure to form large multimers, which is revealed by multimeric analysis or, much more simply, by crossed immunoelectrophoresis. In type IIA, the bleeding time is usually prolonged, and the factor VIII level is decreased or normal. Other types of von Willebrand's disease appear to be exceedingly rare. The recognition of type IIB is considered important because

Table 42-3   Hereditary Conditions Associated with
Decreased Platelet Aggregation

Glanzmann's thrombasthenia

Essential athrombia

Storage pool defect (decreased content of ADP)

  Chédiak-Higashi syndrome

  Thrombocytopenia with absent radii (TAR syndrome)

  Wiskott-Aldrich syndrome

  Hermansky-Pudlak syndrome

Aspirinlike defect

  Cyclo-oxygenase deficiency

  Thromboxane synthetase deficiency

Inborn errors of metabolism

  Homocystinuria

  Wilson's disease

  Glycogen storage disease, type I

Connective tissue abnormalities

  Ehlers-Danlos syndrome (collagen[a])

  Pseudoxanthoma elasticum (collagen[a])

  Osteogenesis imperfecta (collagen[a])

  Marfan's syndrome

  Constitutional abnormality of collagen (patient's collagen only[a])

Afibrinogenemia

Bernard-Soulier syndrome (ristocetin[a])

von Willebrand's syndrome (ristocetin[a])

Swiss-cheese platelets

Gray platelet syndrome

SOURCE: Reprinted with permission from Triplett DA, Harms CS, Newhouse P, et al: *Platelet Function, Laboratory Evaluation and Clinical Application.* Chicago, American Society of Clinical Pathologists, 1978.

[a] The abnormal aggregation patterns are obtained only when this aggregating reagent is used

---

it does not respond to desmopressin (de-amino-d-arginine-vasopressin or DDAVP). In this form of the disease, the bleeding time is prolonged, and von Willebrand's antigen is usually reduced, while its activity as measured by quantitative ristocetin-induced platelet aggregation (RIPA) is somewhat lower than that of the antigen. The diagnostic feature is that a concentration of ristocetin too low to induce aggregation in normal platelet-rich plasma will do so in the patient's platelet-rich plasma. In this form of the disease, the largest multimers appear to be lacking, and it resembles another very rare form (pseudo–von Willebrand's disease or platelet-type von Willebrand's disease), in which there is believed to be abnormal platelet receptors. The laboratory findings in type IIB and the platelet-type are similar, showing enhanced responsiveness of platelet-rich plasma to lower-than-normal concentrations of ristocetin. Direct binding of von Willebrand's factor to the patient's platelets with aggregation in absence of another agonist, however, has been demonstrated in the platelet-type. More recently, a form of von Willebrand's disease has been described similar to type IIA but characterized by the presence of a normal multimeric pattern and normal crossed immunoelectrophoresis. The laboratory and clinical findings of von Willebrand's disease are summarized in Table 42–4.

Acquired forms of von Willebrand's disease have been reported. These forms may result from development of an autoantibody against von Willebrand's factor appearing in a previously healthy individual without any apparent cause or in an individual with systemic lupus erythematosus. Acquired von Willebrand's disease may also occur in lymphoma or multiple myeloma due to the presence of an abnormal protein that in some way inhibits a hypothetical physiologic counterpart of ristocetin.

Qualitative abnormalities of platelets are encountered in the myeloproliferative disorders (especially essential thrombocythemia) and, to a lesser extent, in polycythemia vera, myeloid metaplasia, and chronic myelogenous leukemia. Mild abnormalities are found in uremia, cirrhosis, scurvy, and the dysproteinemias (Table 42–5). By far, however, the most common acquired cause is ingestion of aspirin and other medications. Evaluation of these disorders proceeds as follows:

1. Hematologic evaluation, with particular attention to platelet numbers and morphology.

2. Screening tests for bleeding abnormality, including the activated partial thromboplastin time (APTT), prothrombin time (PT), bleeding time, platelet count, and the clot retraction test, which is performed as part of whole-blood clotting and clot observation tests. The hemophilioid or coagulation type of abnormality is excluded if the APTT and prothrombin time are normal. If results

Table 42–4   Clinical and Laboratory Findings in von Willebrand's Disease

---

Autosomal dominant trait but sometimes recessive

Features of both coagulation and purpuric type of bleeding

Ristocetin-induced platelet aggregation absent or reduced; however in many mild cases, normal aggregation may be seen when ristocetin is added directly to the patient's platelet-rich plasma (nonquantitative RIPA)[a], although quantitative RIPA is reduced

Von Willebrand's antigen usually decreased; if normal, the antigen may have an abnormal mobility on crossed immunoelectrophoresis

Factor VIII usually 6% to 60%, but may be normal or very low

Bleeding time prolonged in about 33% of cases

Immediate and delayed rise in factor VIII after transfusion of preparations containing vWf (eg, cryoprecipitate) indicating de novo synthesis of factor VIII

Levels of both vWf and factor VIII may increase to normal values or even higher in mild cases following stress, exercise, pregnancy, administration of DDAVP, or certain diseases such as hepatitis

Normal platelet aggregation with ADP, epinephrine, and collagen

ABBREVIATIONS: RIPA = ristocetin-induced platelet aggregation; DDAVP = de-amino-d-arginine-vasopressin; ADP = adenosine diphosphate.

[a] There is enhanced responsiveness to low concentrations of ristocetin in type II B

---

of one or both of these tests are prolonged, specific assays are performed (see chapter 43). If the factor VIII level is found to be decreased or at the lower limits of normal, von Willebrand's disease must be excluded. If the bleeding time test result is normal and a qualitative platelet abnormality is suspected, the test may be repeated 2 hours after ingestion of 10 grains of aspirin (aspirin tolerance test), but this should be performed only when all other types of coagulopathies have been excluded.

3. Platelet aggregation tests, which are nonquantitative, are necessary for the diagnosis of von Willebrand's disease and the qualitative platelet disorder. If ristocetin-induced platelet aggregation is abnormal and the aggregation patterns with ADP, col-

Table 42-5   Acquired Conditions Associated with Decreased Platelet Aggregation

---

Myeloproliferative disorders

   Polycythemia vera

   Myeloid metaplasia

   Hemorrhagic thrombocythemia

   Paroxysmal nocturnal hemaglobinuria

   Di Guglielmo syndrome

   Chronic myelocytic leukemia (?)

   Acute myelomonocytic leukemia

   Sideroblastic anemias

Immunoproliferative disorders

   Waldenström's macroglobulinemia

   Plasma cell myeloma

Cirrhosis

Uremia

Asthma (epinephrine[a])

Platelets in idiopathic thrombocytopenic purpura

Drug-induced conditions

Tuberculosis (approximately 15% of cases)

Scurvy

SOURCE: Reprinted with permission from Triplett DA, Harms CS, Newhouse P, et al. *Platelet Function. Laboratory Evaluation and Clinical Application.* Chicago, American Society of Clinical Pathologists, 1978, pp 43–44.

[a] Abnormal aggregation pattern observed only when this reagent is used

---

lagen, epinephrine, and arachidonic acid are normal, the patient has von Willebrand's disease or, rarely, Bernard-Soulier disease. A quantitative ristocetin aggregation test is then performed, using the patient's plasma and normal freshly washed or formalin-fixed platelets. This test gives a measure of the von Willebrand's factor and is referred to as vWf_{Rist}. It is normal in Bernard-Soulier disease, because normal platelets are used in the test, and the defect in this condition resides in the platelets, while the plasma is normal. This is the reverse of von Willebrand's disease, in which the vWf_{Rist} is reduced.

4. Determination of von Willebrand's antigen (vWd_{Ant}). Occasionally, von Willebrand's disease, which in the mild form is relatively common, may coexist with an intrinsic qualitative platelet disorder.

5. If von Willebrand's antigen is normal or only slightly reduced and von Willebrand's factor, as determined by ristocetin-induced aggregation, is very low, the patient has the relatively rare variant type IIA of von Willebrand's disease. This is confirmed by either crossed immunoelectrophoresis when an antigen of abnormal mobility is found or by multimeric analysis.

Hematologic Findings

General features are usually unremarkable, and apart from the Bernard-Soulier syndrome where giant platelets are seen, abnormal platelets are seen only rarely on the smear.

Peripheral Blood Smear Morphology. The number of platelets in the peripheral blood should be estimated, and the presence of any large platelets should be noted. Unless there has been significant bleeding, the red and white cells will be normal. A direct platelet count should be performed.

Bone Marrow Examination. Characteristic changes in bone marrow are seen with acquired platelet defects secondary to myeloproliferative disorders or in association with the dysproteinemias of immune proliferative disorders.

Other Laboratory Tests

42.1   Platelet Aggregation Tests

Purpose. Platelet aggregation tests are used to detect abnormalities in platelet function (Figure 42–1). Such defects, which may be hereditary or result from the ingestion of certain drugs, can be the cause of bleeding in certain patients.

Principle. When an aggregating agent is added in the cuvette of an aggregometer to platelet-rich plasma, which is turbid, the platelets clump, permitting more light to pass through the plasma. The aggregometer is basically a photo-optical instrument, and the amount of light transmitted through the cuvette is recorded on a strip recording chart.

Specimen. Platelet-rich plasma prepared from whole blood anticoagulated with sodium citrate is used. The responsiveness of the platelets to aggregating agents is influenced by the time elapsing from collection, and the tests should be completed within 1 to 3 hours of collection. The temperature at which the platelet-rich plasma is stirred before aggregation studies as well as the temperature at which the actual aggregation tests are carried out have a significant influence on the rate and extent of aggregation. Platelets stored at room temperature are more sensitive to ADP than are platelets stored at 37° C.

Procedure. Platelet-rich plasma is obtained by the slow centrifugation of whole blood anticoagulated with sodium citrate; this procedure is carried out in plastic tubes at room temperature, and at no time should the plasma be cooled. The aggregating agents used are ADP, collagen suspensions (which may be obtained commercially or prepared by homogenizing tissue obtained at operation), epinephrine, and ristocetin (Figure 42–2); some laboratories also use thrombin. A blank value is obtained by using platelet-poor plasma from the patient. The platelet-rich plasma is placed in the cuvette and warmed to 37° C, the aggregating agent is added, and the contents of the cuvette are stirred constantly by means of a small Teflon stirring rod.

Interpretation. The results with each aggregating agent may be recorded as the slope of the curve, the absolute magnitude of the transmittance change, or the percentage change of the transmittance or of the optical density. In most laboratories, however, the results are not reported in a quantitative manner but merely in descriptive terms. The results are dependent on the concentration of the aggregating agents, which should be stated in the report. With relatively low doses of ADP (1 μg/mL), 2 waves of aggregation are seen. The first, or primary, wave is induced by the ADP added to the patient's plasma, while the secondary wave is attributed to release of relatively large amounts of intrinsic ADP from the storage pool within the platelets. With even lower concentrations of ADP (0.5 μg/mL), the release reaction does not occur, the platelets disaggregate, and only a primary wave is seen, while with relatively large doses of ADP a single

Figure 42–2 Platelet aggregation studies: normal tracing. The strength of (ADP) was 1 μg/mL. Note that the initial steep slope of the primary or reversible wave with this strength of ADP begins to flatten out and is rapidly followed by the second steep slope of the second irreversible wave.

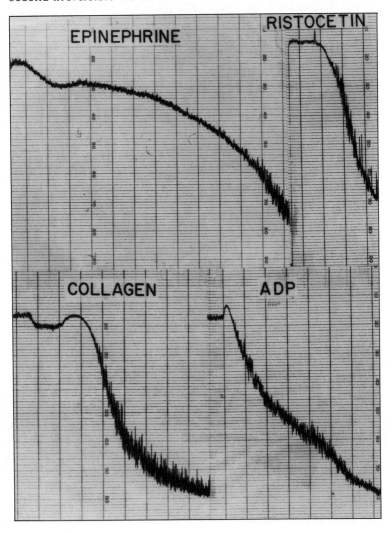

broad wave is seen. A biphasic response is seen with epinephrine in about 50% to 80% of healthy persons. As collagen acts by inducing release of ADP, a primary wave is not seen. In thrombasthenia, there is no aggregation with any concentration of ADP, epinephrine, or collagen, but aggregation is seen with

Figure 42–3   Platelet aggregation studies: thrombasthenia. No aggregation with epinephrine, (ADP), or collagen; normal aggregation with ristocetin.

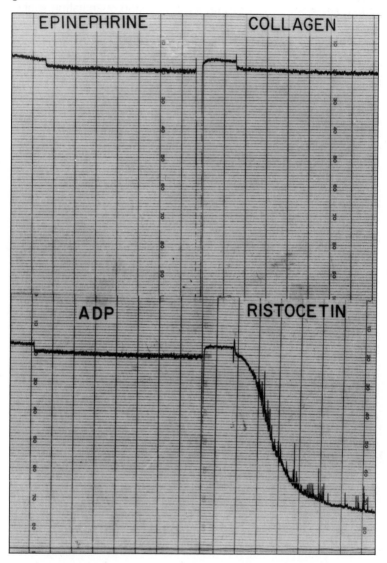

ristocetin (Figure 42–3). In Bernard-Soulier disease, there is normal aggregation with ADP, epinephrine, or collagen but no aggregation with ristocetin. The findings are similar to von Willebrand's disease (Figure 42–4), although it is far more common to find reduced rather than absent aggregation with ristocetin.

Figure 42–4 Platelet aggregation studies: von Willebrand's disease. Note absence of aggregation with ristocetin. A total lack of aggregation with this reagent is seen only in severe cases. In mild cases, aggregation of ristocetin is variable and quantitation is necessary. A similar pattern is seen in the very rare condition, Bernard-Soulier disease. ADP indicates adenosine diphosphate.

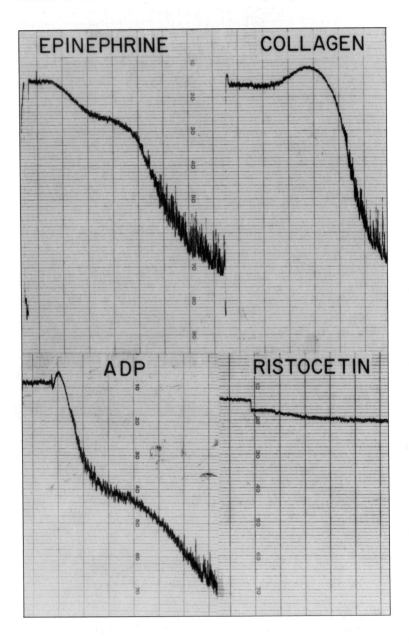

Figure 42–5   Platelet aggregation studies: storage pool disease. Note the absence of secondary wave with epinephrine and ADP and no aggregation with collagen. Platelets react normally with ristocetin. Similar tracings may be seen in platelet membrane defects or after ingestion of drugs, such as aspirin and many others.

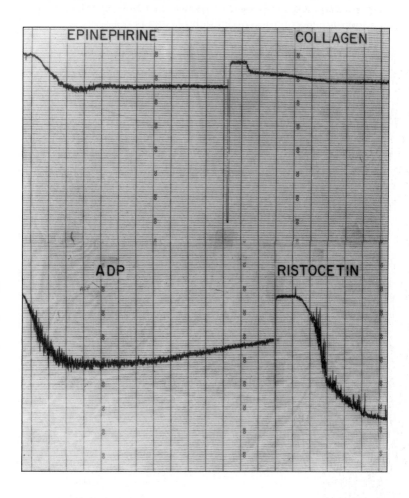

In storage pool disease and in release defects (aspirin-catalyzed disorders), the secondary waves with ADP and epinephrine are absent (Figure 42–5), and there is reduced or absent aggregation with collagen; ristocetin aggregation is normal.

More subtle changes may be clinically significant when ristocetin is used as the aggregating agent, and the slope should be compared with that of the control. A normal tracing with ristocetin does not exclude a moderate deficiency of von Willebrand's factor. Thus, when this disease is suspected, a quantitative ristocetin aggregation test must be performed. In addition to the usual concentration of ristocetin, a lower concentration (0.5 mg/mL final concentration) should also be used in the nonquantitative test to detect the rare type IIB, von Willebrand's disease. In this condition, aggregation occurs with the lower concentration of ristocetin, while aggregation with the normal control platelet-rich plasma is not seen.

Notes and Precautions.   Specimens left for more than 3 hours at room temperature may lose their ability to aggregate. Platelets stored at 0° C sometimes undergo spontaneous aggregation. Occasionally, platelets of healthy individuals who have apparently not taken any drugs appear abnormal. Whenever an abnormal result is obtained, the test should be repeated on another specimen collected some days later.

42.2   Von Willebrand Factor Quantitative Assay (Quantitative Ristocetin Aggregation)

Purpose.   The test is used to measure the biologic activity of the von Willebrand's factor. It is decreased in von Willebrand's disease and in certain acquired disorders.

Principle.   The ability of the patient's plasma to aggregate normal platelets in the presence of ristocetin is compared with that of normal pooled plasma.

Specimen.   Plasma used for the performance of the APTT test is satisfactory; the plasma may be stored for several weeks at $-20°$ C without losing activity.

Procedure.   Serial dilutions of plasma in saline are prepared, and an aliquot of each is added to a fixed amount of a saline suspension of washed platelets in the cuvette of an aggregometer. Ristocetin is then added and the slope of the wave determined (maximum change in light transmittance). By plotting slope against dilution of the plasma on log-log paper, a straight line is obtained. A dilution of the patient's plasma is tested, and the equivalent dilution of normal plasma that would give the same slope is read from the straight-line curve, eg, if a 1:5 dilution of the patient's plasma gives the same slope as a 1:10 dilution of the normal plasma, the activity of vWf in the patient's plasma is 50% that of the normal control subject.

Interpretation. A decrease in von Willebrand's factor in a patient with a lifelong history of bleeding is pathognomonic of von Willebrand's disease. Acquired deficiencies caused by antibodies against von Willebrand's factors and certain paraproteins may also result in a decrease in von Willebrand's factor.

42.3 Immunoprecipitation Assay for von Willebrand Antigen

Purpose. The immunoprecipitation assay is used for the diagnosis of von Willebrand's disease. In this disease, von Willebrand's factor antigen is usually decreased.

Principle. A precipitating rabbit antibody against von Willebrand's factor is used to quantitate von Willebrand's factor. The immunoassay is usually performed by the Laurell technique, which is an electroimmunodiffusion method for the quantitation of proteins in which rocket-shaped anodic immunoprecipitates are formed. The height of the rocket is proportional to the concentration of von Willebrand's factor.

Specimen. The patient's plasma or serum may be used, but the former is preferable. Plasma collected for the APTT test is satisfactory.

Procedure. The antibody is mixed with liquid agarose, which is then poured onto a plate and allowed to solidify by cooling. Holes are punched on one side of the plate, which is then placed in an electrophoresis chamber. Serial dilutions of the standard, normal pooled plasma (1:2, 1:4, 1:8, etc, in saline), and a 1:2 dilution of the plasma being tested are prepared and placed in the wells. Electrophoresis of the sample is then performed, and when the run is completed, the plate is examined. The rocket-shaped immunoprecipitates are sometimes hard to see, but the visibility can be increased by immersing the plates in tannic acid for a few minutes.

Interpretation. A value below 50% is consistent with von Willebrand's disease, and values between 50% and 60% are borderline. If the quantitative ristocetin aggregation test shows abnormal results, and the antigen is normal, cross immuno-electrophoresis is indicated. Alternatively, multimeric analysis may be used, but this procedure is technically more difficult and time-consuming. Von Willebrand's factor antigen and von Willebrand's factor, as determined by quantitative ristocetin aggregation, are both increased by exercise, by hepatitis, and during pregnancy, and a corresponding increase is seen in patients with von Willebrand's disease. Thus, in these conditions, normal values do not preclude the disease.

Notes and Precautions. The determination of von Willebrand's antigen, often referred to as factor VIII related antigen, should be distinguished from the determination of the factor VIII antigen. The latter is the antigen corresponding to the factor VIII coagulant protein, which is decreased in at least 90% of patients with hemophilia A. The test to determine factor VIII antigen is currently available in only a few laboratories.

References

1. Baugh BF, Hougie C: Characterization of a new mode of defective ristocetin-induced platelet aggregation. *J Lab Clin Med* 1981; 97:864–880.
2. Czapek EE, Deykin D, Salzman E, et al: Intermediate syndrome of platelet dysfunction. *Blood* 1978; 52:103–113.
3. Holmberg L, Nilsson IM: von Willebrand's disease. *Clin Haematol* 1985; 14:461–488.
4. Ruggeri Z, Zimmerman TS: Platelets and von Willebrand disease. *Semin Haematol* 1985; 22:203–218.
5. Triplett DA, Harms CS, Newhouse P, et al: *Platelet Function: Laboratory Evaluation and Clinical Application.* Chicago, American Society of Clinical Pathologists, 1978.
6. Weiss HJ: Abnormalities of factor VIII and platelet aggregation: Use of ristocetin in diagnosing the von Willebrand syndrome. *Blood* 1975; 45:403–417.

43

Hereditary Coagulation Disorders

Hereditary coagulation disorders resulting from a deficiency or abnormality of a clotting factor are characterized by delayed bleeding following trauma. Hemophilia A and hemophilia B comprise >95% of these disorders.

Pathophysiology

When a small vessel is punctured or cut, a hemostatic plug formed from aggregated platelets seals the hole, and the plug is subsequently reinforced by fibrin. In conditions in which the formation of fibrin is abnormal, the plug may be relatively weak and unstable and liable to break down, sometimes several days following the injury. Based on the degree of severity of symptoms for the same level of reduced activity, factors VIII and IX appear to be the 2 most important procoagulant factors required for normal hemostasis. Factor XI deficiency is either very mild or asymptomatic while factor V, VII, or X deficiencies are intermediate in severity. Deficiencies of the contact factors, other than factor XI, are not associated with any hemostatic abnormalities, which may be explained by the presence of bypass mechanisms. Thus, the reaction product of tissue factor and factor VIIa can convert in vitro factor IX to factor IXa, thereby bypassing the contact mechanism, but this does not explain why some patients with factor XI deficiency bleed.

Clinical Findings

The characteristic clinical features of a bleeding disorder caused by an abnormality of a blood clotting factor (features that distinguish them from platelet disorders) are outlined in Table 40–1.

The great majority of hereditary disorders of the coagulation type are relatively benign, and bleeding only occurs when the hemostatic mechanism is severely challenged. A history of easy bruising and excessive bleeding after minor surgery, such as tonsillectomy or tooth extraction, usually exists. Such bleeding is troublesome but rarely life-threatening. Hemarthroses are usually seen only in severe cases but may occur in mild cases following joint injuries. The clinical differentiation of this type of disorder from a purpuric state is usually not clear-cut, but a history of bleeding from a wound or injury starting after an interval of several hours or days suggests a coagulation type rather than a purpuric disorder. The lifelong nature of the bleeding disorder is usually sufficient to permit categorization of the disorder as a hereditary rather than acquired one. Acquired disorders of clotting are considered in chapter 44.

Approach to Diagnosis

Hemarthroses in a male patient may be considered the hallmark of a severe coagulation disorder. If this is sex linked, the patient has either hemophilia A or hemophilia B; exceptions to this rule are rare. All that is then needed to establish the diagnosis is a specific assay of factor VIII and, if the results are normal, an assay for factor IX. Purpura is rare in a coagulation disorder and suggests either von Willebrand's disease or the coexistence of thrombocytopenia or a qualitative platelet disorder.

Evaluation of hereditary coagulation disorders proceeds as follows:

1. Hematologic evaluation to exclude thrombocytopenia and anemia.

2. Screening tests for a bleeding disorder, including APTT, PT, thrombin time, and bleeding time determinations. The necessity for and nature of subsequent studies depend on the results of these tests (Tables 43–1 and 43–2). Thus, if the bleeding time is prolonged and the PT and APTT are normal, tests for a qualitative platelet disorder or von Willebrand's disease should be performed (chapter 41). The clinical and laboratory findings that enable the differentiation of mild hemophilia A from von Willebrand's disease are shown in Table 43–3. The majority of patients with a coagulation-type defect have a prolonged APTT,

Table 43–1   Screening Tests in Hereditary Deficiencies of Clotting Factors

Factor	APTT	Prothrombin Time	Thrombin Time
HMW-K (Fitzgerald)	Increased	Normal	Normal
Fletcher	Increased	Normal	Normal
XII, XI, IX	Increased	Normal	Normal
VIII	Increased	Normal	Normal
V, X	Increased	Increased	Normal
Prothrombin	Increased	Increased	Normal
VII	Normal	Increased	Normal
Hypofibrinogenemia	Increased	Increased	Increased
Dysfibrinogenemia	Increased	Increased	Increased
Factor XIII deficiency	Normal	Normal	Normal

ABBREVIATIONS: APTT = activated partial thromboplastin time.

a normal PT, and a normal bleeding time. In 95% of cases, a deficiency of factor VIII, IX, or XI will be found.

3. If the APTT is prolonged and the PT is normal, specific assays for the intrinsic factors are performed (Figure 43–1). Factor VIII is assayed first; if normal, factor IX is assayed. If all 3 of these factors are normal, the Passovoy defect should be considered. Deficiencies of factor XII, Fletcher factor (prekallikrein), or HMW-kininogen result in a prolonged APTT but do not cause a bleeding tendency. Thus, a deficiency of any one of these 3 contact factors can account for the prolonged APTT but not for the bleeding tendency.

4. If both the APTT and PT are prolonged while the thrombin time is normal, specific assays for factors X and V and prothrombin are performed.

5. If the APTT, PT, and thrombin time are prolonged, dysfibrinogenemia or hypofibrinogenemia should be considered, and a fibrinogen determination should be performed using at least two techniques.

6. If the APTT is normal and the PT is prolonged, a deficiency of factor VII should be considered and a specific assay for this factor performed.

7. If the APTT, PT, and thrombin time are normal, a test for clot solubility in 5 M urea should be performed to exclude a defi-

Table 43–2 Use of Activated Partial Thromboplastin Time, Prothrombin Time, and Bleeding Time as Screening Tests in Lifelong Bleeding Disorders

APTT	PT	Bleeding Time	Further Tests to be Performed
Normal	Normal	Normal or Increased	Platelet function tests, including ristocetin aggregation, vWf factor antigen, VIII assay if APTT is borderline, factor XIII screen
Increased	Normal	Increased	VIII assay, vWf_{Ant} quantitative ristocetin
Increased	Normal	Normal	VIII assay, if normal, IX, then XI; if VIII is low perform vWf_{Ant} and quantitative ristocetin, exclude inhibitor
Increased	Increased	Normal or Increased	Thrombin time, if normal V, X, and prothrombin assays; if thrombin time is prolonged, assay fibrinogen
Normal	Increased	Normal or Increased	VII deficiency

ABBREVIATIONS: APTT = activated partial thromboplastin time; PT = prothrombin time; vWf = von Willebrand's factor.

ciency of the fibrin stabilizing factor (Laki-Lorand factor, or factor XIII).

8. Inhibitor screen. When the APTT is prolonged while the PT is normal, the APTT should be repeated on a mixture of equal parts of the patient's and normal plasma. This test is, however, relatively insensitive and nonspecific, and in all patients with a deficiency of factor VIII a specific test for the presence of an antibody against factor VIII should be performed. In patients with other types of hereditary deficiencies, with the possible exception of factor XIII, the development of an antibody specifically directed against the deficient factor is excessively rare. Accordingly, unless there is some unusual circumstance, such as failure to respond to treatment with the appropriate concentrate, or when the APTT inhibitor screen is positive, a specific search for antibody is not part of the evaluation of hereditary deficiencies of a clotting factor other than factor VIII.

Table 43–3 Differential Diagnosis of von Willebrand's Disease from Hemophilia A

Characteristic	von Willebrand's Disease	Hemophilia A
Inheritance	Autosomal	Sex linked
Hemarthroses or joint damage	Rare	Present in most severe cases
Clinical severity	Usually mild and rarely dangerous or crippling	Mild to severe cases
Bleeding time	May be prolonged	Normal if performed correctly
Factor VIII level	Usually 6% to 50%	0% to 35%
Factor VIII level following stress, exercise, or severe liver disease	May increase severalfold	May also increase severalfold[a]
vWf antigen	<50%	>50%
vWf (ristocetin aggregation)	Abnormal	Normal
Effect of transfusion of concentrates containing vWf and factor VIII[b]	Immediate response, but factor VIII continues to rise for 24–48 hours	Immediate response followed by rapid decay (T½ = 12 hours)

ABBREVIATIONS: vWf = von Willebrand's factor.
[a]In severe cases with less than 1% factor VIII, there is no apparent effect
[b]This should never be used as a diagnostic test

9. Von Willebrand's factor and antigen determinations. In some patients with von Willebrand's disease, the bleeding time may be normal and the clinical and laboratory findings may mimic those seen in mild hemophilia (Table 43–3). It is therefore necessary to perform tests for von Willebrand's disease in all patients with decreased levels of factor VIII in whom there is no clear-cut sex-linked family history.

10. If results of all the above tests are normal, the alpha$_2$-antiplasmin level should be determined. Heterozygotes for this deficiency have levels of 35% to 60% and may bleed excessively, while homozygotes have a severe hemorrhagic diathesis of the coagulation type.

Figure 43–1   Evaluation of patient with lifelong history of bleeding and prolonged activated partial thromboplastin time (APTT).

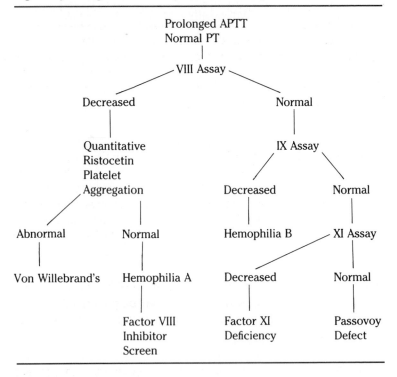

Hematologic Findings

Apart from the exclusion of anemia and thrombocytopenia, the morphology of the formed elements in the blood are usually unremarkable.

Blood Cell Measurements.   Blood counts and red cell morphology can be consistent with a hypochromic anemia in a few patients with very frequent or chronic blood loss.

Other Laboratory Tests

43.1   Assay for Factor VIII

Purpose.   The determination of the level of factor VIII is necessary for the diagnosis of hemophilia A. The level usually correlates well with clinical severity. Assays are also used for monitoring the effect of concentrates. Factor VIII is usually decreased in von Willebrand's disease proportionately to von Willebrand's factor. While hemophilia A carriers also have decreased levels of factor VIII, their von Willebrand's factor is normal. Stress or pregnancy in hemophilia A carriers may cause the factor VIII to rise to normal, but the ratio of von Willebrand's factor to factor VIII remains increased. Factor VIII must be assayed in every patient who has an acquired coagulopathy with a prolonged APTT and a normal PT.

Principle. The ability of dilutions of the patient's plasma to correct the prolonged APTT of plasma deficient in factor VIII is compared with that of normal pooled plasma, eg, if a 1:20 dilution of normal plasma shortens the clotting time of the deficient plasma to the same extent as a 1:5 dilution of the patient's plasma, the patient's plasma has 25% of the activity of the normal plasma.

Specimen. The plasma collected for the APTT test is used. Factor VIII is fairly stable, and the test may be performed on plasma frozen within an hour or two of collection and stored at $-30°$ C.

Procedure. The deficient plasma used is obtained from a patient known to have less than 1% factor VIII. It may be kept for several months if stored at $-70°$ C. Dilutions of normal pooled plasma (1:5, 1:10, 1:20, 1:40, 1:80, 1:160) and the patient's plasma (1:5, 1:10) in saline are prepared. One part of each dilution is added to 1 part of the deficient plasma, and the APTT of the mixture is determined.

Interpretation. The 1:5 dilution of the normal pooled plasma is arbitrarily taken as 100% activity, the 1:10 as 50%, the 1:20 as 25%, and so forth. A straight line is obtained on log-log paper when clotting times are plotted against percentage concentration of normal plasma. The concentrations of normal plasma that would give the same clotting times as the 1:5 and 1:10 dilutions of the patient's plasma are determined from the graph. The percentage concentration obtained with the 1:5 dilution is the actual concentration of factor VIII in the patient's plasma, while the value obtained with the 1:10 dilution has to be multiplied by 2. The mean of the two values is reported. If the value with the 1:10 dilution is significantly higher than that of the 1:5 dilution, an inhibitor should be suspected, but the assay should be repeated to exclude an error in technique. The normal range for factors VIII and IX is 60% to 150%.

Notes and Precautions. The activity of factor VIII may be increased significantly by trace amounts of thrombin that may form if the blood is collected too slowly or if it is incompletely mixed with the anticoagulant. Factor VIII is also sometimes increased in disseminated intravascular coagulation (DIC), presumably because of thrombin activation, as well as by exercise. Running for 5 minutes may double or even triple the level, which may remain high for several hours.

43.2   Assays for Other Factors Involved in Intrinsic Pathway Only

Purpose. Assays for other factors involved in the intrinsic pathway may reveal the cause of a prolonged APTT not attributable to factor VIII.

Principle. The principle is the same as that underlying the one-stage procedure for the factor VIII assay described previously. The relative ability of the patient's plasma to shorten the prolonged APTT of plasma from a patient deficient in the factor being tested is compared with that of pooled normal plasma.

Procedure. The procedure is the same as that described for the assays of factor VIII, using the appropriate deficient plasma in place of factor VIII–deficient plasma. For the assay of Fletcher factor (prekallikrein), the preincubation period in the APTT test after addition of kaolin should not exceed 3 minutes; longer incubation periods cause the APTT of Fletcher factor–deficient plasma to approach the normal value. Accordingly, certain automated instruments in which the preincubation period exceeds 3 minutes cannot be used. In the HMW-K assay, the 1:20 dilution of normal plasma may be as effective in shortening the APTT of the HMW-K–deficient plasma as the 1:5 dilution. Therefore, in performing this assay, it is advisable to start at a 1:20 dilution and to continue up to a 1:320 dilution. The unknown is tested at a 1:5 dilution up to a 1:20 dilution.

Interpretation. The normal range for these factors is 60% to 150%.

Notes and Precautions. The deficient plasma may be obtained from a commercial source. Fletcher factor and HMW-K–deficient plasmas are rare, and, accordingly, few coagulation laboratories are able to perform these assays, although they are technically quite simple. In most instances, however, a provisional diagnosis of these two deficiencies may be made by a process of exclusion. Thus, if the patient has a prolonged APTT, normal PT, normal levels of all the intrinsic factors (including factors XI or XII), and a negative bleeding history, a deficiency of Fletcher factor or HMW-K should be considered. Fletcher factor–deficient plasma shortens progressively on incubation with kaolin (Celite) and may be normal after 8 minutes of preincubation, thereby differing from HMW-K–deficient plasma.

43.3 Assays for Prothrombin and Factors V, VII, and X

Purpose. Assays for prothrombin and for factors V, VII, and X are performed to determine the specific cause(s) of a prolonged PT.

Principle. The principle is the same as that for assays of the factors that were described previously, but the PT is used instead of the APTT.

Specimen. Blood is collected in the same manner as for the assay of factor VIII. The assay for factor V should be performed within 4 hours of collection because it is relatively labile. Assays of factor VII are best performed as soon as possible after collection because it may increase in value when the plasma is stored in the refrigerator.

Procedure. The actual technique using plasma from patients deficient in prothrombin and factors V, VII, or X is very simple; however, these deficient states are very rare, and the deficient plasmas are usually prepared artificially and are available commercially. For example, factor V–deficient plasma is prepared by aging plasma at 37° C. The assays are performed in the same manner as the assays for the intrinsic factors (eg, factor VIII), using the PT instead of the APTT. The ability of the patient's plasma to shorten the prolonged PT of plasma deficient in the factor being assayed is compared with that of normal plasma.

Interpretation. The normal range for prothrombin and for factors V, VII, and X is 60% to 150%.

43.4   Inhibitor Screening Test

Purpose.   The inhibitor screening test is used for detection of inhibitors of clotting, which are usually immunoglobulins.

Principle.   The addition of plasma containing an inhibitor of a factor involved in intrinsic clotting prolongs the APTT of normal plasma.

Specimen.   The same plasma used in the APTT test is used as a specimen.

Procedure.   One part of the plasma being tested is incubated with an equal part of normal plasma. The APTTs of the mixture are determined immediately and after 20 minutes incubation at 37° C.

Interpretation.   When 1 part of plasma congenitally deficient in a clotting factor, such as factor VIII, is mixed with an equal part of normal plasma, the APTT of the mixture is usually ≤5 sec longer than that of the normal plasma alone if this is between 26 and 30 sec. A difference of 6 sec or more is good evidence of an inhibitor, while a difference of 5 sec is equivocal. Most inhibitors are immediate-acting, ie, their action is not enhanced by incubation, but notable exceptions are antibodies to factor VIII.

Notes and Precautions.   The inhibitor screening test is subject to many technical variations, such as differences in the concentration of the sodium citrate used to anticoagulate the normal and patient's plasma. Incubation of normal platelet-poor plasma alone can result in an increase in the APTT because of loss of factor V; on the other hand, if the plasma is not centrifuged at a speed sufficient to sediment most of the platelets, the APTT of the plasma can actually shorten on incubation. An inhibitor can result in spuriously low values of the intrinsic factors; results of such assays must be interpreted with caution when an inhibitor is suspected. The tissue thromboplastin inhibition test (TTI) is not specific for lupuslike anticoagulants and may be abnormal in patients with acquired inhibitors against factor VIII (chapter 44); it is therefore not recommended. The platelet neutralization test (Triplett) is more specific, but the author relies on assays of factors VIII, IX, XI, and XII to exclude a factor VIII inhibitor. If the factor VIII assay results are higher than those of the other factors, the inhibitor is very unlikely to be directed against this factor.

43.5   Factor VIII Antibody Screening Test

Purpose.   Antibodies against factor VIII develop in about 7% of patients with hemophilia A. The titer of the antibody increases after transfusions of plasma or factor VIII concentrates, and their detection is important because the patient's condition may become refractory to treatment. Factor VIII antibodies are an important cause of a severe hemorrhagic diathesis in previously healthy individuals; in patients with a background of an immunological disorder, such as systemic lupus erythematosus, rheumatoid arthritis, and penicillin sensitivity; and in females following parturition. An antibody to factor VIII must be excluded in every patient found during a preoperative workup to have an inhibitor. While the vast majority of inhibitors are of the lupuslike type (chapter 44) and do not give rise to excessive bleeding, surgery in a patient with a factor VIII inhibitor is dangerous and often fatal.

Principle.   If plasma suspected of containing a factor VIII inhibitor is incubated with an equal volume of normal plasma, after a short period of incubation, the factor VIII concentration of the mixture will be significantly lower than the mean of the two.

Specimen.   Plasma collected for the APTT is used as a specimen; the antibodies are remarkably stable and are present in both plasma and serum. The specimen may be adsorbed with aluminum hydroxide and heated to 56° C for 30 minutes without effect on the antibody.

Procedure.   One part of plasma from the patient is mixed with an equal volume of normal pooled plasma (used as the 100% standard). After incubation for 30 minutes at 37° C, the mixture is diluted in a ratio of 1:5 in saline and assayed for factor VIII.

Interpretation.   If the factor VIII concentration of the mixture is ≥35%, the patient does not have an inhibitor, or the inhibitor is too weak to be significant.

Notes and Precautions.   To detect a low-titer inhibitor, it is advisable to obtain plasma several days after, as well as before, replacement therapy.

43.6   Factor VIII Antibody Titer

Purpose.   This test estimates the potency of an antibody against factor VIII.

Principle.   Serial dilutions of plasma containing the inhibitor are incubated with normal plasma for a specified period, and the residual factor VIII is determined. Factor VIII inhibitor titers are commonly expressed in Bethesda units, which are defined as the amount that, when incubated with normal plasma, neutralizes half of the factor VIII in 2 hours.

Specimen.   Blood is collected as for the APTT test or factor VIII assay.

Procedure.   Serial dilutions in saline (1:2, 1:4, etc) of the plasma being tested are incubated with an equal volume of normal plasma for 2 hours at 37° C. The residual factor VIII in each of the incubation mixtures is determined. The inhibitor titer in Bethesda units is the reciprocal of the dilution of the test plasma that gives 50% inhibition; this may be determined by drawing a curve relating activity of residual factor VIII to the reciprocal of the dilution or by a rough approximation made by inspection of the data.

Interpretation.   A hemostatic level of factor VIII can usually be achieved by replacement therapy using human factor VIII concentrates in patients with ≤2 Bethesda units. After four days, however, the inhibitor titer in a hemophiliac is likely to have increased severalfold; in a nonhemophiliac, this increase may not occur.

There is considerable heterogeneity between the factor VIII antibodies of different patients. The antibodies seen in non-hemophiliacs may differ strikingly from those seen in hemophiliac patients. For example, some of the antibodies seen in nonhemophiliacs may only neutralize 80% of the available factor VIII in normal plasma over a period of 12 hours, reaching a plateau, yet when the factor VIII concentration of the mixture is increased to 100% by addition of factor VIII concentrate, the level again falls to only 20%, indicating that the antibody was only partially neutralized. Moreover, if a factor VIII concentrate is given to a patient with a factor VIII antibody, the factor VIII level determined in the laboratory may not be a true reflection of the level at the time the plasma was withdrawn, as destruction occurs in vitro between the time of collection and actual performance of the assay. Other test systems are used to assay factor VIII antibodies, with different definitions of a unit. The results obtained using different test systems are in general poorly correlated; however, each method gives useful information with respect to the relative potency of the antibody in any one patient over a period of time.

Course and Treatment

The specific treatment for the bleeding of hereditary coagulation disorders is to raise the level of the deficient or defective protein above the minimum concentration believed adequate for normal hemostasis, ie, approximately 40% of the mean normal level for most factors; to achieve this level in a patient with a very low baseline value with plasma alone is virtually impossible, so that concentrates have to be used. Concentrates are generally available for the treatment of hemophilia A and hemophilia B. Cryoprecipitate is a good source of both factor VIII and von Willebrand's factor, and each pack is derived from a single unit of blood. The more potent concentrates are derived from multiple donors and carry a much greater risk of infection with the non A, and non B hepatitis virus and also the hepatitis B virus. More than half of the hemophilic patients who received these concentrates developed AIDS. Now, however, the preparations are subjected to various treatments to inactivate the human immunodeficiency virus (HIV). Recently, recombinant factor VIII has been used successfully in clinical trials, while a very high purified preparation derived from human plasma and free of viral contamination is now available, albeit extremely expensive. Factor IX concentrates also contain prothrombin and factors X and VII and may be used in the treatment of deficiencies of these factors. The factor IX concentrates are currently heat-treated and, like factor VIII concentrates, are no longer believed to transmit HIV. Concentrates are not available for the treatment of factor V, XI, or XIII deficiencies but, fortunately, these are rarely required. The dosage schedules depend on the half-life of the factor being replaced, which is roughly 12 hours for factor VIII and 24 hours in the case of factor IX. Replacement therapy is indicated for life-threatening hemorrhages (eg, central nervous system or intraperitoneal bleeds), surgery, and the early treatment of hemarthroses and deep-tissue hematomas. Almost all patients with mild hemophilia and all patients with von Willebrand's disease (with very few exceptions that include the rare type IIB) respond well to the intravenous infusion of Desmopressin[R] (DDAVP), a synthetic analogue of vasopressin given in doses of 0.3 μg/g over a period of 15 to 30 minutes. This drug often induces increases of factor VIII and von

Willebrand's factor, which may be as much as twofold or threefold above the basal level, often without any side effects. Thus, plasma or plasma concentrates are rarely required by these patients. EACA or tranexamic acid are sometimes useful for minor bleeding episodes in the coagulation disorders and are very effective in the treatment of alpha$_2$-antiplasmin deficiency.

References

1. Bloom AL, Giddings JC, Peake IR: The haemophilias, in Poller L (ed): *Recent Advances in Blood Coagulation.* New York, Churchill-Livingstone Inc, 1985, vol 4, pp 91–116.

2. Girolami A, de Marco L, Zanon RDB, et al: Rarer quantitative and qualitative abnormalities of coagulation. *Clin Haematol* 1985; 14:385–409.

3. Hougie C: Circulating anticoagulants, in Poller L (ed): *Recent Advances in Blood Coagulation.* New York, Churchill-Livingstone Inc, 1985, vol 4, pp 63–90.

4. Kasper CK, Dietrich SL: Comprehensive management of haemophilia. *Clin Haematol* 1985; 14:489–512.

5. McGraw RA, Davis LM, Lundblad RL, et al: Structure and function of factor IX: Defects in haemophilia B. *Clin Haematol* 1985; 14:359–383.

6. Miles LA, Plow EF, Donnelly KJ, et al: A bleeding disorder due to a deficiency of alpha$_2$-antiplasmin. *Blood* 1982; 59:1246–1251.

7. Triplett DA: Congenital coagulation factor deficiencies (excluding abnormalities of factor VIII), in Triplett DA (ed): *Laboratory Evaluation of Coagulation.* Chicago, American Society of Clinical Pathologists Press, 1982, pp 53–113.

44

Acquired Coagulation Disorders

The most common causes of acquired deficiencies of clotting factors associated with hemorrhagic manifestations are decreased or abnormal synthesis of clotting factors caused by liver disease and disseminated intravascular coagulation (DIC); the latter is seen in almost every type of severe illness, including metastatic carcinoma and infectious diseases. Vitamin K deficiency is an important but now a relatively uncommon cause of a hemorrhagic diathesis. While lupuslike anticoagulants are encountered very frequently and result in apparent decreases in certain clotting factors, they are not associated with excessive bleeding. On the other hand, antibodies against prothrombin and factors V, VIII, and XIII, although rare, may arise de novo in individuals with no previous hemorrhagic disorder, causing severe bleeding.

Pathophysiology

The liver is the major site of synthesis of clotting factors, and a hemorrhagic diathesis can occur in severe hepatitis or cirrhosis. In these conditions, the vitamin K–dependent clotting factors (ie, prothrombin and factors VII, IX, and X) (see chapter 40) are usually the first to be reduced, followed by factor V. Factor VIII, which is an acute-phase protein, although synthesized in the liver, is at normal or actually increased levels, while von Willebrand's factor, which is synthesized by endothelial cells, is often strikingly increased. In addition to these changes, there may be a defect in the polymerization of fibrin monomer. The fibrinolytic potentiality may be increased because of a decrease in alpha$_2$-antiplasmin, while the capacity to inactivate partially activated products of blood coagulation may be impaired; these 2 factors may account for the fairly common occurrence of DIC in advanced liver disease. Moderate thrombocytopenia, which can be the result of DIC or splenic pooling if splenomegaly is present, may also be found frequently in patients with liver disease. Vitamin K is essential for the normal synthesis of the vitamin K–dependent clotting factors. In its absence, the vitamin K–dependent factors do not bind calcium and, although synthesized in normal amounts, are inactive. Naturally occurring vitamin K is fat-soluble, and bile is essential for its absorption from the gastrointestinal tract. In any condition in which influx of bile into the gut is impeded, a hemorrhagic diathesis may ensue. The absorption of vitamin K occurs in the small intestine and may be deficient in such diseases of the intestinal wall as regional ileitis and nontropical sprue. Because bacterial flora play an important part in the synthesis of vitamin K in the gut, sterilization of the bowel resulting from the oral administration of antibiotics or nonabsorbable sulfonamides, such as succinylsulfathiazole (Sulfasuxidine), may also result in vitamin K deficiency.

The delicate hemostatic balance between the procoagulant factors and the natural inhibitors, which is necessary for the maintenance of the fluidity of the blood, may be disturbed in many disease states (Table 44–1). This can result in the widespread formation of thrombi in the microcirculation, a process referred to as disseminated intravascular coagulation (DIC). This term is usually used to include a paradoxical hypocoagulable state that is the natural sequela of DIC and that is attributable to the consumption of platelets, fibrinogen, and other procoagulant factors in the formation of the thrombi. The bleeding tendency that results is generally purpuric. The thrombi removal, essential for the survival of the patient, is accomplished by fibrinolysis, and this mechanism, although primarily protective, may in itself aggravate the bleeding tendency. The formation of thrombin is believed to be a sine qua non of DIC, but its neutralization is almost instantaneous. Its presence is presumed by the recognition of the products of its action on fibrinogen. These products include fibrinopeptides A and B and fibrin monomer. While some of the fibrin monomers polymerize, forming fibrin, a proportion form soluble complexes with native fibrinogen and with the degradation products that result from the lysis of formed fibrin. The fibrinopeptides have half-lives of only a few minutes, which limits their usefulness as an index of DIC. On the other hand, the soluble fibrin monomer complexes remain in the circulation for

Table 44–1 Causes of Disseminated Intravascular Coagulation

Release of tissue products after necrosis or trauma

  Metastatic carcinoma

  Tissue injury, eg, brain tissue destruction, lung surgery

  Extensive burn

  Heat stroke

Infections

  Gram-negative endotoxinemia
    Meningococcemia
    Septicemia

  Severe gram-positive septicemia

  Rocky Mountain spotted fever

  Viral infections

Obstetric disorders

  Concealed antepartum hemorrhage

  Amniotic fluid embolism

  Retained dead fetus

  Eclampsia

  Hypertonic saline abortion

Hemolytic reactions

Endothelial damage

  Acute systemic vasculitis

  Trauma

Liver disease

  Severe cirrhosis

  Hepatic necrosis

Antigen-antibody reactions

Promyelocytic leukemia

Giant hemangioma

Snake bites

Unknown etiologies

  Thrombotic microangiopathies
    Thrombotic thrombocytopenic purpura
    Hemolytic uremic syndrome

several hours. Fibrinolysis results in the formation of several fibrin degradation products, of which products D and E are the most stable and readily measured.

Fibrin is cross-linked by the action of factor XIIIa (transglutaminase). The major soluble degradation products retain these covalent bonds and are sometimes referred to as "D-dimers." Specific monoclonal antibodies to these cross-linked domains can be prepared and may be used to detect D-dimers; such antibodies do not react with fibrinogen or fibrinogen degradation products, as they lack the covalent bonds. Fibrinogen degradation products appear when urokinase or streptokinase is infused intravenously to convert plasminogen into plasmin and dissolve thrombi. The plasmin may not be neutralized completely by alpha$_2$-antiplasmin and alpha$_2$-macroglobulin and can attack fibrinogen, factor V, and other plasma proteins. If the therapy is efficacious, the thrombus will lyse, and fibrin degradation products with D-dimers will be found as well as fibrinogen degradation products derived from the action of the plasmin on fibrinogen.

One of the consequences of the intravascular fibrin deposition is the fragmentation of red cells by strands of fibrin in the microcirculation resulting in red cell fragmentation with schistocytes, or helmet cells. When associated with a significant hemolytic anemia, it is referred to as "microangiopathic hemolytic anemia." This is prominent in a group of conditions of unknown causes, referred to as "thrombotic microangiopathies" characterized by hyaline microthrombi composed of fibrin and agglutinated platelets in terminal arterioles and capillaries. The thrombotic microangiopathies include thrombotic thrombocytopenic purpura and the hemolytic uremic syndrome, two conditions that have many features in common. Thrombotic microangiopathy is generally considered distinct from DIC because the laboratory findings of DIC are minimal or absent, despite the fact that the histologic findings are pathognomonic for DIC. The distinction is also based on the poor response of this condition to heparin, which is usually ineffective in DIC in general. Accordingly, no validity for the distinction presently exists, and DIC should be considered an integral feature of the thrombotic microangiopathies.

Clinical Findings

The bleeding found in thrombocytopenia and functional disorders of platelets is purpuric, while the bleeding manifestations of acquired deficiencies of coagulation factors are of the coagulation types (Table 40–4). In von Willebrand's disease and DIC, however, features of both types may be present.

Hemorrhagic disease of the newborn (melena neonatorum) caused by deficiency of vitamin K, which was a common disease four decades ago, has been virtually eliminated as a result of prophylactic vitamin K therapy. The bleeding typically occurs during the second to sixth day after delivery. Hemorrhagic disease of the newborn is an exaggeration of physiologic hypoprothrombinemia, a temporary state that reaches its maximum point of bleeding on the second or third day and usually returns to normal within a week. The onset of bleeding is usually abrupt, and the most common presenting symptoms include: melena with hematemesis, umbilical bleeding, epistaxis, submucosal hemorrhages affecting the buccal cavity, and urethral and vaginal bleeding. The disease may also present as excessive bleeding at circumcision or persistent bleeding following a heel prick. Multiple ecchymoses may be found. Petechial hemorrhages are exceptional and suggest thrombocytopenia. Premature infants are particularly prone to excessive bleeding, as immaturity of the liver cells results in decreased synthesis of vitamin K–dependent factors, which is enhanced by vitamin K deficiency. The tissue necrosis that accompanies intracranial hemorrhage in these infants may precipitate DIC and thereby aggravate a preexisting bleeding tendency.

Approach to Diagnosis

If a patient with a severe illness, such as metastatic carcinoma or a fulminant septicemia or viremia, develops purpuric manifestations, the likely cause is DIC (Table 44–1). Fibrinogen is an acute-phase reactant protein and in many of the conditions that can cause DIC, the fibrinogen level may be very high. A significant decrease in the concentration may therefore not be apparent from a single fibrinogen determination, as it may be normal or even high depending on the baseline level. Serial fibrinogen determinations to follow the course of the process should therefore be performed. Factor VIII is also an acute-phase reactant protein and its level may remain above normal in DIC despite a significant fall. Thrombin is believed to cause activation of factor VIII, and a high factor VIII level may also be attributed to this cause. The factor V is usually decreased but rarely sufficiently to raise the PT by more than 1 or 2 sec. Milder depressions of the other factor levels such as factor XIII, also occur, but these changes are of little or no diagnostic value.

A falling platelet count is of considerable diagnostic and prognostic importance and suggests ongoing DIC. The parameter probably used most, however, is the presence of fibrin degradation products, and of these the D-dimer appears to be one of the most specific. Microangiopathic hemolytic anemia is almost diagnostic of DIC.

The response of the PT to the parenteral administration of vitamin K in patients lacking the vitamin K–deficient factors is useful in differentiating hepatocellular diseases from biliary obstruction. In hepatocellular disease, the PT remains prolonged, while it returns to normal in biliary obstruction unless some associated liver parenchymal damage is present. In the case of a previously healthy individual in whom a bleeding diathesis has developed, prolonged PT with otherwise normal liver function test results can often be attributed to accidental ingestion of warfarin sodium (Coumadin). The oral anticoagulants may have a direct toxic effect on the capillary wall, and the type of bleeding seen after an overdose has features of both coagulation and a purpuric type of defect; thus, petechiae may be present, and a hematoma often appears at the site of a clean venipuncture.

The development of a coagulation type of bleeding disorder in an individual with previously normal hemostasis is often manifested by a deep-tissue hematoma and suggests an antibody specifically directed against factor VIII, prothrombin, or, more rarely, one of the other clotting factors. Antibodies against specific factors are encountered far less frequently than antibodies that inhibit clotting without demonstrable specificity for any one of the clotting factors (Table 44–2). This type of nonspecific antibody results in a prolongation of the APTT and, occasionally, the PT, and is perhaps the most frequent cause of a prolongation of the APTT. Patients with a nonspecific antibody rarely bleed excessively, even while undergoing major surgery. As such an antibody was first found in a patient with disseminated lupus erythematosus, it is referred to as the lupuslike inhibitor, even though lupus erythematosus is now known to be a relatively rare cause. The lupuslike antibody may be seen in individuals who are taking hypotensive drugs, such as procainamide and certain tranquilizers, and after viral infections, but is commonly found in individuals in whom no causative factor can be determined. The VDRL test may give a false-positive result. The so-called lupuslike anticoagulant (LLA) probably comprises a heterogeneous group of antibodies with different actions—IgG or IgM that are believed to be targeted against negatively charged phospholipids. When the LLA results in a marked prolongation of the APTT, the APTT of an equal part of the patient's and control plasma usually exceeds that of the control plasma alone by more than 6 sec. The coagulant activities of factors VIII, IX, XI, and XII appear reduced when assayed at a 1:5 dilution, but when assayed at higher dilutions, they usually, but not always, increase significantly. This phenomenon is attributed to "diluting out the inhibitor." Factor VIII usually appears to be reduced the least and factors XI and XII the most. Weak LLAs that result in only a slight prolongation of the APTT are difficult to diagnose. Rarely, an LLA may be associated with a deficiency of prothrombin with normal levels of factors V, VII, and X. This is attributable to an antibody that binds to but does not neutralize prothrombin, with rapid clearance, in vivo, of the antibody-prothrombin complex. Such patients develop a bleeding tendency. An LLA can develop in a patient with a preexisting congenital or acquired coagulation abnormality and give rise to diagnostic problems.

A rare cause of an acquired hemorrhagic diathesis that can result in severe bleeding from raw surfaces is the acquired deficiency of factor X and sometimes factor IX seen in primary amyloidosis. In this condition, the patient responds poorly to the transfusion of plasma concentrates containing these factors.

Evaluation of the acquired coagulation disorders proceeds as follows:

1. Hematologic evaluation, with attention to platelet numbers, red cell changes indicative of DIC, and white cell count and differential.

2. Screening tests for bleeding disorders, including platelet count, bleeding time, APTT, PT, and thrombin time (TT). This battery of tests is useful in differentiating the thrombocytopenic purpuras and the acquired diathesis caused by inhibitors, liver disease, vitamin K deficiencies, or DIC (Table 44–3).

3. In all instances in which the APTT is significantly prolonged, it is now customary to perform it on a mixture of equal parts of normal plasma and the patient's plasma (sometimes referred to as a "50:50 mix"). Failure of the addition of the normal plasma to correct the prolonged APTT is unequivocal evidence of a circulating anticoagulant. This is in contrast to the finding in deficiency states when the APTT value of the 50:50 mix with normal plasma rarely exceeds the APTT of the normal plasma alone by more than 5 sec. One would not expect the APTT of such a mixture to be the same as the normal plasma alone, because it is still partially deficient in one factor. What is referred to in this discussion is not the normal range but the difference between the APTT of the 50:50 mix and that of the normal plasma used in the mixture. Even with the most potent inhibitor, it is unusual not to see some shortening or partial correction. The term "correction" is therefore an arbitrary one. A rough guideline is that a difference of ≥ 7 sec with a normal control not exceeding 35 sec is usually unequivocal evidence of an inhibitor, while values of 5 or 6 sec are equivocal. A value of ≤ 4 sec is considered correction. Correction, however, does not necessarily exclude the presence of an inhibitor. This is particularly applicable when the APTT of the patient's plasma alone is only a few seconds outside the upper limit of the normal range. If one dilutes plasma containing a potent LLA with normal plasma to shorten the APTT

Table 44–2   Acquired Clotting Inhibitors

Type	Clinical Associations	Nature of Antibody
Specific antibodies against factor VIII	Previously healthy elderly persons Patients with some autoimmune disorder Postpartum	IgG, monoclonal
Specific antibodies against factor V	Usually preceded by streptomycin administration May develop after massive blood transfusion	IgG or IgM Polyclonal
Specific antibodies to prothrombin	Usually associated with lupus-like anticoagulants No apparent etiologic agent	IgG
Specific against factor XIII or XIIIa	Therapy with isoniazid	IgG but may not be an immunoglobulin
Specific against vWf	Myeloma	IgG
lupus-like anticoagulant	Drug ingestion viz chlorpromazine Lupus erythematosus No apparent etiologic agent	Usually IgG, sometimes IgM or both

ABBREVIATIONS: APTT = activated partial thromboplastin time; PT = prothrombin time; vWf = von Willebrand's factor.

to approximately 40 sec, the demonstration of the LLA in the resulting plasma mixture on the sole basis of correction by addition of an equal volume of normal plasma will often be very difficult. In the case of some very slow-acting factor VIII inhibitors, correction may also be observed, particularly if the APTT test is performed within a few minutes of preparing the 50:50 mix with normal plasma.

4. If an inhibitor is present or cannot be excluded on the basis of the APTT of the 50:50 mix, and the PT is normal, the presence of an inhibitor directed against factor VIII must be excluded. Our practice is to perform assays of factor VIII, IX, XI, and XII routinely in all such cases. If the factor VIII level appears higher than that of the other factors, a factor VIII inhibitor can be excluded, and the patient is considered to have an LLA without further testing.

Clinical Findings and Course	Laboratory Finding
May be persistent especially in elderly patients; life-threatening bleeding can occur	APTT increased, PT normal, factor VIII decreased Other factors usually normal or only slightly reduced
Bleeding tendency usually disappears in weeks or months	APTT increased, PT increased, factor V decreased, TT normal
Bleeding tendency usually disappears in weeks	APTT increased, PT increased Inhibitor screen positive Prothrombin decreased Factors V, VII and X normal
Bleeding tendency usually disappears in weeks or months	APTT normal; PT normal; clot soluble in 5 M urea
Mild bleeding tendency	Bleeding time increased; ristocetin aggregation decreased; factor VIII normal
Bleeding tendency absent; patients may have thromboembolic manifestations or repeated abortions	APTT increased; PT usually normal; Inhibitor screen positive

On the other hand, if the factor VIII level is significantly decreased, equal to, or lower than that of the other factors, and does not appear to increase when tested at a higher dilution (eg, 1:20), a test for a factor VIII inhibitor is performed (see chapter 43). When both the APTT and PT are prolonged and neither is corrected in the 50:50 mix while the thrombin time is normal, a specific inhibitor against factor V should be considered. If the PT prolongation but not the APTT is corrected in the 50:50 mix, specific assays for prothrombin and factors VII, V, and X should be performed. If they are all normal, the cause of the PT prolongation may be an unusual type of LLA; if prothrombin is the only factor whose level is decreased, then an inhibitor against prothrombin should be considered. Although rarely necessary, the diagnosis of an LLA may be confirmed by the tissue thrombo-

Table 44–3 Use of Screening Tests in Acquired Hemorrhagic Disorders

Disorder	Platelet Count	Bleeding Time
Thrombocytopenic purpura[a]	Decreased	Increased
Liver disease	Normal or Decreased	Normal or Increased
Vitamin K deficiency	Normal	Normal or Increased
Factor VIII antibody	Normal	Normal
Lupus-like inhibitor	Normal	Normal
DIC	Decreased	Increased

ABBREVIATIONS: APTT = activated partial thromboplastin time; PT = prothrombin time; TT = thrombin time; DIC = disseminated intravascular coagulation.

[a]See Chapter 41

plastin inhibition test or the platelet neutralization test. In the thromboplastin inhibition test, the PT of the patient's plasma is determined using dilute brain extract: if an LLA is present, the ratio of the patient's PT to that of the control exceeds 1.2. The platelet neutralization test is based on the ability of washed platelets to shorten the APTT of plasma containing an LLA following incubation with an activating agent and phospholipid. It is more specific than the thromboplastin inhibition test, but even with this test, a positive result is occasionally found in a patient with a factor VIII inhibitor.

5. A search for fibrinogen degradation products and for evidence of fibrin monomer, using the protamine sulfate paracoagulation test and also serial fibrinogen determinations, is useful if the history or screening procedures suggest DIC.

6. Liver function tests are useful in differentiating a prolongation of the PT caused by ingestion of warfarin sodium (Coumadin) from that caused by liver disease or biliary obstruction. If it is suspected that the patient has ingested Coumadin or that some failure of absorption of vitamin K has occurred, the PT test should be repeated 4 to 24 hours after the parenteral administration of this vitamin.

Hematologic Findings

If platelets are absent or markedly reduced, the patient is evaluated for thrombocytopenic purpura (see chapter 41). A moderate reduc-

APTT	PT	TT
Normal	Normal	Normal
Increased	Increased	Normal or Increased
Increased	Increased	Normal
Increased	Normal	Normal
Increased	Normal or Increased	Normal
Normal or Decreased	Normal	Increased

tion, however, is found in DIC and may be associated with schistocytes and spherocytes in the peripheral blood smear.

Peripheral Blood Smear Morphology. A platelet count is performed, and the morphology of red cells (schistocytes, etc) is evaluated.

Bone Marrow Examination. Bone marrow tests are performed only if thrombocytopenia is present (see chapter 41).

Other Laboratory Tests

44.1 The Protamine Plasma Paracoagulation Test (3P Test)

Purpose. The 3P test detects fibrin monomer in plasma and is used for the diagnosis of DIC.

Principle. Soluble complexes of fibrin monomer with FDPs or fibrinogen dissociate on the addition of protamine sulfate and the fibrin monomers and then polymerize, forming a fibrin web.

Specimen. Platelet-poor plasma is used as collected for the APTT test.

Procedure.   Ten drops of plasma are placed in a small glass test tube warmed to 37° C; one drop of 1% protamine sulfate is then added and, after gentle shaking, incubated for 20 minutes.

Interpretation.   Webs or strands of fibrin are considered an un-equivocally positive result, while a finely granular, noncohesive precipitate is usually interpreted as a weakly positive result.

Notes and Precautions.   False-positive results may be obtained if there is difficulty with venipuncture or delay in mixing the blood with anticoagulant because of the formation of small amounts of thrombin in vitro. A test should not be performed on oxalated or heparinized blood, but the administration of heparin to the patient does not interfere with the test.

44.2   Latex Particle Agglutination Tests for Fibrin or Fibrinogen Degradation Products

Purpose.   This test detects the presence of fibrin or fibrinogen degradation products (FDP) and is used in the diagnosis of DIC.

Principle.   Antibodies to FDP are bound to latex particles, which clump in the presence of the antigen. If an antiserum to highly purified fibrinogen fragments D and E is employed in the test (FDP test), a positive result is obtained with fibrinogen and fibrinogen degradation products as well as with fibrin degra-dation products. In another version of the test, a highly specific monoclonal antibody to D-dimers (cross-linked fibrin degra-dation products) is used, and in this type of test (D-dimer test), positive results are obtained only with FDPs.

Specimen.   In the FDP test, only serum may be used. The blood must be obtained by careful and clean venipuncture and placed in a special sample collection tube that contains soybean tryp-sin inhibitor and thrombin or reptilase. After formation of a clot, the tube is incubated at 37° C for approximately 30 minutes before separating the serum by centrifugation. For the D-dimer test, either plasma or serum may be used, but the former is preferred, and no special precautions are needed if serum is used.

Procedure.   In the D-dimer test, the undiluted plasma (or serum), 1:2 dilution in buffer, and 1:4 dilution in buffer are added to the suspension of latex beads on a glass plate. The mixtures are stirred with mixing rods, and the slides are rocked gently to and fro for a precise number of minutes. After this period, the slide is inspected for macroscopic agglutination. Known negative or positive controls are run with each test. The procedure is almost identical in the FDP test, except 1:5 and 1:20 dilutions of the serum in buffer are used. In the FDP test, the normal serum level of degradation products derived from fibrinogen or fibrin is <10 μg/mL, and the reagents are so adjusted that serum with less than this concentration will give no agglutination with either 1:5 or 1:20 dilutions of normal serum. In DIC, the level of fibrinogen or fibrin split products exceeds 10 μg/mL, and in acute cases may exceed 40 μg/mL. The normal plasma concentration of cross-linked fibrin degradation products containing the D-dimer domain is less than 200 ng/mL, and the reagents for this test are so adjusted to give negative readings with this concentration. The concentration of D-dimers can be assayed semiquantitatively by preparing serial dilutions of the specimen and determining the highest dilution titer that remains positive.

Notes and Precautions.   Degradation products of fibrinogen or fibrin may be incorporated into the clots formed in vitro during the preparation of the serum, thereby giving a normal (negative) result or a spuriously low value. As plasma may be used in the D-dimer test but not in the other type of the test, this is a significant advantage. The D-dimer test is sensitive only to fibrin degradation products and cannot be used for monitoring fibrinolytic therapy (eg, streptokinase), in which it is desirable to assay fibrinogen degradation products as well as fibrin degradation products. Both types of tests may give positive results for several days following surgical procedures, presumably caused by lysis of hemostatic plugs or lysis of the fibrin formed in extravasated blood. Positive results in both type of tests are sometimes found in deep-vein thrombosis and pulmonary embolism, but the increases in degradation products are very transient.

Course and Treatment

Specific treatment for the coagulation defect is rarely required in the acquired disorders. The treatment of DIC is directed at the primary cause. Formerly, heparin was widely advocated to halt or impede thrombotic events, but the risks of accentuating the hemorrhagic tendency often exceeded any benefits, and its use is now restricted to the exceptional case, eg, purpura fulminans in which no primary cause for the DIC can be found. No treatment is required for LLAs, which are almost always transient. If the anticoagulant, however, is persistent and associated with repeated abortions, treatment with steroids has been recommended. Factor VIII antibodies developing in nonhemophilic individuals are sometimes treated with immunosuppressive agents (eg, adrenal steroids and cyclophosphamide), but as the antibodies often disappear spontaneously, it is difficult to be certain of the efficacy of this form of therapy. Specific antibodies against other clotting factors almost always disappear spontaneously.

References

1. Bang NV: Disseminated intravascular coagulation, in Triplett DA (ed): *Laboratory Evaluation of Coagulation.* Chicago, American Society of Clinical Pathologists Press, 1982, pp 143–208.

2. Byrnes JJ, Moake JL: Thrombotic thrombocytopenic purpura and the haemolytic-uremic syndrome: Evolving concepts of pathogenesis and therapy. *Clin Haematol* 1986; 15:413–442.

3. Green D, Hougie C, Kazmier FJ, et al: Report of the working party on acquired inhibitors of coagulation: Studies of the 'lupus anticogulant.' *Thromb Haemost* 1983; 49:144–146.

4. Hessel LW, Kluft C: Advances in clinical fibrinolysis. *Clin Haematol* 1986; 15:443–466.

5. Hougie C: Circulating anticoagulants, in Poller L (ed): *Recent Advances in Blood Coagulation.* New York, Churchill-Livingstone Inc, 1985, vol 4, pp 63–90.

6. Prentice CRM: Acquired coagulation disorders. *Clin Haematol* 1985; 14:413–442.

PART 13

Thrombotic Disorders

45

Thrombotic Disease

Thrombosis is defined as the formation of a blood clot in the circulatory system during life. Arterial thrombi, especially those plugging the smallest vessels, are composed predominantly of platelets, while fibrin is the predominant component of venous thrombi. Hypercoagulability, which is a much abused term, should be used only to refer to changes in the blood that are associated with an abnormal tendency toward thrombosis; it should never be used to refer to conditions in which the clotting time is shortened or procoagulant factor levels are increased, unless these changes are known to be associated with an abnormal tendency toward thrombosis. Those patients with uncomplicated lupuslike anticoagulants or deficiencies of factor XII, prekallikrein, or high-molecular-weight kininogen (HMW-K) and long clotting times do not bleed excessively and therefore do not have a "hypocoagulable" state. Similarly, in most conditions in which there are increases in procoagulant factors or shortened APTT (eg, after exercise, in late pregnancy, with oral contraceptive usage [The belief that oral contraceptives predisposed to thromboembolic disease was primarily based on retrospective statistical studies of women diagnosed as having thromboembolic disease *subsequent* to the widespread publicity given to a possible association. It has since been shown that these results can be explained by diagnostic bias. The overall death rates from thromboembolic disease actually dropped dramatically in nonpregnant women of fertile age at the time the pill was first introduced (*Fertil*

Table 45–1   Features of Vitamin K–Dependent Proteins

	Protein C	Protein S
Molecular Weight	62,000 daltons	69,000 daltons
Plasma Concentration	4 μg/mL	35 μg/mL
Activation	Zymogen activated by thrombin-thrombomodulin complex	None required
Function	Inactivation of Va VIIIa	Cofactor of APC Anchor for C4b binding protein
Inactivation	APC inhibitor	Thrombin cleavage

ABBREVIATIONS: APC = activated protein C.

Steril 1981; 35:275, and *Am Heart J* 1973; 85:538)], there is no evidence of hypercoagulability, as defined above, despite a widespread belief to the contrary.

Pathophysiology

Hemostasis is a very complex process in which endothelial surfaces seem to play a pivotal role in maintaining the fluidity of the blood. The coagulation cascade is just one facet of a very complex mechanism that is modulated by many regulatory mechanisms. Some of these mechanisms only come into play in vivo and are therefore difficult to study. Good examples are proteins C and S, two vitamin K–dependent proteins synthesized by the liver (Table 45–1). Neither has any apparent role in in vitro blood coagulation; nevertheless, they are potent anticoagulants. Protein C is converted to an active form (protein Ca) and this activation is mediated by a receptor, thrombomodulin, which is present on endothelial surfaces. The thrombomodulin forms a stoichiometric complex with thrombin on the endothelial surface, and this complex activates protein C, which in turn inactivates factors V and VIII, especially the active forms of these proteins. Protein S appears to be a cofactor of protein Ca and circulates in a bound and free form.

Antithrombin III is another naturally occurring anticoagulant that binds to and inactivates several intermediates of the cascade, including thrombin. Its action is greatly enhanced by heparin. While there is some dispute as to whether there is a natural herparin circulating in the blood, proteoglycans with actions similar to commercial heparin extracted from animal lung can be found in endothelial cells.

Following a thrombotic attack, platelets aggregate more readily in response to ADP and other agonists and also show an increased tendency to adhere to one another and glass surfaces. It has been suggested that such increased adhesiveness or enhanced ability to aggregate found in an otherwise normal individual is evidence of a thrombotic predisposition, but such claims are virtually impossible to substantiate or refute. Platelets, however, undoubtedly play a pivotal role in thrombosis, especially in the microvasculature.

While the intermediates of blood coagulation formed during the buildup of a thrombus are generally very unstable and rapidly excreted or removed by the reticuloendothelial system, there are some which persist long enough in the circulation to be quantitated. These include fibrinopeptides A and B, which are cleaved from fibrinogen by the action of thrombin and soluble fibrin monomers.

The formation of fibrin is essential in wound healing as well as hemostasis, but its removal, as soon as it has served its purpose, is equally important. This removal is accomplished by the fibrinolytic enzyme system that, like the coagulation system, is composed of activators and inhibitors in delicate balance. Moreover, this system, which is part of the overall hemostatic mechanism, functions cooperatively with the coagulation system. Both may be triggered by the same mechanism, and the formation of fibrin greatly enhances activation of fibrinolysis. The fibrinolytic enzyme system has not been studied as intensively as the coagulation cascade but, in recent years, an explosive burgeoning of knowledge of this process has occurred. Nevertheless, despite all that is now known, current concepts still remain rudimentary.

Well-characterized components of the system (Table 45–2) include the active serine protease plasmin, which is derived from the inactive zymogen, plasminogen, which, unlike plasmin, circulates in the plasma; alpha$_2$-antiplasmin, an inhibitor that neutralizes free plasmin almost instantaneously; tissue plasmin activator; another activator best known as urokinase but more recently referred to as urinary plasminogen activator u-PA; at least two inhibitors of the activators referred to as PAI-1 and PAI-2, histidine-rich glycoprotein (HRG); and protein C.

The fibrinolytic system may be initiated by the coagulation cascade or by tissue injury. As soon as fibrin is formed, it binds plasminogen, plasminogen activators, and alpha$_2$-antiplasmin. Plasminogen activation occurs in the fibrin clot, but any plasmin formed may be neutralized by alpha$_2$-antiplasmin, which is present in the clot at equivalent molar concentration as the fibrin-bound plasminogen. Such is the state of equilibrium that when clots are formed in vitro they do not lyse under normal conditions. In the circulation, however, plasminogen activators are released from endothelial surfaces in contact with the clot and are absorbed onto the thrombus so that the equilibrium then favors fibrinolysis. In congenital or acquired states in which the activity of the fibrinolytic inhibitor alpha$_2$-antiplasmin is decreased, excessive clot lysis occurs at a site of injury, and the hemostatic plugs break down prematurely with bleeding. Apart from local manifestations, however, such individuals do not show any general evidence of increased fibrinolytic activity. When a fibrin clot prepared from plasma deficient in alpha$_2$-antiplasmin or normal plasma is added to plasma containing normal amounts of this protein, the clot prepared from the alpha$_2$-antiplasmin–deficient plasma, but not that prepared from the normal plasma, will lyse. On the other hand, a clot prepared from normal plasma does not lyse when placed in either plasma that is deficient in alpha$_2$-antiplasmin or in normal plasma. This illustrates that the relatively small amount (about one-fifth) of alpha$_2$-antiplasmin cross-linked to fibrin is more efficient in the prevention of spontaneous clot lysis than the remaining much larger part in the circulation. Fibrin plays an integral role in the interplay between tissue plasmin activator, plasminogen, and alpha$_2$-antiplasmin, and tissue plasmin activator has little effect on plasminogen in the absence of fibrin. The affinity of plasminogen for fibrin is attributable to lysine-rich binding sites and is inhibited by lysine, epsilon-aminocaproic acid (EACA), and tranexamic acid. Even a hundredfold increase of free tissue plasmin activator activity, such as occurs in good responders after strenuous exercise or injection of DDAVP (chapter 42), does not result in the presence of free plasmin in the blood. Kallikrein formed during the initial contact phase of blood coagulation converts precursor urinary plasminogen activator or urokinase (which is present in plasma) from a single chain form to a manyfold more active two-chain form.

Of the classic triad of Virchow (ie, endothelial damage, stasis, and changes in blood constituents), endothelial damage is by far the most important factor in arterial thrombosis. Because platelets adhere to damaged endothelium, thrombosis may be considered the natural sequela of arterial disease; by far, the most common cause of this is atherosclerosis. Thrombotic episodes, usually arterial and involving the smaller vessels, are frequent in the myeloproliferative disorders, especially polycythemia vera when the platelet count is very high.

In contrast to arterial thrombosis, in venous thrombosis, stasis plays a far more important role. Thus, even in normal individuals, venous thrombosis in the lower extremity occurs with surprising frequency whenever the leg is immobilized for a number of hours, eg, during a long plane journey, but the fibrinolytic system almost

Table 45–2   Components of the Fibrinolytic Enzyme System

Protein	Site of Synthesis or Source	Concentration in Plasma	
		mg/mL	M
Plasminogen	Liver	200	2 μM
Histidine-rich glycoprotein (HRG)		100	1.5 μM
Tissue-plasminogen activator (t-PA)	Endothelial cells	.005	70 pM
Urokinase- or urinary-plasminogen activator (u-PA)	Several cell lines but probably not endothelial cells	.008	150 pM
Plasminogen activator Inhibitor-1	Endothelial cells, platelets, hepatoma cells	.05	1 nM
Plasmogen activator Inhibitor-2	Placenta, leukocytes, histocytes	<.005	<100

ABBREVIATIONS: HRG = histidine-rich glycoprotein; PA = plasminogen activator; DDAVP = de-amino-d-arginine-vasopressin or desmopressin acetate.

always removes the thrombi before any signs or symptoms become apparent. Unsuspected pulmonary emboli have been found at autopsy in almost two thirds of a group of hospitalized patients. While endothelial damage is probably present to some degree, it has lesser etiological importance than is the case in arterial thrombosis. Abnormalities or decreases in activity in the natural anticoagulants, protein C, protein S, or antithrombin III may be associated with an increased incidence of venous but not arterial thrombosis, while the therapeutic infusions of antifibrinolytic agents or activated clotting factors have resulted in massive venous thrombosis. This may explain why altering the equilibrium between procoagulants and anticoagulants by anticoagulant drugs is generally more useful in the treatment of venous than in arterial thrombosis.

Severe disturbances of the hemostatic balance may result in the formation of thrombi in the flowing blood. This is referred to as disseminated intravascular coagulation (DIC). It is most frequently found in conditions in which tissue is damaged by injury or infection and in metastatic cancers. In this last condition, necrosis may be a factor, but, in addition, certain tumor cells produce abnormal proteins with potent coagulant properties. DIC may be paradoxically

MW × 1000	Comments
92	Precursor of plasmin; 50% forms reversible complex with HRG
75	Competitive inhibitor of plasminogen for which it has high affinity
68	Most is complexed to PA-Inhibitor 1; high concentrations released from endothelial cells by occlusion, exercise, DDAVP, adrenalin, etc
54	Role in thrombosis uncertain, believed important in peri-cellular proteolytic reactions (eg, tumor invasion inflammatory processes)
54	Inhibits t-PA and two-chain u-PA
47	Inhibits u-PA

associated with bleeding manifestation as was discussed in Chapter 44.

Clinical Findings

The symptoms of arterial thrombosis or embolism are dependent on the size of the vessel, the state of the vessel wall, the degree and length of time of occlusion, adequacy of a collateral circulation, and the organ involved. If the thrombus or embolus occludes the retinal artery, permanent loss of sight may result; on the other hand, occlusion of a small branch of a renal artery may be asymptomatic. The consequences of venous thrombosis are, as a rule, not as severe as those of arterial thrombosis. Thus, thrombi in the lower calf veins are often asymptomatic and can be the source of emboli that lodge in one or more branches of the pulmonary artery. Because deep venous thrombosis is so frequently symptomless, a high index of suspicion is usually required for its recognition, and the differential diagnosis is, more often than not, difficult. The diagnosis often can be established only by arteriography or venography; noninvasive techniques, such as impedance phlebography, are also useful.

Approach to Diagnosis

Obesity, diabetes, smoking, and hypertension are associated with an increased risk of atherosclerosis as well as arterial and venous thrombosis. It is generally accepted that a high cholesterol–high-density lipoprotein ratio carries an increased risk of atheroma and therefore of arterial thrombosis. Venous thrombosis is particularly common after surgical procedures associated with tissue injury, after fractures of the neck of the femur, and in the postpartum period; in these conditions, immobilization of the lower limbs is also an important causative factor. Whenever one or more of these conditions is present, a special hematological workup is rarely indicated. On the other hand, when a predisposing cause is absent, the venous thrombosis occurred at a very early age or at an unusual site (eg, axillary vein); there have been several episodes; or there is a family history of venous thrombosis, the possibility of a hereditary or primary hypercoagulable state should be considered. The diagnostic evaluation of such proceeds as follows:

1. Hematological evaluation with particular reference to platelet count and smear.

2. Determination of the APTT and, if prolonged, a search for a lupuslike anticoagulant (see chapter 44). Thrombin time and fibrinogen determination. If the thrombin time is abnormal and the patient has not received heparin or the fibrinogen level is abnormal a dysfibrinogenemic state should be considered.

3. Antithrombin III determination.

4. Proteins C and S determinations.

5. Plasminogen determination.

6. Abnormalities of tissue plasim activator, plasminogen activator inhibitors, or heparin cofactor II have been reported in a few familial cases, but these determinations are currently performed in only a very small number of research laboratories.

Hematologic Findings

Localized thrombotic events, such as coronary thrombosis or femoral vein thrombosis, are not usually associated with striking changes in the peripheral blood count, and the platelet count is usually within normal limits. While some of the changes seen in DIC (see chapter 44) may be present, they are rarely pronounced.

Other Laboratory Tests

45.1   Antithrombin III Determination

Purpose.   Antithrombin III determinations are usually performed to detect a hypercoagulable state associated with venous thrombotic episodes and may be useful in patients who appear to be hyporesponsive to heparin.

Principle.   A known amount of thrombin is added to the patient's plasma, and the residual thrombin activity is determined. Antithrombin III may also be measured by the Laurell immunoelectrophoretic rocket technique or radial diffusion methods using specific antibodies.

Specimen.   Citrated plasma is used in those methods that utilize synthetic substrates. In the clotting assay methods, either citrated plasma or serum may be used, but plasma should be defibrinated.

Procedure.   A known amount of thrombin is added to the plasma in the presence of heparin; after a timed interval, an aliquot is removed and added to a specific synthetic chromogenic or fluorescent thrombin substrate. In the chromogenic method, colored *p*-nitroaniline is liberated from the colorless substrate by the thrombin and measured spectrophotometrically; in the fluorescent method, a fluorescent compound is released and measured in a fluorometer.

Interpretation.   The normal range appears to be a relatively narrow one (82% to 114% based on a normal pool). The level is slightly decreased by oral contraceptives; it is also decreased in the last trimester of pregnancy, but the levels rarely fall below 75% of normal. Such minor decreases have no clinical relevance. Prolonged use of heparin can result in marked decreases in antithrombin III whose level may fall following a thrombotic event, especially in DIC. Low values are associated with liver disease. In the hereditary deficiency states, the levels are usually in the 40% to 65% range. In approximately 10% of cases of antithrombin III deficiency, the antigen level may be normal, so that a functional measurement should be performed, at least initially, to exclude these variant types.

Notes and Precautions. Serum gives values approximately 30% lower than plasma.

45.2   Protein C Determination

Purpose. This test is performed to detect hypercoagulable states associated with venous thrombotic episodes.

Principle. Protein C in plasma is activated by a thrombin-thrombomodulin complex, or a specific snake venom. The activated protein C (protein Ca) is then assayed by its ability to prolong the APTT of normal plasma (clotting assay) or to cleave a specific synthetic substrate. Specific antibodies are available commercially, and antigenic determinations can be performed using Laurell immunoelectrophoresis.

Specimen. Citrated plasma is used.

Procedure. In one procedure, the protein C is separated from inhibitors by absorption and elution from barium citrate; thrombin is added to the eluate to activate the protein C, and the thrombin is then neutralized by an excess of antithrombin III. The activated protein C in the eluate is then assayed by its ability to prolong the APTT of normal plasma. In other procedures that are less cumbersome but require special reagents, the protein C in the plasma is activated directly with a thrombomodulin-thrombin complex or a specific snake venom (Protac). The activated protein C is then assayed either by a clotting method or an amidolytic assay using a chromogenic substrate.

Interpretation. The normal range is 70% to 130%. The level is reduced in hepatocellular disease, and even a moderate disturbance of liver function may reduce the level to as low as 30%. Hereditary protein C deficiency is transmitted in an autosomal recessive manner, and heterozygotes have levels of 30% to 65%; however, most heterozygotes with levels above 50% do not have a thrombotic tendency. Homozygotes apparently do not survive infancy. A normal antigenic level does not exclude heterozygosity because there are rare variants in which there is synthesis of an abnormal protein. As protein C is a vitamin K–dependent protein with a very short half-life, it is depressed early during oral anticoagulant therapy. Patients with familial protein C deficiency who are receiving warfarin and have a stable prothrombin time have a reduced ratio of plasma protein C antigen to plasma factor X antigen. The ratio of protein C activity to protein C antigen is reduced by warfarin therapy even in the absence of a hereditary abnormality of protein C. The protein C level is reduced in DIC and is lower in serum than plasma. Newborn infants who are receiving warfarin and have a stable prothrombin time have physiological low levels that rise slowly during postnatal life; the levels are even lower in premature infants.

45.3   Protein S Determination

Purpose.   Protein S acts as a cofactor for protein C and should be assayed whenever an assay of protein C is indicated.

Specimen.   Citrated plasma.

Principle.   Immunological methods are currently used, as biological assays are difficult to perform and are performed only in a few centers. The Laurell method is the immunological technique usually used in most laboratories.

Interpretation.   Heterozygotes with levels between 30% and 60% of the normal range may have recurrent venous thrombotic episodes.

45.4   Plasminogen Determination

Purpose.   This test is usually performed to monitor fibrinolytic therapy, with tissue plasmin activator (t-PA) or urokinase (u-PA). It is also used to distinguish hereditary from acquired deficiencies of alpha$_2$-antiplasmin; in the former, plasminogen is normal, but in acquired states (eg, liver disease, DIC), plasminogen and alpha$_2$-antiplasmin are reduced in parallel.

Principle.   Plasminogen is converted to its active form, plasmin, by addition of an activator; the plasmin is then assayed by the release of a colored marker or fluorescent molecule from a small synthetic peptide substrate. Specific antibodies are available commercially, and immunologic assays can be used.

Specimen.   Citrated plasma.

Procedure.   Streptokinase or urokinase is usually added to the plasma, converting inactive plasminogen to plasmin. The plasmin is then assayed by removing an aliquot and adding a small synthetic peptide substrate bound either to a fluorescent molecule or to a p-nitroanilide compound. The release of fluorescence is measured by a fluorometer, while the release of the colored p-nitroaniline compound from the colorless substrate is followed by measurement of OD at 405 nm in a spectrophotometer.

Interpretation.   The normal plasminogen level is 2.4 to 4.4 CTA units/mL. Striking decreases are found in primary and secondary fibrinolysis (DIC). Plasminogen levels are decreased in liver disease and may be very low or absent following treatment with tissue plasmin activator, urokinase or streptokinase.

Notes and Precautions.   The test cannot be performed on patients who have received fibrinolytic inhibitors (eg, EACA or AMICAR) or on specimens containing these types of inhibitors. Antigenic assays give higher values than functional methods, probably because of the action of natural inhibitors in the latter. Several different substrates, such as fibrin or casein, may be used but have been almost completely replaced in routine coagulation laboratories by methods utilizing synthetic chromogenic or fluorescent substrates.

45.5   Alpha$_2$-antiplasmin Determination

Purpose.   An alpha$_2$-antiplasmin determination is performed in patients with an acquired or inherited bleeding diathesis who have normal bleeding times, normal platelet function, and normal levels of the known coagulation factors.

Principle.   A known amount of plasmin is added to the patient's plasma and, after a short interval, the amount of residual plasmin is measured. The method for determining the plasmin level is essentially the same as that described under the assay for plasminogen in which a fluorescent or chromogenic substrate is used. The percentage of plasmin inhibited provides a measure of the alpha$_2$-antiplasmin. Alpha$_2$-antiplasmin may also be measured by immunological methods.

Specimen.   Citrated plasma.

Procedure.   Aliquots of a standardized and stable preparation of human plasmin are added to the patient's and control plasmas and also to a saline control. After exactly 1 minute, the mixture containing the plasmin is then added to a fluorescent or chromogenic synthetic substrate as described under the assay procedure for plasminogen. The residual plasmin is the difference between the values obtained for the plasma sample under test and the control containing saline instead of plasma. A normal range has to be established for each laboratory and is usually 80% to 120%.

Interpretation. Heterozygotes for hereditary alpha$_2$-antiplasmin deficiency that usually have levels between 25% and 60% of normal may bleed excessively following surgery. In acquired deficiencies, which are seen in liver disease and in thrombotic states, especially DIC, plasminogen activity is depressed concomitantly.

Notes and Precautions. Alpha$_2$-antiplasmin determinations cannot be performed on patients who are receiving fibrinolytic inhibitors (eg, EACA).

References

1. Bachmann F: in Verstraete M, Vermylen J, Lijnen HR, et al (eds): *Fibrinolysis, Thrombosis and Haemostasis,* International Society on Thrombosis and Haemostasis, Leuven University Press, 1987; pp 227–265.
2. Mannucci PM, Tripodi A: Laboratory screening of inherited thrombotic syndromes. *Thromb Haemost* 1987; 57:246–251.
3. Miles LA, Plow EF, Donnelly KJ, et al: A bleeding disorder due to deficiency of alpha$_2$-antiplasmin. *Blood* 1982; 59:1246–1251.

Anticoagulant Therapy

46

Control of Anticoagulant Therapy and Thrombolytic Therapy

Anticoagulant therapy is designed to inhibit the formation of thrombi and prevent the extension and propagation of formed thrombi. The goal of thrombolytic therapy is to dissolve or lyse a recent thrombus. Antiplatelet therapy is a form of anticoagulant therapy aimed at reducing the ability of platelets to adhere to one another (aggregate) or to stick to the damaged endothelium (adhesiveness) and thereby inhibit thrombosis.

Pathophysiology

Endothelial damage is by far the most important factor in arterial thrombosis. As this damage is almost always induced by atherosclerosis, measures designed to reverse or halt this process may be considered antithrombotic. Platelets adhere to the damaged endothelial lining, forming the foundation for the eventual buildup of a thrombus; moreover, platelets can form aggregates in the circulation that may be large enough to block a small artery. In venous thrombosis, in contrast to arterial thrombosis, endothelial damage is not an essential component; stasis, by impeding the removal of activated products by the flowing blood from the site of the thrombus, is relatively more important. Thus, immobilization of the lower limb, particularly in bedridden patients or following surgery or delivery, may precipitate venous thrombosis.

The oral anticoagulants comprise derivatives of coumadin and include warfarin and a closely related compound, phenindione (Dindevan). They all inhibit the synthesis of vitamin K–dependent proteins by the liver. The vitamin K–dependent proteins involved in coagulation are the procoagulants, prothrombin and factors VII, IX, and X, and the anticoagulants, proteins C and S. The normal biosynthesis of these proteins requires vitamin K. In the absence of vitamin K, an inactive molecule is synthesized. Vitamin K is essential for a posttranslational event in which glutamic acid residues are carboxylated. The oral anticoagulants are all vitamin K antagonists. As the half-lives of the various vitamin K–dependent factors differ, they decrease at different rates. Factor VII and protein C have half-lives of less than 10 hours and are the first to fall and reappear on cessation of drug therapy, while prothrombin has the longest half-life (3 days) and is the last to fall and reappear.

The other type of anticoagulant widely used is heparin, a heterogenous substance consisting of glycosaminoglycans of widely varying but high average molecular weight. Several low-molecular-weight heparins and analogues are now available. Heparin, which is negatively charged, binds to antithrombin III and sterically modifies this molecule so that its ability to bind to and inactivate thrombin and factors IX and X are greatly enhanced; it is rapidly neutralized by protamine sulfate, which is positively charged. Heparin is usually administered intravenously and may be administered subcutaneously but not intramuscularly.

The original rationale for oral anticoagulant therapy was that as changes in the constitutents in the blood appear to have a role in venous thrombosis, merely reducing the concentration of procoagulants should prevent or at least impede thrombosis. Unfortunately, this argument can no longer be used because some patients who have long clotting times (eg, patients with lupuslike anticoagulants or a deficiency of factor XII) may actually have an increased risk of thrombosis. It may also be argued that while oral anticoagulant therapy reduces the concentration of prothrombin and factors VII, IX and X, it also reduces proteins C and S activity; thus, the hemostatic balance may be maintained, albeit at a lower level. Clearly, one cannot equate in vitro clotting to in vivo events, however rational this may appear. In contrast to anticoagulant therapy with either oral anticoagulants or heparin, antifibrinolytic agents have a relatively rapid action and can be monitored closely, and the breakup and dissolution of a fresh thrombus can be visualized; accordingly, there can be no question of the efficacy of this form of therapy. Treatment with antifibrinolytic agents, which include urinary-plasminogen activator or urokinase (u-PA), streptokinase, and tissue-plasminogen activator (t-PA), may result in bleeding from sites at which venipuncture was performed some days earlier, indicating dissolution of the hemostatic plugs and the effectiveness of these agents.

When the degree of anticoagulation with oral anticoagulants exceeds a level considered toxic, hematuria is almost invariable, and purpura is a frequent complication. Similarly, a patient receiving heparin is likely to bleed from an open wound, and while there can be no question that both oral anticoagulants and heparin are potent drugs with powerful hemostatic effects, this is not evidence that the drugs are effective anticoagulants. The question of whether their benefits outweigh the risks of hemorrhage and other complications still has to be answered. The current use of heparin and oral anticoagulants to treat those conditions for which they are generally recommended is based on clinical impressions and animal experiments with some support, not all favorable, from clinical trials. Much of the evidence of their efficacy is scanty—opinion rather than fact—nevertheless, their use has become embedded in established clinical practice. The problem with clinical trials is that as the frequency of thromboembolic disease is low, almost all of the trials have been multicentered. As there are no standard or uniform methods of controlling therapy, attempts to compare results obtained from different hospitals are rarely valid, although there have been some recent efforts to introduce some measure of standardization.

Clinical Indications

Anticoagulant therapy is recommended for the treatment of venous thrombosis with or without evidence of pulmonary embolism. It is used, although less often than in the past, in the short-term management of patients with acute myocardial infarction, particularly if the infarction is transmural. A recent clinical trial also supports its use in the long-term management of these patients. Oral anticoagulants have been advocated for prophylactic use in patients with fractured hips and total hip replacements. In these conditions and in patients who have undergone surgery, low-dose heparin has also been recommended, but the evidence of efficacy seems unconvincing. The use of anticoagulants is accepted in the management of patients with prosthetic heart valves, arterial or venous grafts, and mitral valve disease with fibrillation. The short-term use of anticoagulants in the management of acute stroke is not recommended because of the difficulties of distinguishing a stroke from hemorrhage; moreover, if the diagnosis of a thrombotic occlusion is established, the risk of hemorrhage in the infarcted area still exists. On the other hand, anticoagulants are sometimes used in patients who have had transient ischemic attacks.

Method of Administration

Anticoagulant therapy in patients with acute venous thrombosis usually consists of concurrent administration of heparin and warfarin. Heparin is best given by intravenous drip starting with a bolus of 5,000 or 10,000 units, followed by 1,000 units hourly. It may also be given intermittently with a 10,000 unit bolus and 5,000 units every 4 hours, but this is less satisfactory than the continuous infusion method. Warfarin is given in amounts of 10 mg daily for the first 2 days. The heparin is then stopped for at least 3 hours, and the PT test is performed; if the time is considered satisfactory, heparin therapy is discontinued and warfarin alone is administered. Minidose heparin is given subcutaneously in 3 daily doses of 5,000 units at intervals of 8 hours.

Method of Control

The effect of heparin can be monitored by a wide variety of methods, but the method usually used is the APTT. It is usually recommended that the APTT be maintained between 1.5 to 2 times the normal value for an optimal effect. The type and content of phospholipid in the reagent used in the APTT test has, however, an important effect on the result of this test, and some reagents are far more sensitive than others to the presence of heparin. The above recommendation is, therefore, quite arbitrary and has no real scientific basis. If the heparin is administered by intravenous drip at a constant rate, once equilibrium is reached, the time at which the sample is taken is unimportant. If the heparin is administered intermittently at intervals of 4 to 6 hours or longer, however, the best time to draw the sample is 3.5 hours after the preceding dose or immediately before the next dose is due. There is usually no point in performing the test within 2 hours of administering the drug.

Withdrawing blood from an indwelling catheter often gives erroneous results, even if the catheter is first flushed with saline. On the other hand, if the blood is collected directly by venipuncture, a large hematoma may form despite reasonable care. For these reasons, heparin therapy is often used without any laboratory control; this is particularly true in the case of low-dose regimens ("miniheparin") and when heparins of low molecular weight are used.

Blood levels do not correlate with the degree of anticoagulation with oral anticoagulants. The dose must be regulated entirely according to the results of the one-stage PT test or one of the modifications of this test—oral anticoagulants must never be administered without such control measures. Only recently has there been any measure of agreement as to an efficacious or therapeutic range at which the PT should be maintained because of the absence of a uniform or standard way of performing the one-stage PT test (see chapter 40). The reason for this is that different tissue extracts or, as they are usually called, "tissue thromboplastins" can give quite different PTs with different pathologic plasmas, although the normal control times may be the same. Even extracts prepared by the same method from the same tissue do not always give identical results with a pathologic plasma, although the differences are minimized. In general, acetone extracts give shorter times with pathologic plasmas than saline extracts, while human brain extracts, now rarely used, give longer times than rabbit brain extracts. When the test was first devised by Dr Armand Quick, it was believed to measure prothrombin specifically, provided the concentration of fibrinogen was above a certain critical level, and the results were often recorded in terms of percent prothrombin activity. With the subsequent discovery of factors V, VII, and X, which, with prothrombin, are also measured by the test, this method of reporting became invalid. It then became a common practice to omit the "prothrombin" and record the results merely in terms of percent activity, but this begs the question "What activity?", particularly as the vitamin K factors depressed by the oral anticoagulants do not decrease at the same rate, and different tissue extracts used in the test have varying sensitivities to each of the factors influencing the test. For example, certain lung extracts may be relatively insensitive to deficiencies in factor VII. The level of factor IX does not generally affect the PT, but bovine brain and, to a lesser extent, rabbit brain react differently than human brain to the presence of certain abnormal factor IX molecular variants. For example, in hemophilia B_M, in which such a variant is present, the PT is prolonged with animal brain extracts but not with human brain. Results should never be recorded in percent values as this can be misleading; a result of 25% activity in one laboratory might well be found to be 50% in another, even though the same thromboplastin reagent is used. This is because the calibration curve from which the percent activity is derived may be obtained by diluting the normal pooled plasma with either saline or plasma from which the vitamin K–dependent factors have been removed by absorption with $BaSO_4$ or $Al(OH)_3$. If the saline dilution curve is used, the percent activity will be found to be significantly lower. Not only is there no scientific validity for referring to the activity in terms of percent, but such a result may be misleading unless the method and the diluent used to obtain the "activity" curve is stated on the report, and this is rarely, if ever, done. Furthermore, some laboratories report in percent values obtained by expressing the ratio of normal time to that of the patient's time as a percentage.

It is now customary to merely record the patient's time together with that of the normal control, and often the ratio of the patient's time to that of the control is also stated. Ideally, results of a test used to monitor oral anticoagulant therapy should reflect only changes in the vitamin K–dependent factors. In the prothrombin-proconvertin (P&P) test (formerly believed to measure only prothrombin and factor VII, or proconvertin, but now known to measure factor X, which was discovered later), this was accomplished by diluting the test plasma and the pooled control plasma with $BaSO_4$ or $Al(OH)_3$-absorbed plasma instead of saline, thereby providing a constant amount of factor V and fibrinogen, which are not decreased by oral anticoagulants. In the thrombotest procedure, the tissue factor reagent contained a source of fibrinogen and factor V. The thromboplastin used in the P&P test was a saline extract of human brain and in the thrombotest procedure a carefully standardized ox brain extract. While the use of these modifications was a big step toward standardization, for technical and economic reasons they were never very popular and are now available in only a few medical centers.

A recent advance has been the adoption of a WHO international reference thromboplastin preparation. Each new batch of thromboplastin can be calibrated against the primary WHO reference material by determining with each thromboplastin the PTs of plasmas from many different patients whose conditions have been stabilized with long-term oral anticoagulant therapy. The unknown preparation of thromboplastin will be found to give the same, longer (higher ratios) or shorter (shorter ratios) times with the pathological plasmas than those obtained with the standard thromboplastin, but a consistent and reproducible pattern will be obtained. These results are used to calculate the relative sensitivity of the unknown preparation compared to the standard. From this value, an international normalized ratio (INR), defined as the PT ratio that would have been obtained if WHO international reference thromboplastin had been used, can be determined for any ratio obtained with the unknown thromboplastin.

The calibration should be performed by the manufacturer on each new lot of thromboplastin, and a table enabling conversion to the equivalent INR should be included in the product insert. The laboratory report should always state the INR as well as the technique and source of thromboplastin. Only then can a result be interpreted by a physician at another institution without having to first consult the pathologist performing the test. In the past, many physicians strived to maintain the ratio at 2, but with some reagents, this represented an excessive degree of anticoagulation and resulted in a relatively high incidence of hemorrhagic manifestations, while with other reagents, this ratio provided relatively little protection

Table 46–1   Prothrombin Time Ratios

Clinical State	Recommended INR	Equivalent Ratio with a Commercial Rabbit Brain Thromboplastin
Prophylaxis of deep vein thrombosis including high risk surgery (2.0 to 3.0 for hip surgery and fractured femur operations)	2.0 to 2.5	1.3 to 1.5
Treatment of deep vein thrombosis, pulmonary embolism, and transient ischemic attacks	2.0 to 3.0	1.3 to 1.7
Recurrent deep vein thrombosis and pulmonary embolism	3.0 to 4.5	1.3 to 2
Arterial disease including myocardial infarction		
Arterial grafts		
Cardiac prosthetic valves and grafts		

NOTE: British Society of Hematology Guidelines for Anticoagulant Therapy

ABBREVIATIONS: INR = international normalized ratio.

against thrombosis. In guidelines issued by the British Society of Hematology, the therapeutic ranges in terms of INR are shown (Table 46–1); equivalent ratios obtained with the commercial preparation of acetone-extracted rabbit brain used in the laboratory have been added. As manufacturers may change their formulation from time to time while different batches of the same formulation may have different sensitivities, the name of the preparation is not given. The recommended range of 2 to 3 with the reference standard corresponds to actual times of 24 to 36 sec, while the equivalent times are 14 to 20 sec with the commercial preparation, assuming that the normal for both is 12 sec. In this example, the reference standard is more sensitive than the commercial preparation, and the closer a commercial preparation approaches the sensitivity of the WHO standard or exceeds it, the better it will be. The INR range of 3 to 4.5 recommended by the British Society of Hematology for recurrent deep-vein thrombosis is associated with a relatively high incidence of bleeding manifestations, and the patients should therefore be

Table 46–2   Well-Known Drugs Interacting with Oral Anticoagulants

Enhance Warfarin Effect	Decrease Warfarin Effect
Cimetidine	Vitamin K
Nonsteroidal anti-inflammatory agents	Barbituates
Allopurinol	Carbamazepine (Tegretol^R)
Anabolic steroids	Rifampin
Phenyloin (Dilantin)	
Tricyclic antidepressants	
Trimethroprim-sulphamethoazole (Bactrim™)	

very carefully monitored for gross hematuria or other signs of bleeding.

Many drugs inhibit or enhance the effect of the oral anticoagulants, and recent ingestion of such a drug should be suspected whenever the PT changes unexpectedly in a patient whose condition was previously stabilized. A partial list of drugs known to enhance or inhibit the effect of the oral anticoagulants is shown in Table 46–2. In an individual in whom dietary vitamin K intake is marginal, sterilization of the gut by an antibiotic can result in increased sensitivity to vitamin K.

Thrombolytic Therapy

The systemic intravenous infusion of streptokinase has been used for at least three decades to dissolve arterial or venous clots. Streptokinase, however, is a bacterial product derived from streptococci and, as many individuals have significant titers of antistreptokinase antibodies as a result of a previous streptococcal infection, this complicates therapy and may also result in severe side effects. Until recently, urokinase and tissue plasminogen activators were derived only from human sources and were scarce and very expensive; however, with the increasing availability of bioengineered products, their use is likely to become more widespread. These products, as well as streptokinase, may be infused locally by an arterial catheter directly adjacent to arterial thrombi. Such local infusions do not require monitoring. As soon as fibrinolytic therapy is discontinued, the patient should undergo anticoagulation with heparin, because the patient's plasminogen will be depleted and any new thrombi that form will be resistant to natural or induced lysis by plasminogen activators. The systemic use of fibrinolytic agents may be controlled by the APTT, fibrinogen concentration, thrombin time, or euglobulin lysis time, but no generally accepted protocol exists. Fibrinogen determinations are useful, and a level below 100 mg/dL is cause for concern. The APTT, PT, and thrombin time are also determined, but they are not easy to interpret if the patient is receiving heparin. Fibrin split product activity is increased while plasminogen and alpha$_2$-antiplasmin activities decrease, but their assay is not necessary for the control of these patients. The euglobulin lysis time, which is shortened by increases in plasminogen activators, is another test that is sometimes used for monitoring these patients, but it is a crude test, and the results are difficult to interpret.

Drugs and Platelet Function

Aspirin is now used extensively to treat arterial thromboembolic disease and prevent occlusion of arterial grafts and formation of thrombi on prosthetic heart valves. It reduces thromboxane production for the lifetime of the platelet, thereby decreasing platelet aggregation. On the other hand, it also diminishes the production of prostacyclin by the endothelium, albeit for a relatively shorter time (see chapter 42), thereby enhancing aggregation. Extensive studies have been performed to evaluate the possibility that low-dose aspirin therapy might be used selectively to inhibit platelet thromboxane synthesis without affecting vascular prostacyclin production. A single dose of 150 to 300 mg of aspirin inhibits production of both, while a single dose of 40 mg has a substantially greater effect on platelet thromboxane than on vascular prostacyclin formation. A daily dose as low as 20 mg, however, suppresses both platelet thromboxane and endothelial cell prostacyclin synthesis. In clinical trials, the daily dose has varied from as low as 80 mg ("baby aspirin") to as high as 2,000 mg.

The other drug that has been used as an antithrombotic agent is dipyridamole (Persantine), but it does not alter platelet function as measured by routine laboratory methods. It is believed to increase the concentration of cyclic AMP thereby inhibiting the release reaction (see chapter 42). Dipyridamole has been used alone or in combination with aspirin. In one study, therapy with the combination of dipyridamole and aspirin was found to reduce mortality by 18% in a 36-month follow-up of patients surviving their first myocardial infarction. This reduction in survival was barely an improvement over the use of aspirin alone. Antiplatelet therapy is not monitored by laboratory testing.

References

1. Douglas AS, Bennett B, Ogston D: Antithrombotic therapy, in Biggs R, Rizza CR (eds): *Human Blood Coagulation, Haemostasis and Thrombosis.* Boston, Blackwell Scientific Publications Inc, 1984, pp 489–541.

2. Evatt BL: Monitoring of oral anticoagulant therapy, in Triplett DA (ed): *Laboratory Evaluation of Coagulation.* Chicago, American Society of Clinical Pathologists Press, 1982, pp 245–269.

3. Gerard JM, Friesen LL: Platelets, in Poller L (ed): *Recent Advances in Blood Coagulation,* New York, Churchill Livingstone, 1985, vol 4, pp 139–168.

4. Hyers TM, Hull Rd, Weg JG: Antithrombotic therapy for venous thromboembolic disease. *Chest* 1986; 89:26–35. ACCP-NHLBI Nat Conf on Antithrombotic Therapy.

5. Poller L: Advances in oral anticoagulant treatment, in Poller L (ed): *Recent Advances in Blood Coagulation.* New York, Churchill-Livingstone Inc, 1985, pp 191–214.

6. Poller L: Laboratory control of oral anticoagulants. *Br Med J* 1987; 294:1184.

7. Thomas DP: Heparin. *Clin Hematol* 1986; 10:81–92.

8. Triplett DA: Heparin: Clinical use and laboratory monitoring, in Triplett DA (ed): *Laboratory Evaluation of Coagulation.* Chicago, American Society of Clinical Pathologists Press, 1982, pp 271–313.

APPENDIX

Hematology Reference Values

Table 1 Hematology Reference Values in Adults

	Men
Test	Conventional Units
Hemoglobin	13–18 g/dl
Hematocrit	40%–52%
Red cell count	4.4–5.9 × 10⁶/μl
White cell count	3.8–10.6 × 10³/μl
MCV	80–100 fl
MCH	26–34 pg
MCHC	32–36 g/dl
Platelet count	150–440 × 10³/μl
Reticulocyte count	0.8%–2.5%
Reticulocyte count	18000–158000/mm³
Sedimentation rate[a]	0–10 mm/h
Zeta Sedimentation Rate	40–52

Values modified from:

Wintrobe MM: *Clinical Hematology,* ed 8, Philadelphia, Lea and Febiger, 1984. Henry JB: *Clinical Diagnosis and Management by Laboratory Methods,* ed 17, Philadelphia, W.B. Saunders, 1984. Miale JB: *Laboratory Medicine: Hematology,* ed 6, St. Louis, Mosby, 1982. Williams WJ, Beutler E, Erslev AJ, Lichtman MA: *Hematology,* ed 3, New York, McGraw-Hill Book Co., 1983.

[a] May be age dependent, according to method

Table 2 Hematology Reference Values in Adults

	Men
Test	Conventional Units
Serum Iron	70–201 μg/dl
Total Iron Binding Capacity	253–435 μg/dl
Ferritin	20–250 ng/ml
Serum B₁₂	200–1000 pg/ml
Serum Folate	2–10 ng/ml
Red Cell Folate	140–960 ng/ml
Hemoglobin A₂	1.5%–3.5%
Hemoglobin F	<2%

Values modified from:

Wintrobe MM: *Clinical Hematology,* ed 2, Philadelphia, Lea and Febiger, 1984. Henry JB: *Clinical Diagnosis and Management by Laboratory Methods,* ed 17, Philadelphia, W.B. Saunders, 1984. Miale JB: *Laboratory Medicine: Hematology,* ed 6, St. Louis, Mosby, 1982. Williams WJ, Beutler E, Erslev AJ, Lichtman MA: *Hematology,* ed 3 New York, McGraw-Hill Book Co., 1983.

Men	Women	
SI	Conventional Units	SI
130–180 g/L	12–16 g/dl	120–160 g/L
0.40–0.52	35%–47%	0.35–0.47
4.4–5.9 × 10^{12}/L	3.8–5.2 × 10^6/μl	3.8–5.2 × 10^{12}/L
3.8–10.6 × 10^9/L	3.6–11.0 × 10^6/μl	3.6–11.0 × 10^9/L
80–100 fl	80–100 fl	80–100 fL
26–34 pg	26–34 pg	26–34 pg
320–360 g/L	32–36 g/dl	320–360 g/L
150–440 × 10^9/L	150–440 × 10^3/μl	150–440 × 10^9/L
0.008–0.025	0.8%–4.0%	0.008–0.025
18–158 × 10^9/L	18000–158000/mm^3	18–158 × 10^9/L
0–10 mm/h	0–20 mm/h	0–20 mm/h
40–52	40–52	40–52

Men	Women	
SI	Conventional Units	SI
12.7–35.9 μmol/L	62–173 μg/dl	11–30 μmol/L
45.2–77.7 μmol/L	253–435 μg/dl	45.2–77.7 μmol/L
20–250 μg/L	10–200 ng/ml	10–200 μg/L
150–750 pmol/L	200–1000 pg/ml	150–750 pmol/L
4–22 nmol/L	2–10 ng/ml	4–22 nmol/L
550–2200 nmol/L	140–960 nmol/l	550–2200 nmol/L
0.015–0.035	1.5%–3.5%	0.015–0.035
<0.02	<2%	<0.02

Table 3 Hematology Reference Values During the First Month of Life in the Term Infant

Value	Cord Blood	Day 1
Hb (g/dL)	16.8	18.4
Hematocrit (1/1)	0.53	0.58
Red cells ($\times 10^{12}$/L)	5.25	5.8
MCV (fL)	107	108
MCH (pg)	34.0	35.0
MCHC (g/dL)	31.7	32.5
Reticulocytes (%)	3–7	3–7
Nucleated RBC ($\times 10^9$/L)	500	200
Platelets ($\times 10^9$/L)	290	192

From Oski F, Naiman JL: *Hematologic Problems in the Newborn*, ed 2, Philadelphia, W.B. Saunders Co., 1972.

Table 4 White Blood Cell Differential Count Reference Values in Adults

Cell Type	Conventional Units Relative
Segmented Neutrophils	50%–70%
Bands	2%–6%
Lymphocytes	20%–44%
Monocytes	2%–9%
Eosinophils	0%–4%
Basophils	0%–2%

Day 3	Day 7	Day 14	Day 28
17.8	17.0	16.8	15.6
0.55	0.54	0.52	0.45
5.6	5.2	5.1	4.7
99	98	96	91
33.0	32.5	31.5	31.0
33.0	33.0	33.0	32.0
1–3	0–1	0–1	0–1
0–5	0	0	0
213	248	252	240

Conventional Units	SI	
Absolute Counts	Relative	Absolute Counts
2400–7560/µl	0.5%–0.7%	2.40–7.56 × 10^9/L
96–648/µl	0.02%–0.06%	0.09–0.648 × 10^9/L
960–4752/µl	0.2%–0.44%	0.96–4.75 × 10^9/L
96–972/µl	0.02%–0.09%	0.096–0.972 × 10^9/L
0–432/µl	0.00%–0.04%	0.00–0.432 × 10^9/L
0–216/µl	0.00%–0.02%	0.00–0.216 × 10^9/L

Table 5 Differential Counts of Bone Marrow Aspirates from 12 Healthy Men

Cell Type	Mean (%)	Observed Range (%)	95% Confidence Limits (%)
Neutrophilic series (total)	53.6	49.2–65.0	33.6–73.6
Myeloblasts	0.9	0.2–1.5	0.1–1.7
Promyelocytes	3.3	2.1–4.1	1.9–4.7
Myelocytes	12.7	8.2–15.7	8.5–16.9
Metamyelocytes	15.9	9.6–24.6	7.1–24.7
Band	12.4	9.5–15.3	9.4–15.4
Segmented	7.4	6.0–12.0	3.8–11.0
Eosinophilic series (total)	3.1	1.2–5.3	1.1–5.2
Myelocytes	0.8	0.2–1.3	0.2–1.4
Metamyelocytes	1.2	0.4–2.2	0.2–2.2
Band	0.9	0.2–2.4	0–2.7
Segmented	0.5	0–1.3	0–1.1
Basophilic and mast cells	0.1	0–0.2	
Erythrocytic series (total)	25.6	18.4–33.8	15.0–36.2
Pronormoblasts	0.6	0.2–1.3	0.1–1.1
Basophilic	1.4	0.5–2.4	0.4–2.4
Polychromatophilic	21.6	17.9–29.2	13.1–30.1
Orthochromatic	2.0	0.4–4.6	0.3–3.7
Lymphocytes	16.2	11.1–23.2	8.6–23.8
Plasma cells	1.3	0.4–3.9	0–3.5
Monocytes	0.3	0–0.8	0–0.6
Megakaryocytes	0.1	0–0.4	
Reticulum cells	0.3	0–0.9	0–0.8
M:E ratio	2.3	1.5–3.3	1.1–3.5

From Wintrobe MM: *Clinical Hematology*, ed 8, Philadelphia, Lea Febiger, 1984.

Index

Authorship of individual chapters is indicated by large boldface line entries. Numbers in *italics* refer to pages on which Tables or Figures appear. Numbers in **boldface** refer to pages on which Tests appear.

nase (G6PD), *128*

fluorescent screening test for, **132-133**

quantitative assay, **134**

in acquired hemolytic anemia, drug related, 200

Glucose-6-phosphate dehydrogenase (G6PD) deficiency, *93*, *95*, *96*, 189, *271*. *See also* Acquired hemolytic anemia, drug related

approach to diagnosis of, 131

clinical findings in, 130-131, *131*

course of, 136

drugs and chemicals causing hemolytic anemia in, *130*

drugs associated with hemolysis in, *191*

hematologic findings in, 132

pathophysiology of, 127-130

treatment of, 136

Glucose-6-phosphate dehydrogenase (G6PD) testing. *See* Glucose-6-phosphate dehydrogenase, fluorescent screening test for; Glucose-6-phosphate dehydrogenase, quantitative assay

Glucose-phosphate isomerase, *120*

deficiency of. *See* Hereditary nonspherocytic hemolytic anemia

γ-Glutamyl cysteine synthetase deficiency, 129, *129*, 136

Glutathione peroxidase deficiency, 129, *129*

Glutathione reductase, *128*

deficiency of, 129, *129*

Glutathione reductase assay, **134-135**

Glutathione stabilizing enzyme deficiency, *93*

Glutathione synthetase deficiency, 129, *129*, 136. *See also* Hereditary nonspherocytic hemolytic anemia

Glutathione testing. *See* Reduced glutathione assay

Glyceryl guaiacolate ether, *560*

Glycogen storage disease, *564*

Glycolysis, 119-121, *120*

Gold, *60-61*

Gout, *234*

Graft-versus-host disease, *60*, *242*

Granulocyte antibody test, **267-**

268

in neutropenia, 267-268

Granulocytes, 3

functional defects of

approach to diagnosis of, 272

blood cell measurements in, 272

bone marrow examination in, 273

clinical findings in, 272

conditions associated with, *271*

course of, 275

hematologic findings in, 272-273

myeloperoxidase stain in, 274

nitroblue tetrazolium dye test in, 273-274

pathophysiology of, 270-272

peripheral blood smear morphology in, 273

treatment of, 275

marginal pool, 2

monoclonal antibody markers in, *290-291*

Granulocytosis. *See* Neutropenia

Granulomatous disorder, *425*

Gray platelet syndrome, *564*

GSH. *See* Reduced glutathione

Hairy cell leukemia, 407-418, *410-411*, *415*, *444*

Halothane, *61*

Ham's presumptive test, in paroxysmal nocturnal hemoglobinuria, 166

Ham's test for acid hemolysis, **212-213**

Hand-Schüller-Christian disease, *257*

Haptoglobin testing. *See* Serum haptoglobin quantitation

Hashish, *560*

Hay fever, *243*

Heart failure, *308*

Heart valve prosthesis, *93*, *97*, 101

Heat stroke, *593*

Heavy-chain disease

approach to diagnosis of, 495-496, 509-510

Bence-Jones protein test in, 500-501

beta-2-microglobulin quantitation in, 507-508

over; Hemoglobin, synthesis disorders
high oxygen affinity, *221*
Hemoglobin S, 139, *139*. *See also* Sickle cell anemia
solubility test for, **151-152**
Hemoglobin testing. *See* Acid elution test for fetal hemoglobin in red cells; Alkali denaturation test for fetal hemoglobin; Carboxyhemoglobin testing; Fetal hemoglobin quantitation; Hemoglobin electrophoresis; Hemoglobin H inclusion body test; Isopropanol stability test; Plasma hemoglobin quantitation; Quantitation of hemoglobin A_2 by chromatography; Solubility test for hemoglobin S; Urine hemoglobin quantitation; Urine hemoglobin test
Hemoglobinuria, 106-107
Hemolysin testing. *See* Donath-Landsteiner test
Hemolysis, intravascular, 95, *96-97*
Hemolysis testing. *See* Acid hemolysis test; Ham's test for acid hemolysis; Sucrose hemolysis test
Hemolytic anemia, *20*, *251*, *329*, *545*. *See also* Accelerated erythrocyte turnover
acquired. *See* Acquired hemolytic anemia
approach to diagnosis of, *29*
autoimmune. *See* Autoimmune hemolytic anemia
chronic, *77*
cold autoantibody, *169*
hereditary nonspherocytic. *See* Hereditary nonspherocytic hemolytic anemia
warm autoantibody, *169*
Hemolytic disease of newborn. *See* Acquired hemolytic anemia, fetomaternal incompatibility
Hemolytic uremic syndrome, *93*, 101, *593*
Hemopexin, in accelerated erythrocyte turnover, *99*, 106
Hemophilia, 529, *530-533*. *See also* Bleeding disorder; Hereditary coagulation disorder

approach to diagnosis of, *581*
Hemosiderin testing. *See* Urine hemosiderin test
Hemosiderosis, *337*
Heparin, *234*, *242*, *559*, 621, 623. *See also* Anticoagulant therapy
Heparin-induced thrombocytopenia test, **552**
Hepatic fibrosis, *337*
Hepatic necrosis, *593*
Hepatic vein obstruction, *337*
Hepatitis, *60*, 287-288, *283*, *288*, *337-338*, *516*, 591
Hepatoma, *223*
Hereditary coagulation disorder
activated partial thromboplastin time in, *579-580*
approach to diagnosis of, 578-582, *579-582*
assay for clotting factors in intrinsic pathway only in, 584-585
bleeding time test in, *580*
blood cell measurements in, 582
clinical findings in, 578
course of, 589-590
factor V assay in, 585
factor VII assay in, 585
factor VIII antibody screening test in, 587
factor VIII antibody titer in, 588-589
factor VIII assay in, 582-584
factor X assay in, 585
hematologic findings in, 582
inhibitor of clotting screening test in, 586-587
pathophysiology of, 577
prothrombin assay in, 585
prothrombin time in, *579*
thrombin time in, *579*
treatment of, 589-590
Hereditary nonspherocytic hemolytic anemia (HNSHA), *131*
approach to diagnosis of, 122-123
blood cell measurements in, 123
clinical findings in, 121-122
course of, 126
fluorescent screening test for pyruvate kinase deficiency in, 124-125
glycolytic pathway deficiencies

that cause, *121*
hematologic findings in, 123-124
isopropanol stability test in, 126
osmotic fragility test in, 126
pathophysiology of, 119-121
peripheral blood smear morphology in, 123
red cell enzyme assays in, 125-126
treatment of, 126
Hermansky-Pudlak syndrome, *564*
Heterophile antigen, *297-298*
Heterophile screening test, **299-303**
in infectious mononucleosis, 299-303
Hetrol test, 299-303, *300-301*
Hexokinase, *120*
deficiency of. *See* Hereditary nonspherocytic hemolytic anemia
Hexose monophosphate shunt, *128*
hereditary disorders of, 127-136
Histamine, *234*
in polycythemia, *227*
Histamine testing. *See* Serum histamine quantitation; Urine histamine quantitation
Histidine-rich glycoprotein, 607-611, *610-611*
Histiocytic lymphoma, *206*
Histiocytosis X, 452
Histoplasmosis, *314*, *320-321*
HLA-DR marker, *382*
HNSHA. *See* Hereditary nonspherocytic hemolytic anemia
Hodgkin's disease, *66*, *206*, *242*, *251*, *257*, *308*, *337*, *393*, *425*, *516*
approach to diagnosis of, 478-479
blood cell measurements in, 479-480
bone marrow examination in, 480
classification of, 475-478, *476*
clinical findings in, 475
course of, 481
hematologic findings in, 479-480
laparotomy in, 481
lymphocyte depletion, *476*, 477
lymphocyte predominance, 476-477, *476*, *483-484*
mixed cellularity, *476*, 477, *484*

nodular sclerosis, *476*, 477-478, *485-486*
pathophysiology of, 474-475
peripheral blood smear morphology in, 480
radiologic studies in, 480
staging of, *478-479*
treatment of, 481
Homocystinuria, *564*
Hougie, Cecil, author of chapters **40-46**
Howell-Jolly bodies, *4-5*
Human immunodeficiency virus (HIV) infection, *320-321*. *See also* AIDS
anti-HIV serology in, 318-322
Hydronephrosis, *221*, *223*
Hydroxychloroquine sulfate, *560*
Hypercholesterolemia, *15*
Hypergranular promyelocytic leukemia, *351*, *366*
Hypersensitivity reaction, *251*
Hypersplenism, *261*
approach to diagnosis of, 330
blood cell measurements in, 331
bone marrow examination in, 331
chromium-51 labeling in, 331-333
clinical findings in, 330
course of, 333
hematologic findings in, 331
pathophysiology of, 328-330, *329*
peripheral blood smear morphology in, 331
treatment of, 333
Hypertension, portal, 52. *See also* Liver disease, with portal hypertension
Hypoalbuminemia, *15*
Hypochromic anemia
causes of, *32*
peripheral blood smear morphology in, 33, *34*
Hypofibrinogenemia, *15*
Hypophosphatasia, congenital, *239*
Hypophosphatemia, *393*
Hypoplastic anemia, 55-58
approach to diagnosis of, 62
blood cell measurements in, 63
bone marrow examination in, 63
clinical findings in, 62

course of, 64-65
hematologic findings in, 62-63
pathophysiology of, 59-61
peripheral blood smear morphology in, 63
treatment of, 64-65
Hypothyroidism, *20*, 51

Ibuprofen, *559*
Icterus, neonatal, *131*
Idiopathic thrombocytopenic purpura (ITP), *239*, *393*, *567*
IM. *See* Infectious mononucleosis
Immunocytoma, *444*, 446
Immunoelectrophoresis. *See* Serum protein immunoelectrophoresis; Urine protein immunoelectrophoresis
Immunoglobulin
characteristics of normal, 489, *490-491*
structure of, 488-489, *489*
Immunoglobulin A, *490-491*
Immunoglobulin D, *490-491*
Immunoglobulin E, *490-491*
Immunoglobulin G, *490-491*
Immunoglobulin G antibody, *298*
Immunoglobulin M, *490-491*
Immunoglobulin M antibody, *298*
Immunoglobulin testing, *See*
Platelet associated immunoglobulin detection; Serum immunoglobulin E measurement; Serum immunoglobulin quantitation
Immunologic cell marker study, **378-380**
in acute lymphoblastic leukemia, 378-380, *379*, *381-382*
in acute myeloblastic leukemia, 360-361
in chronic lymphocytic leukemia, 403-404
Immunologic phenotyping, in non-Hodgkin's lymphoma, 459-460, *460*
Immunoprecipitation assay for von Willebrand antigen, **575-576**
in functional platelet disorders, 573-574
Immunoproliferative disorder, *516*, *See also* Heavy-chain disease; Light-chain myeloma; Macroglobulinemia; Multiple myeloma
clinical findings in, *492-493*
hematologic findings in, *494-495*
laboratory findings in, *492-493*
Inclusion, red cell, in hemoglobin H disease, 157
Inclusion body testing. *See* Hemoglobin H inclusion body test
Indirect bilirubin test, in megaloblastic anemia, *84-85*
Indomethacin, *206*, *262*, *559*
Infectious agents, testing for. *See* Infectious serology; Serologic tests for infectious agents
Infectious lymphocytosis, *283*
Infectious mononucleosis (IM), *20*, *93*, *206*, *239*, *283*, 287-288, *288-289*, *314*, *329*, *393*, 461, *462*
antibodies in, *298*
anti-EBV serology in, 303-306
approach to diagnosis of, 297-298
blood cell measurements in, 299
bone marrow examination in, 299
clinical findings in, 296-297
course of, 306
differential absorption test in, *302*, 303
hematologic findings in, 299
heterophile screening test in, 299-303
pathophysiology, 286
peripheral blood smear morphology in, *295*, 299
treatment of, 306
Infectious serology, **287-289**
in reactive disorders of lymphocytes, 287-289, *288*
Influenza, *60*
Inhibitor of clotting screening test, **586-587**
Insecticide, *60*
Interleukin-1 (IL-1), 44-46, *45-46*
Interleukin-2 (IL-2). *See* CD25 marker
Intermediate lymphocytic lymphoma, *444*, 446
Intrinsic factor antibody test, in megaloblastic anemia, 86
Iron-59 labeling, **108**
Iron deficiency anemia, *21*, *41*
in alcoholism, 52

peripheral blood smear morphology in, 279
treatment of, 279
Leukoerythroblastosis, conditions associated with, *425*
Light-chain disease
approach to diagnosis of, 495-496
Bence-Jones protein test in, 500-501
beta-2-microglobulin quantitation in, 507-508
blood cell measurements in, 497
bone marrow examination in, 497-498
bone roentgenogram in, 508
chromosome analysis in, 508
clinical findings in, 490-494, *492-493*
erythrocyte sedimentation rate in, 505-506
gene rearrangement in, 508
hematologic findings in, 497-498
pathophysiology of, 488-490
peripheral blood smear morphology in, 497
renal function tests in, 507
serum calcium quantitation in, 507
serum immunoglobulin quantitation in, 503-504
serum protein electrophoresis in, 498-503, *499, 503*
serum viscosity in, 506-507
urine protein electrophoresis in, 500-501
urine protein immunoelectrophoresis in, 501-503, *503*
Liver biopsy, **342**
in liver disease with portal hypertension, 342
Liver disease, *20. See also* Alcoholism
with portal hypertension. *See also* Cirrhosis
approach to diagnosis of, 338
blood cell measurements in, 339
bone marrow examination in, 340
clinical findings in, 338
course of, 343
hematologic findings in, 338-340

liver biopsy in, 342
liver function tests in, 340-341, *340*
pathophysiology of, 336-338
peripheral blood smear morphology in, 339-340
radiologic imaging in, 342-343
treatment of, 343
Liver fluke, *234, 242*
Liver function tests, **340-341**
in liver disease with portal hypertension, 340-341, *340*
in non-Hodgkin's lymphoma, 459
Löffler's syndrome, *243*
Lupus erythematosus, *545*
Lymphadenitis, viral, *462*
Lymphadenopathy
dermatopathic, *462*
without lymphocytosis
angiotensin-converting enzyme test in, 324
anti-HIV serology in, 318-322
approach to diagnosis of, 315-316
blood cell measurements in, 316
bone marrow examination in, 316
causes of, *314*
chest roentgenogram in, 325
clinical findings in, 313-315
course of, 325
diagnostic methods for, *320-321*
hematologic findings in, 316
lymph node biopsy in, 323-324
lymph node culture in, 322-323
pathophysiology of, 313
serologic tests for infectious agents in, 316-318
skin tests in, 325
treatment of, 325
Lymphangiectasia, intestinal, *308*
Lymph node biopsy, **323-324**
in chronic lymphocytic leukemia, 405
in eosinophilia, 249
in lymphadenopathy without lymphocytosis, 323-324
Lymph node culture, **322-323**
Lymphoblastic lymphoma, *444, 448-450, 448, 470-471*

Lymphocytes, 3-4
 monoclonal antibody markers
  in, *290-291*
 reactive disorders of, 282-283
  approach to diagnosis of,
   285-286
  blood cell measurements in,
   286
  bone marrow examination in,
   286
  causes of, *283*
  characteristics of, *289*
  clinical findings in, 285
  course of, 293
  hematologic findings in, 286
  infectious serology in, 287-
   289, *288*
  pathophysiology of, 284-285
  peripheral blood smear morphology in, 286
  T- and B-cell markers of lymphocytes, 289-293, *290-291*
  treatment of, 293
Lymphocyte testing. *See* B-cell
 markers of lymphocytes; T-
 cell markers of lymphocytes
Lymphocytic leukemia, *206*
Lymphocytic lymphoma, *204*, 205,
 206
Lymphocytosis. *See* Lymphocytes,
 reactive disorders of
Lymphogranuloma venereum, *314*,
 320-321
Lymphoma, *20*, *77*, *314*, *329*. *See
 also* specific types of lymphoma
 evaluation of occult, **216**
  in autoimmune hemolytic
   anemia, 216
  non-Hodgkin's. *See* Non-Hodgkin's lymphoma
Lymphopenia
 approach to diagnosis of, 309
 blood cell measurements in,
  310
 bone marrow examination in,
  310
 causes of, *308*
 clinical findings in, 307-309
 course of, 311-312
 hematologic findings in, 309-310
 pathophysiology of, 307
 serum immunoglobulin testing
  in, 310-311
 T-cell quantitation in, 311

 treatment of, 311-312
Lymphosarcoma cell leukemia
 (LCL), *283*, 408-409, *410-411*,
 416, 445

Macrocytes, *4-5*
Macrocytic anemia
 classification of, *23-24*
 differential diagnosis of, 22-23,
  25
Macrocytosis, *15*
Macroglobulinemia, *567*
 approach to diagnosis of, 495-
  496, 509
 Bence-Jones protein test in,
  500-501
 beta-2 microglobulin quantitation in, 507-508
 blood cell measurements in,
  497
 bone marrow examination in,
  497-498
 bone roentgenogram in, 508
 chromosome analysis in, 508
 clinical findings in, 490-494,
  492-493
 erythrocyte sedimentation rate
  in, 505-506
 gene rearrangement in, 508
 hematologic findings in, 497-
  498
 pathophysiology of, 488-490
 peripheral blood smear morphology in, 497
 renal function tests in, 507
 serum calcium quantitation in,
  507
 serum immunoglobulin quantitation in, 503-504
 serum protein electrophoresis
  in, 498-500, *499*
 serum protein immunoelectrophoresis in, 501-503, *503*
 serum viscosity in, 506-507
 urine protein electrophoresis in,
  500-501
 urine protein immunoelectrophoresis in, 501-503, *503*
Malaria, *93*, *96*, *169*, *257*, *329*
Malignant histiocytosis, *444*, 452-
 453, *468*
Mantle zone lymphoma, *444*, 446
Marfan's syndrome, *564*
Mast cells
 biochemistry of, *253*

histochemistry of, *253*
Maternal antibody screening and identification, **182-183**
  in acquired hemolytic anemia, fetomaternal incompatibility, 182-183
May-Hegglin anomaly, 276-279, *278*
MCH. *See* Mean corpuscular hemoglobin
MCHC. *See* Mean corpuscular hemoglobin concentration
MCV. *See* Mean corpuscular volume
Mean corpuscular hemoglobin concentration (MCHC), 9-10, *10*
Mean corpuscular hemoglobin (MCH), 10, *10*
Mean corpuscular volume (MCV), 10, *21*
Mean platelet volume, 9
Measles, 207, *283*
Mefenamic acid, *192-193, 559*
Megaloblastic anemia
  approach to diagnosis of, 78-79
  blood cell measurements in, 79
  bone marrow examination in, 80, *89*
  clinical findings in, 78
  course of, 88
  dU suppression test in, 87
  gastrin test in, 86-87
  hematologic findings in, 79-80
  indirect bilirubin test in, *84-85*
  intrinsic factor antibody test in, 86
  lactate dehydrogenase quantitation in, *82-83*
  parietal cell antibody test in, 86
  pathophysiology of, 72-78
  peripheral blood smear morphology in, 79-80, *89*
  red blood cell folate quantitation in, *82-83*, 85-86, *86*
  Schilling test in, 87
  serum folate quantitation in, 81-85, *81-82, 86*
  serum iron quantitation in, *82-83*
  serum vitamin B_{12} quantitation in, 80-81, *82-83, 86*
  total iron-binding capacity in, *82-83*
  treatment of, 88
Megaloblastic madness, 78

Melanoma, *462*
Meningococcemia, *593*
Methemalbumin, serum, in accelerated erythrocyte turnover, *99*, 106
Methemoglobin, *221*
Methemoglobinemia, hereditary, 141
Methicillin, *192-193*
Methotrexate, 77, 84, *337*
Methylene blue, *130, 191*
Microangiopathy, thrombotic, *593*
Microcytes, *4*
Microcytic anemia
  classification of, *26-27*
  differential diagnosis of, 24-25
Microcytosis, *15*
Microgranular promyelocytic leukemia, 353
Mixed small and large cell lymphoma, 446, *466*
Monoblasts, 7
Mono-Chek test, 299-303, *300-301*
Monoclonal antibody
  CD1 (Leu 6, OKT6, T6) marker, *290, 381*
  CD2 (Leu 5, OKT11, T11) marker, *290, 381*
  CD3 (Leu 4, OKT3, T3) marker, *290, 292, 381*
  CD4 (Leu 3, OKT4, T4) marker, *290, 292, 381*
  CD5 (Leu 1, OKT1, T1) marker, *290, 381*
  CD6 (T12, T411, TU33) marker, *381*
  CD7 (3A1, 4A, Leu 9) marker, *381*
  CD8 (Leu 2, OKT8, T8) marker, *290, 292, 381*
  CD9 (BA2, J2) marker, *381*
  CD10 (BA3, J5, Leu 17) marker, *290, 381*
  CD11 (Leu 15, Mo1, Mo5, OKM1) marker, *290-291, 381*
  CD15 (Leu M1, My1, x-hapten) marker, *381*
  CD16 (Leu 11, VEP13) marker, *381*
  CD19 (B4, Leu 12) marker, *290, 381*
  CD20 (B1, Leu 16) marker, *290, 381*
  CD21 (B2, CR2) marker, *381*